Study smarter with the online videos and animations at MediaCenter.Thieme.com!

Simply visit MediaCenter.thieme.com and, when prompted during the registration process, enter the code below to get started today.

2JQJ-FWXP-WJ5R-VLVS

	WINDOWS	MAC	TABLET
Recommended Browser(s) **	Recent browser versions on all major platforms and any mobile operating system that supports HTML5 video playback ** *all browsers should have JavaScript enabled*		
Flash Player Plug-in	Flash Player 9 or Higher* * *Mac users: ATI Rage 128 GPU does not support full-screen mode with hardware scaling*		Tablet PCs with Android OS support Flash 10.1
Recommended for optimal usage experience	Monitor resolutions: • Normal (4:3) 1024×768 or Higher • Widescreen (16:9) 1280×720 or Higher • Widescreen (16:10) 1440×900 or Higher DSL/Cable internet connection at a minimum speed of 384.0 Kbps or faster WiFi 802.11 b/g preferred.		7-inch and 10-inch tablets on maximum resolution. WiFi connection is required.

Connect with us on social media

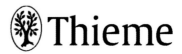

Color Atlas of Brainstem Surgery

Robert F. Spetzler, MD
Department of Neurosurgery
Barrow Neurological Institute
St. Joseph's Hospital and Medical Center
Phoenix, Arizona

M. Yashar S. Kalani, MD, PhD
Department of Neurosurgery
Barrow Neurological Institute
St. Joseph's Hospital and Medical Center
Phoenix, Arizona

Peter Nakaji, MD
Department of Neurosurgery
Barrow Neurological Institute
St. Joseph's Hospital and Medical Center
Phoenix, Arizona

Kaan Yağmurlu, MD
Department of Neurosurgery
Barrow Neurological Institute
St. Joseph's Hospital and Medical Center
Phoenix, Arizona

With 1700 Figures

Thieme
New York · Stuttgart · Delhi · Rio de Janeiro

Executive Editor: Timothy Hiscock
Managing Editor: Sarah Landis
Director, Editorial Services: Mary Jo Casey
Production Editor: Barbara A. Chernow
International Production Director: Andreas Schabert
Senior Vice President, Editorial and E-Product Development: Vera
    Spillner
International Marketing Director: Fiona Henderson
International Sales Director: Louisa Turrell
Director of Sales, North America: Mike Roseman
Senior Vice President and Chief Operating Officer: Sarah Vanderbilt
President: Brian D. Scanlan
Typesetting by Toppan Best-set Premedia Limited
Cover art by Kristen Larson Keil, MS, CMI

Library of Congress Cataloging-in-Publication Data

Names: Spetzler, Robert F. (Robert Friedrich), 1944- author. |
    Kalani, M. Yashar S., author. | Nakaji, Peter, author. | Yağmurlu, Kaan,
    author.
Title: Color atlas of brainstem surgery / Robert F. Spetzler, M. Yashar
    S. Kalani, Peter Nakaji, Kaan Yağmurlu.
Description: New York : Thieme, [2017] | Includes bibliographical
    references and index.
Identifiers: LCCN 2016050689 (print) | LCCN 2016051551 (ebook) |
    ISBN 9781626230279 (alk. paper) | ISBN 9781626230286 (ebook) |
    ISBN 9781626230286
Subjects: | MESH: Brain Stem–surgery | Neurosurgical Procedures |
    Atlases Classification: LCC RD594 (print) | LCC RD594 (ebook) |
    NLM WL 17 | DDC 617.4/81–dc23
LC record available at https://lccn.loc.gov/2016050689

© 2017 Thieme Medical Publishers, Inc.
Thieme Medical Publishers, Inc.
333 Seventh Avenue, New York, NY 10001 USA
+1 800 782 3488, customerservice@thieme.com

Thieme Publishers Stuttgart
Rüdigerstrasse 14, 70469 Stuttgart, Germany
+49 [0]711 8931 421, customerservice@thieme.de

Thieme Publishers Delhi
A-12, Second Floor, Sector-2, Noida-201301
Uttar Pradesh, India
+91 120 45 566 00, customerservice@thieme.in

Thieme Publishers Rio de Janeiro, Thieme Publicações Ltda.
Edifício Rodolpho de Paoli, 25o andar
Av. Nilo Peçanha, 50 – Sala 2508
Rio de Janeiro 20020-906 Brasil
+55 21 3172 2297

Printed in China by Everbest Printing Investment   **5 4 3 2 1**

ISBN 978-1-62623-027-9

Also available as an ebook:
eISBN 978-1-62623-028-6

Important note: Medicine is an ever-changing science undergoing continual development. Research and clinical experience are continually expanding our knowledge, in particular our knowledge of proper treatment and drug therapy. Insofar as this book mentions any dosage or application, readers may rest assured that the authors, editors, and publishers have made every effort to ensure that such references are in accordance with **the state of knowledge at the time of production of the book**.

Nevertheless, this does not involve, imply, or express any guarantee or responsibility on the part of the publishers in respect to any dosage instructions and forms of applications stated in the book. **Every user is requested to examine carefully** the manufacturers' leaflets accompanying each drug and to check, if necessary in consultation with a physician or specialist, whether the dosage schedules mentioned therein or the contraindications stated by the manufacturers differ from the statements made in the present book. Such examination is particularly important with drugs that are either rarely used or have been newly released on the market. Every dosage schedule or every form of application used is entirely at the user's own risk and responsibility. The authors and publishers request every user to report to the publishers any discrepancies or inaccuracies noticed. If errors in this work are found after publication, errata will be posted at www.thieme.com on the product description page.

Some of the product names, patents, and registered designs referred to in this book are in fact registered trademarks or proprietary names even though specific reference to this fact is not always made in the text. Therefore, the appearance of a name without designation as proprietary is not to be construed as a representation by the publisher that it is in the public domain.

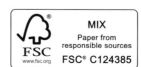

This Atlas is dedicated to all my patients who have entrusted their care into my hands.
They have been my greatest inspiration and teachers.

Robert F. Spetzler, MD

To my wife Kristin.

M. Yashar S. Kalani, MD, PhD

To my residents and fellows, ever toiling upward in the night.

Peter Nakaji, MD

To my mother, Huriye Meral, and to my father, Edip, who always supported me unconditionally and
encouraged me in all avenues of my life. Also, in loving memory of Dr. Albert L. Rhoton, Jr.,
who was the greatest mentor and teacher and who will always be a source of inspiration to me.

Kaan Yağmurlu, MD

Contents

Video Contents

Animation Contents

Foreword

No one has done more than Robert Spetzler to advance the idea that the brainstem is *not* inviolable, inoperable territory. When I was a resident at Barrow Neurological Institute in the 1990s, he began to prove this point, and patients flocked to Barrow from around the world. Other neurosurgeons, it seemed, believed that brainstem surgery was impossible, and so they referred their patients to someone brave enough to believe that it was. That extensive referral network, combined with a large Latino patient population in whom cavernous malformations were prevalent, fueled the discovery that the microsurgical resection of brainstem cavernous malformations was safe and even advisable in many patients. The convergence of a stream of cases and a master neurosurgeon practicing both high-level microsurgery and skull base surgery, at a time when other centers were moving toward endoscopic and endovascular techniques, shaped a new discipline within vascular neurosurgery. Brainstem cavernous malformation surgery began with simple concepts such as the two-point method to select the right approach to expose the lesion. This discipline adapted complex skull base surgical approaches developed for tumors to the simpler pathology of cavernous malformations. Brainstem microsurgery applied technology such as intraoperative navigation for submerged lesions, tractography for pathologies that deviate neural pathways, and micro-instruments that bring precision and light to deep, dark surgical corridors. In the end, our perception of the brainstem as an impenetrable monolith was transformed, and we appreciated it instead as a complex labyrinth with zones that could tolerate safe entry.

After hundreds of cases and innumerable contributions to the literature by Dr. Spetzler and his disciples, both at Barrow Neurological Institute and beyond, the microsurgical resection of brainstem cavernous malformations has become an accepted management option in centers around the world whose specialists are well versed in the techniques described in this book. This book is a singular achievement that describes the nuanced anatomy of the brainstem, the complex surgical approaches to the skull base, and the pioneering experience of Dr. Spetzler. The insights of a master neurosurgeon, and the meticulous work of his coauthors Drs. Kalani, Nakaji, and Yağmurlu, are presented through case examples and stunning illustrations by the virtuoso artists in Neuroscience Publications at Barrow Neurological Institute.

This *Color Atlas of Brainstem Surgery* is destined to become a classic on the shelf of every cranial neurosurgeon.

As I reflect on Dr. Spetzler's legacy and his contributions to brainstem surgery at this, the twilight of his brilliant neurosurgical career, the parallels to Charles Drake and vertebrobasilar aneurysm surgery are striking. In his era, Drake was the recipient of a steady stream of difficult aneurysm cases and London, Ontario, became the crucible of discovery for posterior circulation aneurysm surgery. He amassed an experience that has never been replicated, and he advanced the idea that the posterior circulation was *not* an inviolable territory for aneurysm surgery. Furthermore, he inspired a generation of young neurosurgeons to refine the techniques for basilar aneurysm surgery and to practice them around the world. The same can be said of the unique experience with brainstem surgery amassed by Dr. Spetzler, which has made Phoenix, Arizona, a crucible of discovery for brainstem surgery. The pearls embedded in this atlas will similarly inspire future generations of neurosurgeons to perform safe, curative surgery on the brainstem.

It is worth stating that brainstem surgery is not for the faint of heart or the unsteady of hand. Brainstem cavernous malformations and arteriovenous malformations are particularly challenging, and the line between success and failure is razor thin. Although this book is a testament that brainstem surgery can be safe and curative, it is also a reminder that brainstem surgery can be morbid and sometimes fatal. The pages of this book will undoubtedly inspire the reader to perform this surgery, but they do not contain the intangibles required for its success. I have learned many of these techniques throughout the years I have spent working with Dr. Spetzler, from the judicious selection of patients for surgery to the thoughtful construction of operative strategy, the dexterous dissection to reach the targets, the keen recognition of localizing anatomy, and the judgment to know how aggressively to dissect and when to stop. Learning the special art of brainstem surgery begins with the careful study of books like this one, but it continues by observing master neurosurgeons in action who possess and practice these intangibles.

Michael T. Lawton, MD
San Francisco, CA

Preface

The brainstem, until quite recently, was considered inviolable because of its tightly packed tracts and deep nuclei. Thus, patients with pathology in this region were generally managed conservatively, and their fates were often left to the natural history of their diseases. Early surgery was confounded by inadequate visualization, incomplete understanding of brainstem anatomy, lack of appropriate instrumentation, and poor results from attempted resection of brainstem pathology, particularly the failed surgical attempts to treat infiltrating gliomas.

However, improvements over time in imaging, instrumentation, patient monitoring, operating microscopes, and especially neuronavigation have led to the obvious recognition that the brainstem is just another part of the central nervous system. The natural evolution of tentative steps based on previous successes has led us to understand that the brainstem is not inviolate to surgical manipulation but instead requires proven avenues for safe resection. Brainstem cavernous malformations, whose repeated hemorrhages often demand surgical intervention, have been our greatest teachers as we sought to define safe corridors in this eloquent region. With neuronavigation enabling the neurosurgeon to delineate both a target and a path, lesions deep in the brainstem that were not visible on the surface became reasonable targets for excision. As our experience in operating in the brainstem accrued, the safest entry routes became better defined. This atlas draws on the lessons learned from more than a thousand operations in and around the brainstem conducted by the senior author, and we hope that it proves to be of benefit to our colleagues and their patients.

Many factors influence the decision about whether to operate on a specific patient, including the patient's age and medical condition, the severity of symptoms, the number of hemorrhages, the extent of accessibility, and the experience of the neurosurgeon. The associated venous anomaly frequently requires an approach from a more direct to an alternative route because experience has taught us to preserve these large veins. Although the brainstem is technically surgically accessible, it remains an extremely eloquent structure that demands rigorous decision-making when considering surgery. For example, a patient with a small asymptomatic pontine cavernous malformation in the midline below the floor of the fourth ventricle should never be considered for resection. Alternatively, a patient with a large lateral pontine cavernous malformation that has resulted in clinically significant neurologic deficits will likely receive dramatic benefit from its surgical removal.

This atlas builds on the legacy of many previous atlases. As neurosurgeons, we tend to be visually oriented. Being able to see the anatomy through artists' illustrations and animations, clinical images, operative photographs, and intraoperative videos enables us to better grasp the intricacy of the anatomic relationships and the delicate corridors that are necessary for exposure. As one might expect, this atlas approaches the brainstem regionally. Thus, the reader will find a logical and accessible map to the separate subdivisions of the brainstem, each of which has its own special anatomic and surgical considerations. The thoughtful reader will find much illumination from these shared, hard-learned lessons. We began with the assertion that the nuances found herein will translate to many more areas of neurosurgery than brainstem surgery alone. It is our sincere hope that you, the neurosurgeon, will gain from this knowledge to the ultimate benefit of your patients. We invite you to turn the pages, open your mind, and enter into the hallowed halls of the brainstem.

Robert F. Spetzler, MD
M. Yashar S. Kalani, MD, PhD
Peter Nakaji, MD
Kaan Yağmurlu, MD
Phoenix, Arizona

Acknowledgments

No book of this magnitude could come to fruition without the ceaseless efforts of our talented and hard-working support staff in Neuroscience Publications. They include our editorial coordinators, Rogena Lake and Samantha Soto, who handled manuscript intake and formatting, and who maintained an ongoing record of the project. We thank our production editor, Jaime-Lynn Canales, whose meticulous attention to detail enabled her to keep track of more than 1,700 clinical images, photographs, and illustrations through numerous iterations. She also handled copyright and permissions for all the figures used in the atlas. To our medical editors Mary Ann Clifft, Dawn Mutchler, and Lynda Orescanin, we express appreciation for their skill in polishing our prose and ensuring consistency across the sections of the book and throughout the cases. We thank our video editor Marie Clarkson, who sifted through hours of intraoperative videos to select the intraoperative images used in the side-by-side illustrations in the cases and trimmed the videos to our specifications, then edited our recorded narrative explanations of them. She also edited the narration for the superb animations created by Michael Hickman and Joshua Lai. Above all, we thank our lead medical illustrator Kristen Larson Keil, who so admirably guided—throughout her pregnancy and after her maternity leave—a team of contract artists and in-house illustrators that included Peter Lawrence and Mark Schornak, the manager of Neuroscience Publications. Ms. Keil's artistic talent is showcased in countless illustrations throughout this atlas, particularly in the illustration she prepared for the cover. She and the other illustrators relied not only on their inherent artistic talent but also on their intensive training and their in-depth understanding of anatomy to create beautifully detailed medical illustrations of the anatomy, pathology, and neurosurgical techniques that we describe in depth. They also prepared detailed side-by-side line drawings interpreting the intraoperative photographs to clearly illustrate our step-by-step approach to each case.

Intraoperative photographs showing the positioning of patients for operations were provided by medical photographer Gary Armstrong.

We thank our families for their patience and ongoing support, and our colleagues here and elsewhere—including our current and former residents and fellows—for their input. We also thank our patients, without whom a book such as this would not be possible.

Finally, we thank the team at Thieme Medical Publishers, which includes Timothy Hiscock, Sarah Landis, Barbara Chernow, and their many colleagues. Only with their encouragement and assistance could this book have been produced.

1 Anatomy

Internal Anatomy of the Brainstem

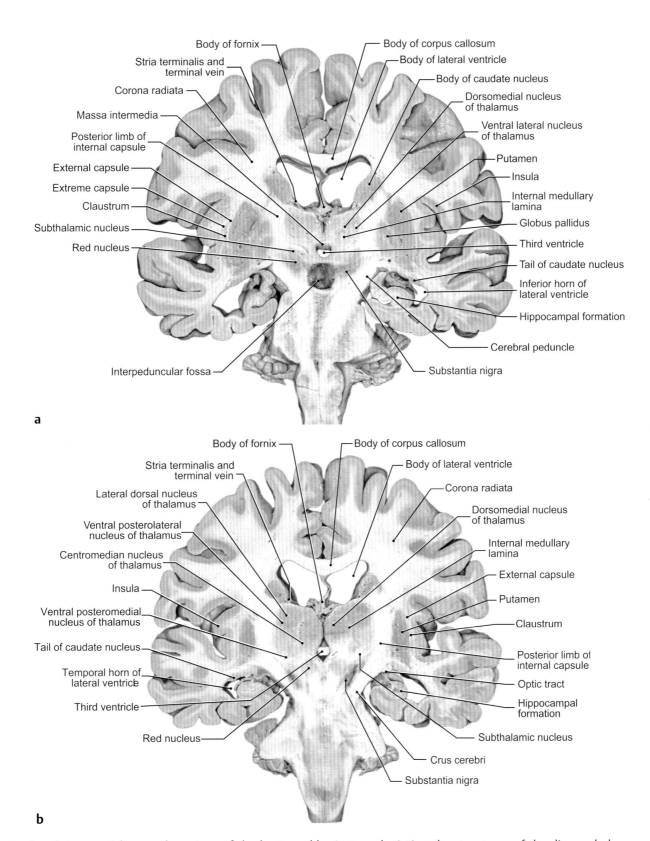

Figure 1.1. (a–e) Sequential coronal sections of the brain and brainstem depicting the structures of the diencephalon.

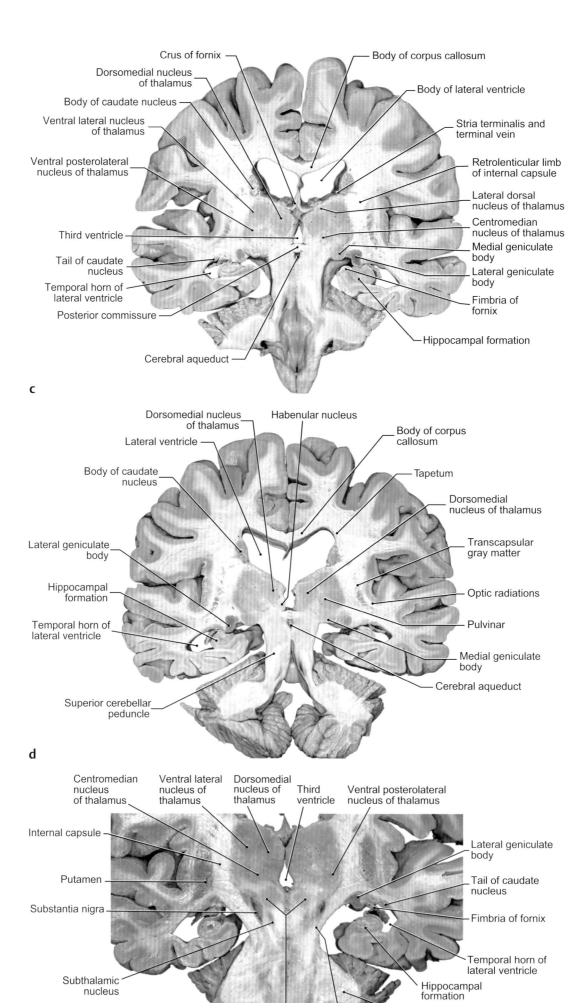

Figure 1.1. (*Continued*)

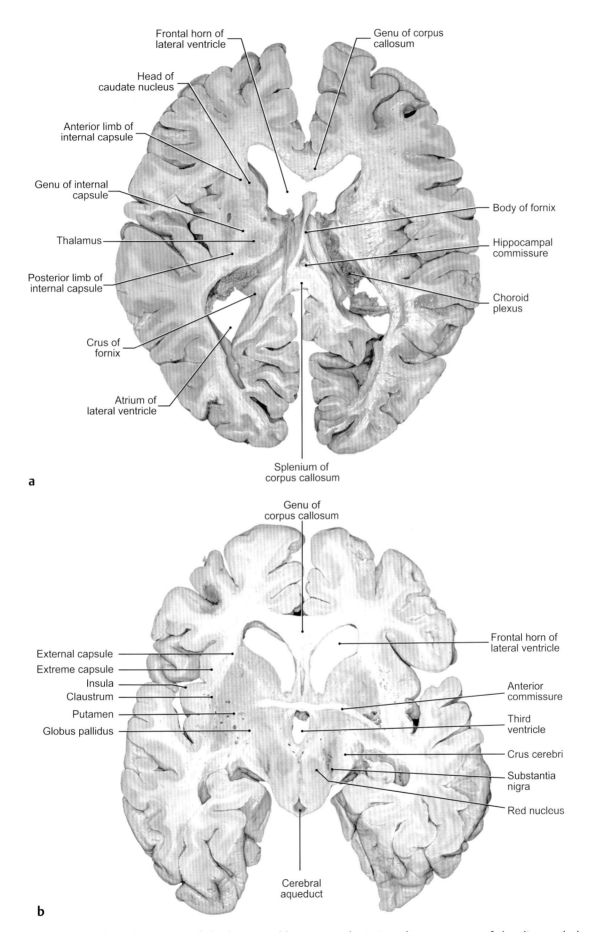

Figure 1.2. (a–d) Sequential axial sections of the brain and brainstem depicting the structures of the diencephalon.

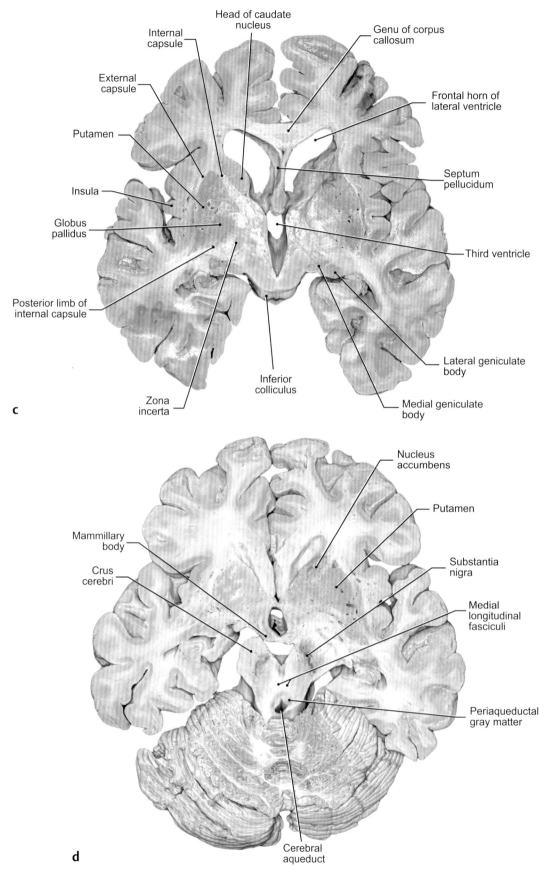

Figure 1.2. (*Continued*)

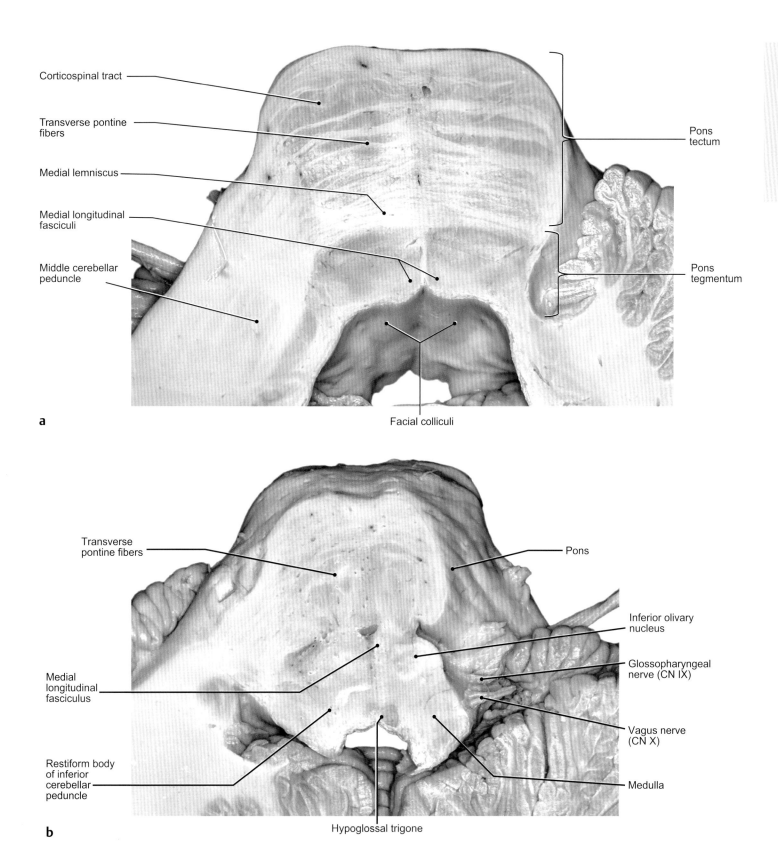

Corticospinal tract

Transverse pontine fibers

Medial lemniscus

Medial longitudinal fasciculi

Middle cerebellar peduncle

Pons tectum

Pons tegmentum

Facial colliculi

a

Transverse pontine fibers

Medial longitudinal fasciculus

Restiform body of inferior cerebellar peduncle

Pons

Inferior olivary nucleus

Glossopharyngeal nerve (CN IX)

Vagus nerve (CN X)

Medulla

Hypoglossal trigone

b

Figure 1.3. (a,b) Axial sections of the brainstem depicting structures of the pons and medulla oblongata. CN, cranial nerve.

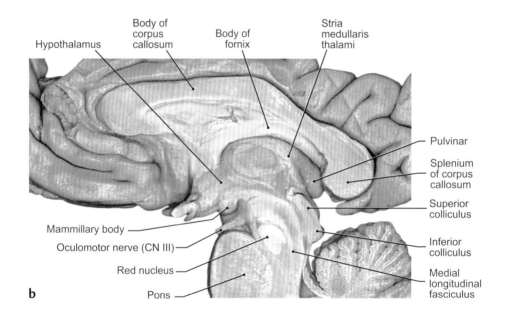

Third ventricle

Medial lemniscus

Corticospinal tract

Trigeminal nerve (CN V), intrapontine segment

Abducens nerve (CN VI)

Glossopharyngeal nerve (CN IX)

Pulvinar

Splenium of corpus callosum

Pineal gland

Superior colliculus

Inferior colliculus

Dentate nucleus

Vestibulocochlear nerve (CN VIII)

Vagus nerve (CN X)

a

Hypothalamus

Body of corpus callosum

Body of fornix

Stria medullaris thalami

Mammillary body

Oculomotor nerve (CN III)

Red nucleus

Pons

Pulvinar

Splenium of corpus callosum

Superior colliculus

Inferior colliculus

Medial longitudinal fasciculus

b

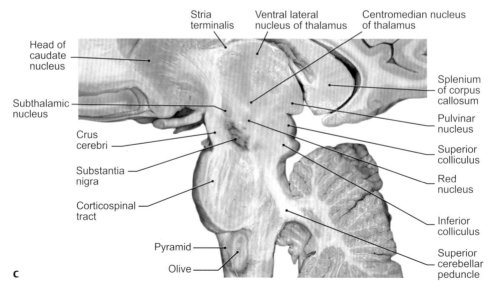

Head of caudate nucleus

Subthalamic nucleus

Crus cerebri

Substantia nigra

Corticospinal tract

Pyramid

Olive

Stria terminalis

Ventral lateral nucleus of thalamus

Centromedian nucleus of thalamus

Splenium of corpus callosum

Pulvinar nucleus

Superior colliculus

Red nucleus

Inferior colliculus

Superior cerebellar peduncle

c

Figure 1.4. (a–c) Sequential sagittal sections of the brain and brainstem depicting critical structures of the diencephalon.

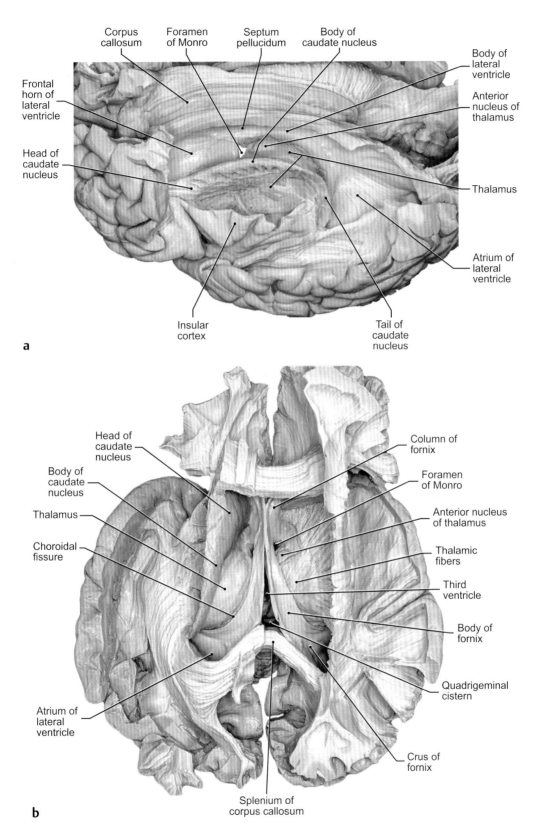

Figure 1.5. (a) Superolateral, **(b)** superior, **(c)** inferior, and **(d)** medial views showing the relationship of the thalamus, the lateral ventricle, and the third ventricle relative to adjacent structures.

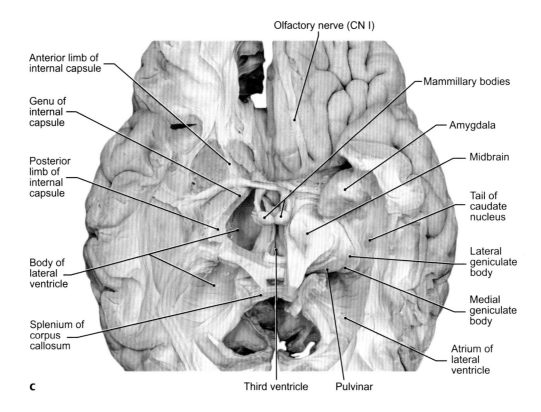

Olfactory nerve (CN I)

Anterior limb of internal capsule

Genu of internal capsule

Posterior limb of internal capsule

Body of lateral ventricle

Splenium of corpus callosum

Mammillary bodies

Amygdala

Midbrain

Tail of caudate nucleus

Lateral geniculate body

Medial geniculate body

Atrium of lateral ventricle

c

Third ventricle   Pulvinar

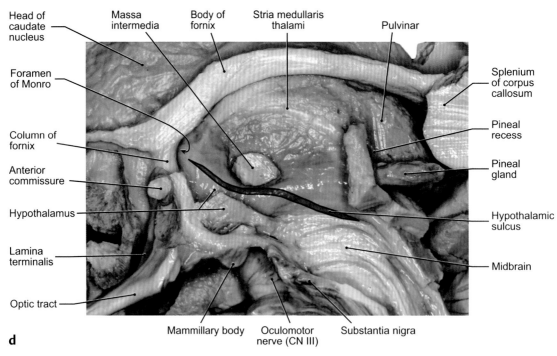

Head of caudate nucleus

Massa intermedia

Body of fornix

Stria medullaris thalami

Pulvinar

Foramen of Monro

Column of fornix

Anterior commissure

Hypothalamus

Lamina terminalis

Optic tract

Splenium of corpus callosum

Pineal recess

Pineal gland

Hypothalamic sulcus

Midbrain

d

Mammillary body   Oculomotor nerve (CN III)   Substantia nigra

Figure 1.5. (*Continued*)

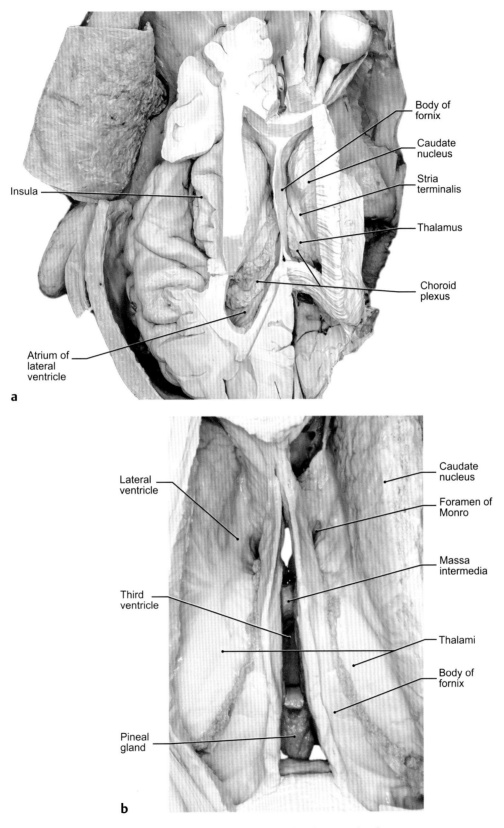

Figure 1.6. (a,b) The relationship of the thalamus to the lateral and third ventricles from a superior view.

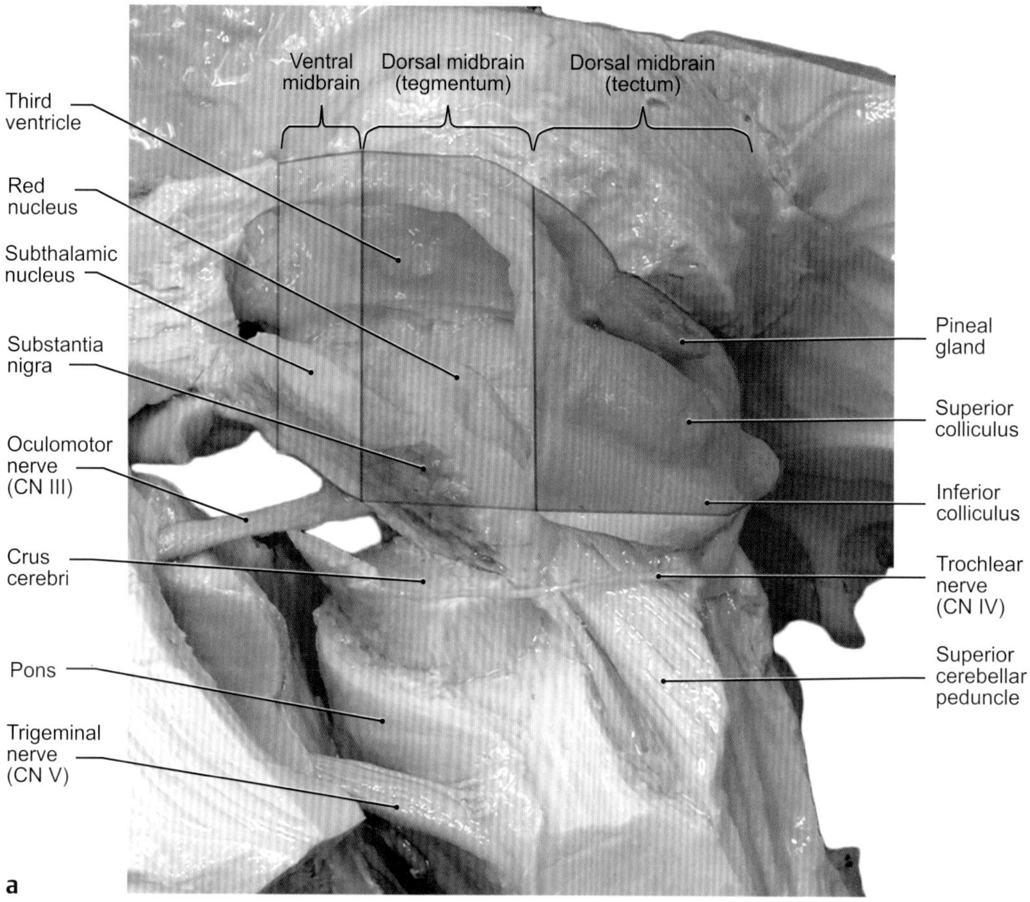

Ventral midbrain

Dorsal midbrain (tegmentum)

Dorsal midbrain (tectum)

Third ventricle

Red nucleus

Subthalamic nucleus

Substantia nigra

Oculomotor nerve (CN III)

Crus cerebri

Pons

Trigeminal nerve (CN V)

Pineal gland

Superior colliculus

Inferior colliculus

Trochlear nerve (CN IV)

Superior cerebellar peduncle

a

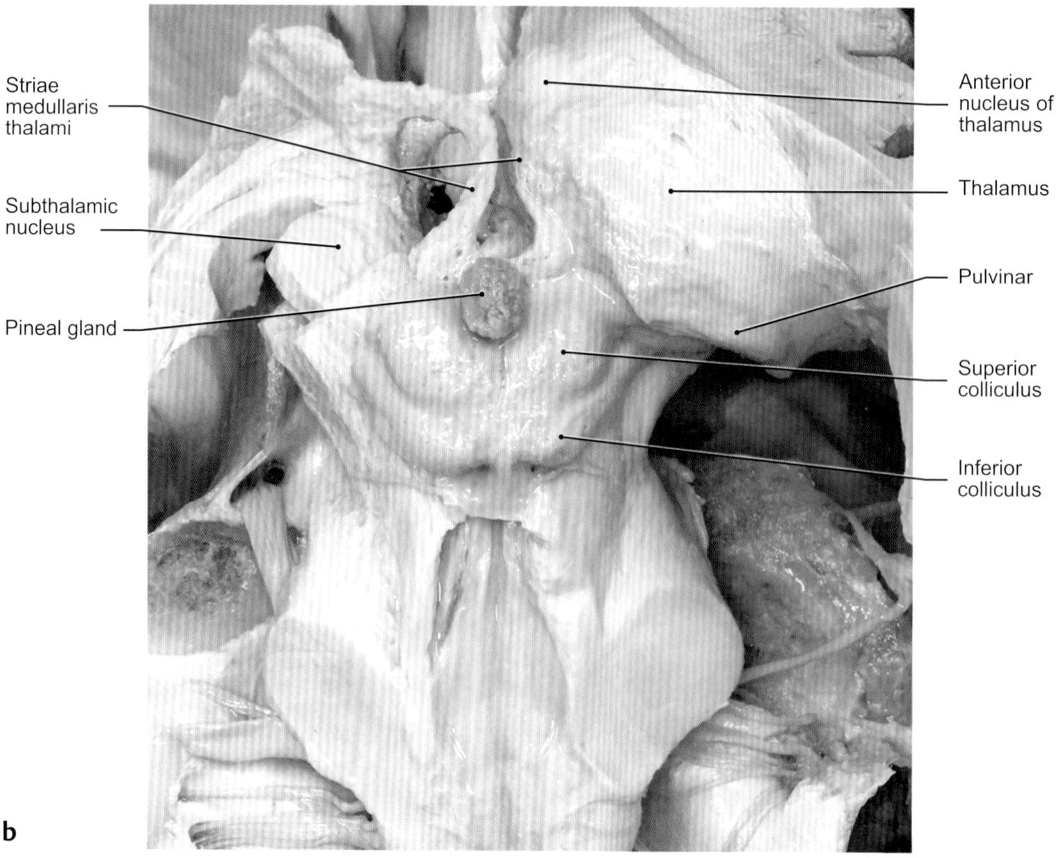

Striae medullaris thalami

Subthalamic nucleus

Pineal gland

Anterior nucleus of thalamus

Thalamus

Pulvinar

Superior colliculus

Inferior colliculus

b

Figure 1.7. (a) Lateral, **(b)** posterior, and **(c)** superior views showing the relationship of the thalamus to midbrain structures.

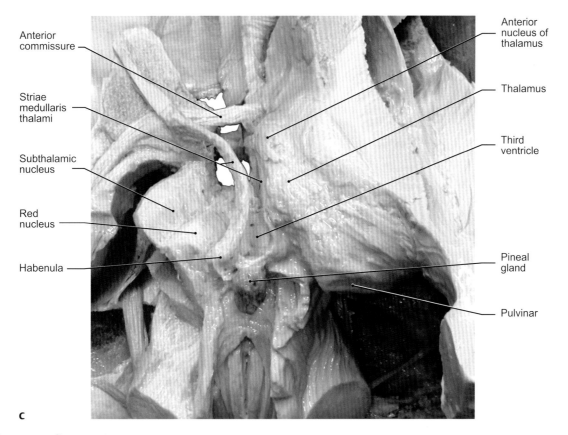

Anterior commissure

Striae medullaris thalami

Subthalamic nucleus

Red nucleus

Habenula

Anterior nucleus of thalamus

Thalamus

Third ventricle

Pineal gland

Pulvinar

c

Figure 1.7. (*Continued*)

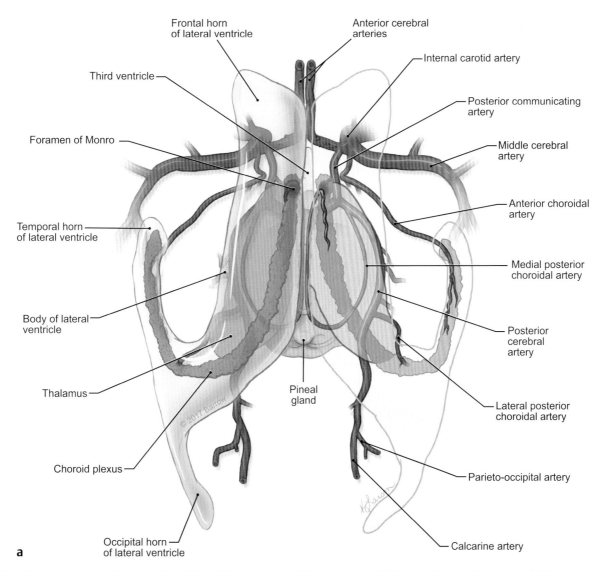

Frontal horn of lateral ventricle

Anterior cerebral arteries

Third ventricle

Internal carotid artery

Posterior communicating artery

Foramen of Monro

Middle cerebral artery

Anterior choroidal artery

Temporal horn of lateral ventricle

Medial posterior choroidal artery

Body of lateral ventricle

Posterior cerebral artery

Thalamus

Lateral posterior choroidal artery

Pineal gland

Choroid plexus

Parieto-occipital artery

Occipital horn of lateral ventricle

Calcarine artery

© 2017 Barrow

a

Figure 1.8. Superior view of the relationship of the cerebral **(a)** arteries and **(b)** veins to the lateral and third ventricles.

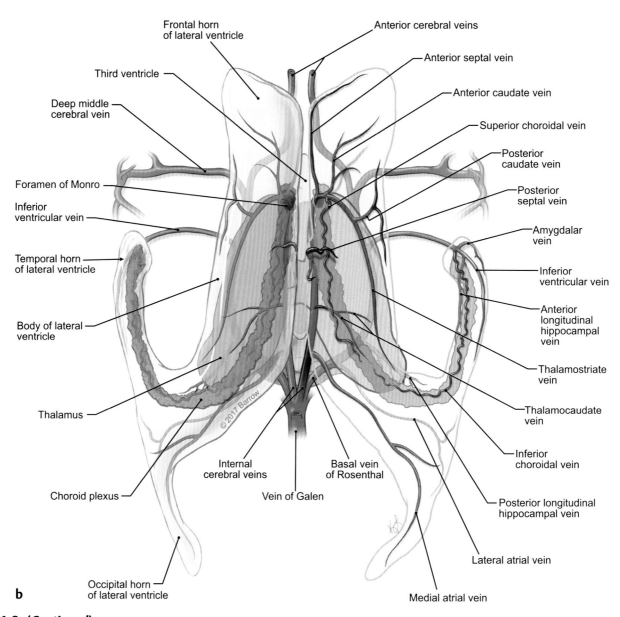

b

Figure 1.8. (*Continued*)

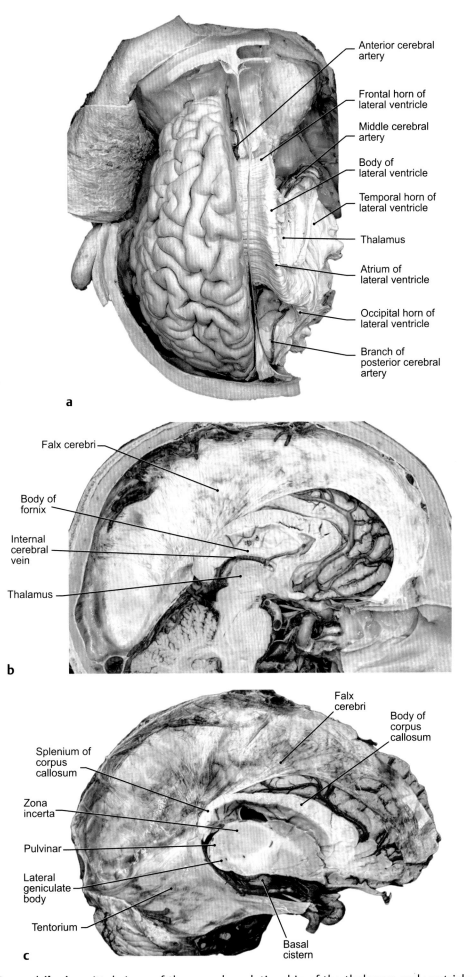

Anterior cerebral
artery

Frontal horn of
lateral ventricle

Middle cerebral
artery

Body of
lateral ventricle

Temporal horn of
lateral ventricle

Thalamus

Atrium of
lateral ventricle

Occipital horn of
lateral ventricle

Branch of
posterior cerebral
artery

a

Falx cerebri

Body of
fornix

Internal
cerebral
vein

Thalamus

b

Falx
cerebri

Body of
corpus
callosum

Splenium of
corpus
callosum

Zona
incerta

Pulvinar

Lateral
geniculate
body

Tentorium

Basal
cistern

c

Figure 1.9. (a) Superior and **(b,c)** sagittal views of the vascular relationship of the thalamus and ventricles.

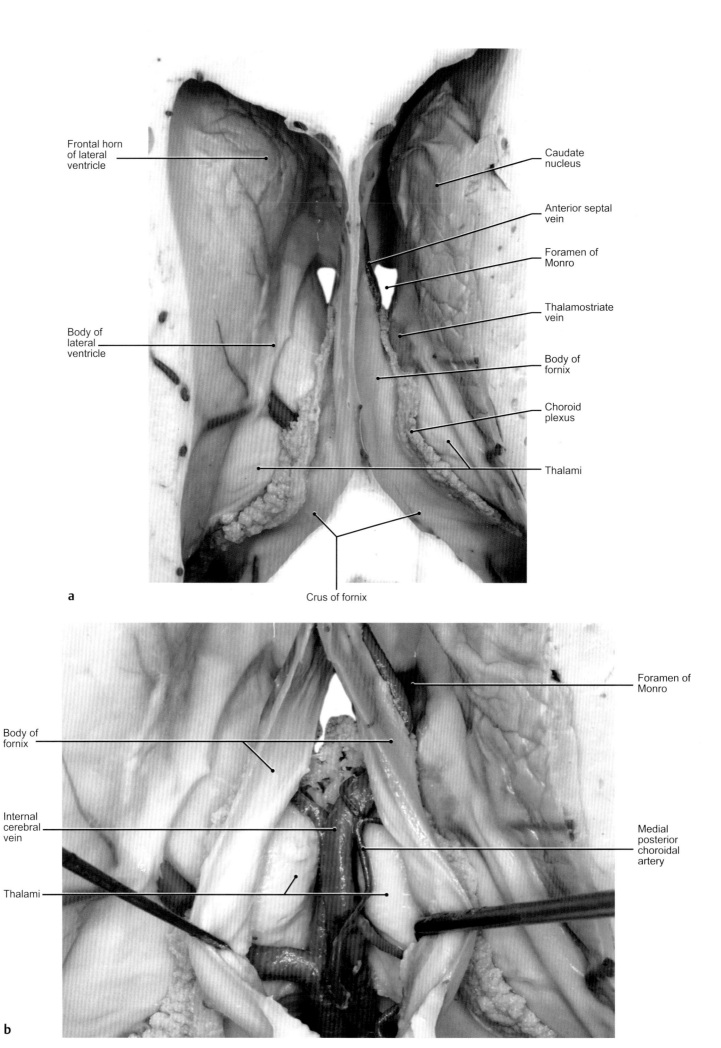

Frontal horn
of lateral
ventricle

Caudate
nucleus

Anterior septal
vein

Foramen of
Monro

Thalamostriate
vein

Body of
lateral
ventricle

Body of
fornix

Choroid
plexus

Thalami

Crus of fornix

a

Foramen of
Monro

Body of
fornix

Internal
cerebral
vein

Medial
posterior
choroidal
artery

Thalami

b

Figure 1.10. **(a)** Superior view of the venous relationship of the lateral and third ventricles. **(b)** Superior view showing the separation of the body of the fornix to expose the third ventricle and vascular structures.

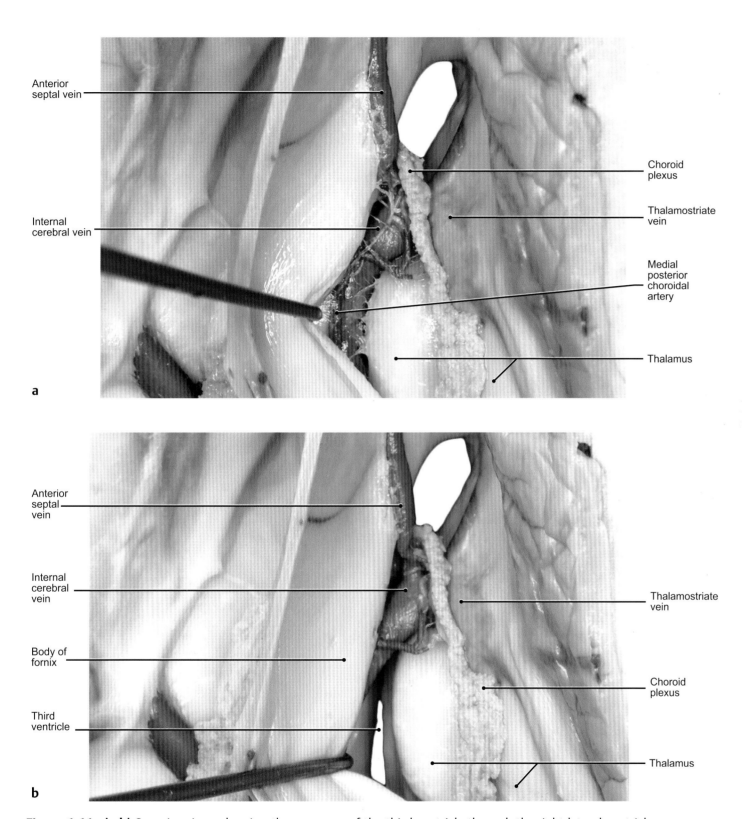

Figure 1.11. **(a,b)** Superior views showing the exposure of the third ventricle through the right lateral ventricle.

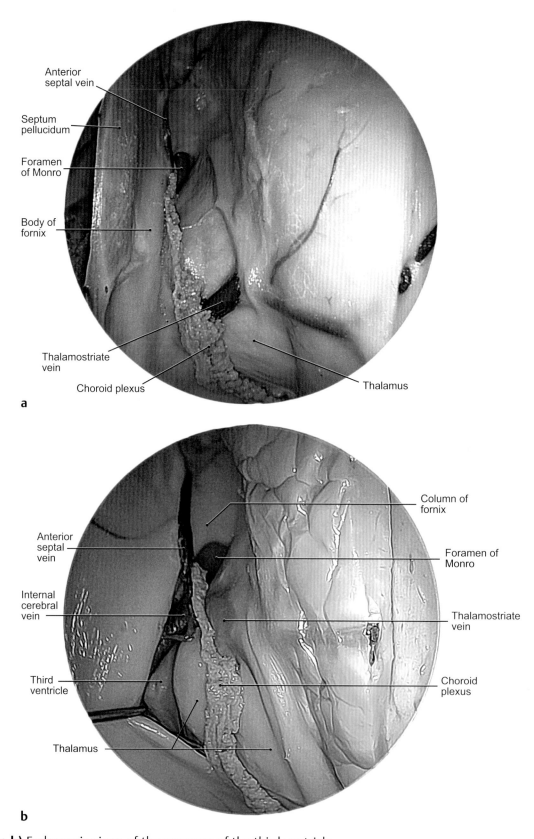

Figure 1.12. (a,b) Endoscopic views of the exposure of the third ventricle.

Surface Anatomy of the Brainstem

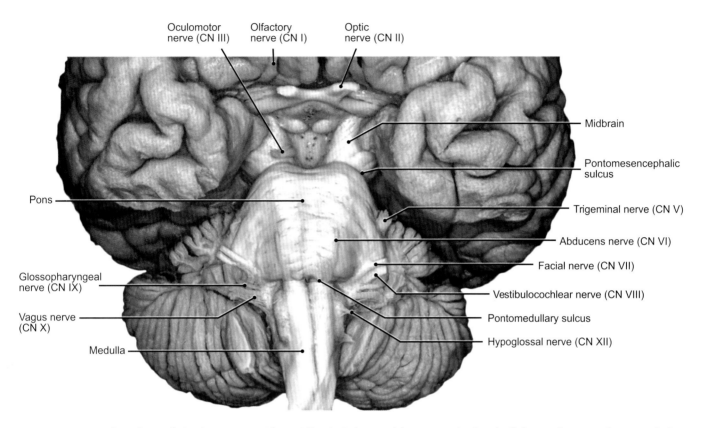

Figure 1.13. Ventral surface of the brainstem. The midbrain is located between the level of the optic tract above and the pontomesencephalic sulcus below. The pons is bordered by pontomesencephalic and pontomedullary sulci. The medulla is situated below the level of the pontomedullary sulcus and transitions into the spinal cord at the level of the first cervical nerve rootlets.

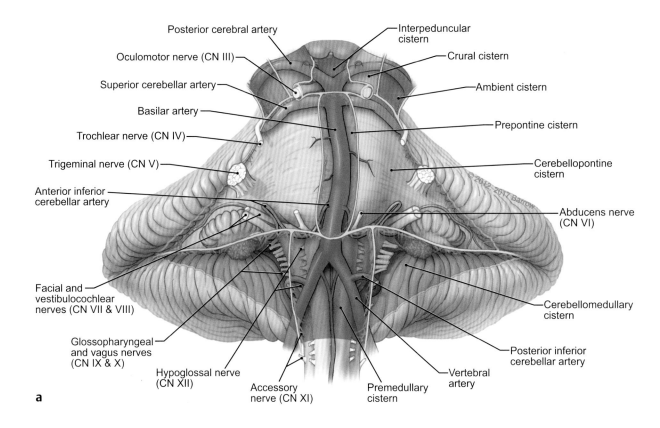

a

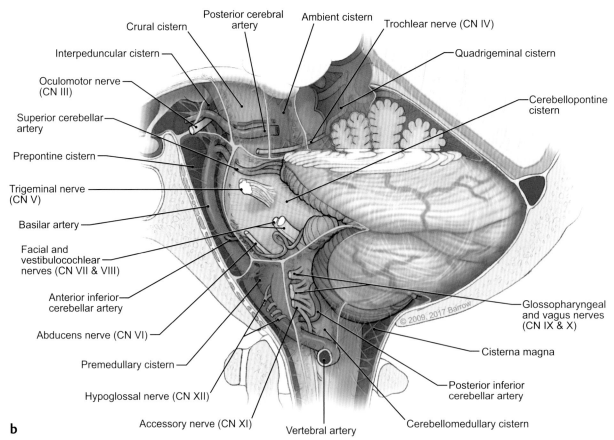

b

Figure 1.14. The brainstem and the cisterns that are associated with the cranial nerves. **(a)** Ventral view and **(b)** lateral view.

Fiber Tracts of the Brainstem

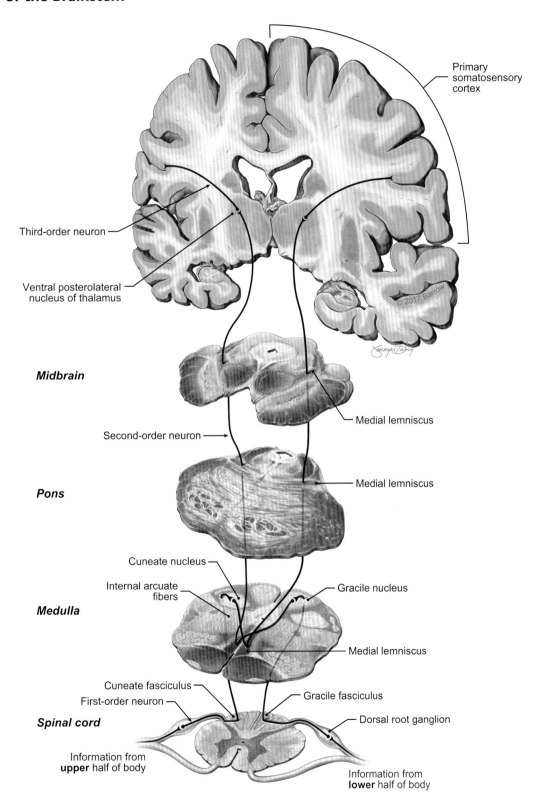

Figure 1.15. Dorsal column–medial lemniscus pathway. The dorsal column–medial lemniscus pathway is the major sensory pathway relaying vibration, proprioception, fine touch, and two-point discrimination from the skin and joints. First-order neurons of this pathway that are located in the dorsal root ganglion send their axons via the gracile fasciculus (information from the lower half of the body) and the cuneate fasciculus (information from the upper half of the body) to the level of the second-order neurons, which are located in the gracile nucleus and cuneate nucleus in the medulla. A subset of these second-order neurons decussates in the medulla, and hence these fibers, which form the medial lemniscus, are named the internal arcuate fibers. Second-order neurons send axons to the ventral posterolateral nucleus of the thalamus, where they synapse with third-order neurons, which then relay information to the postcentral gyrus (not shown).

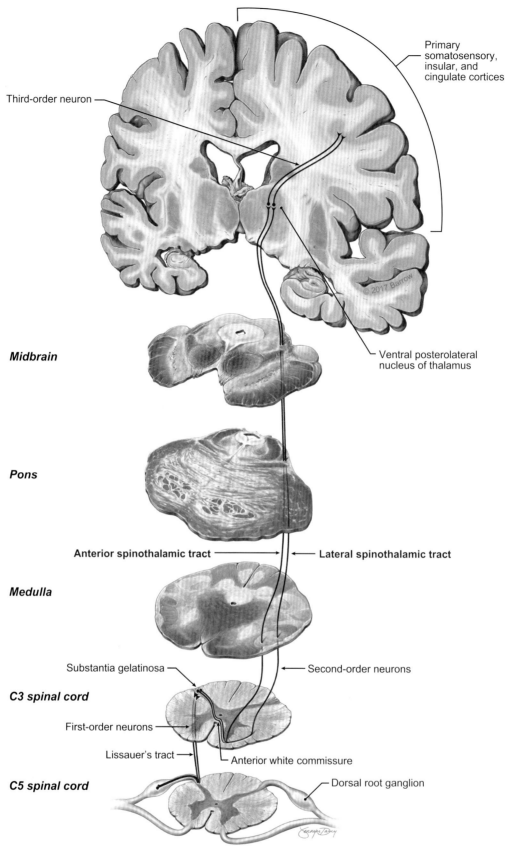

Third-order neuron

Primary somatosensory, insular, and cingulate cortices

© 2017 Barrow

Midbrain

Ventral posterolateral nucleus of thalamus

Pons

Anterior spinothalamic tract ——————— ←—— Lateral spinothalamic tract

Medulla

Substantia gelatinosa

Second-order neurons

C3 spinal cord

First-order neurons

Lissauer's tract ——→ —— Anterior white commissure

C5 spinal cord

Dorsal root ganglion

Figure 1.16. Anterolateral system. The anterolateral system, also known as the spinothalamic system, is one of the major sensory pathways. This pathway consists of two adjacent pathways: the anterior spinothalamic tract, which is responsible for carrying crude touch, and the lateral tract, which carries pain and temperature sensation. Unlike the corticospinal and medial lemniscus pathways, this tract decussates in the spinal cord instead of the brainstem. Neurons in the dorsal root ganglion send ascending fibers, or descending fibers migrate caudally for one or two levels via Lissauer's tract and then synapse with second-order neurons, called tract cells, in the substantia gelatinosa or nucleus proprius. The axons of the second-order neurons decussate via the anterior white commissure, usually one or two levels above the point of entry, and migrate via the spinal cord to the rostral ventromedial medulla. These second-order neurons then connect with third-order neurons in the medial dorsal, ventral posterolateral, and ventral medial posterior nuclei of thalamus. From this point, the information is passed to the primary somatosensory, insular, and cingulate cortices.

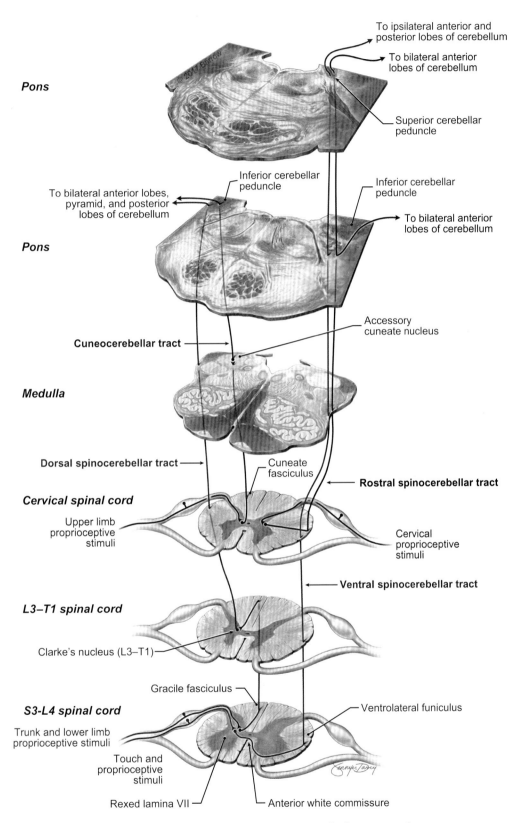

Figure 1.17. Spinocerebellar tract. The spinocerebellar tract is a proprioception tract that transmits signals from the spinal cord to the cerebellum ipsilaterally. The tract is divided into a ventral spinocerebellar tract, a rostral spinocerebellar tract, a dorsal spinocerebellar tract, and a cuneocerebellar tract. Proprioceptive stimuli are received from the Golgi tendon organs and muscle spindles, which have their cell bodies located in the dorsal root ganglion and constitute the first-order neurons in the circuit. These fibers then pass through Rexed laminae I–VI to synapse with second-order neurons in Rexed lamina VII. For the dorsal and cuneocerebellar tracts, the sensory neurons synapse in Clarke's nucleus in layer VII at L3–T1 and then send axons via the spinal cord to the medial zones in the cerebellum using the inferior cerebellar peduncle. For the ventral and rostral spinocerebellar tracts, the sensory neurons synapse in layer VII of S3–L4 and most of these neurons cross to the contralateral lateral funiculus through the anterior white commissure and the superior cerebellar peduncle. In the cerebellum, the bulk of these fibers ultimately cross over again to the ipsilateral side.

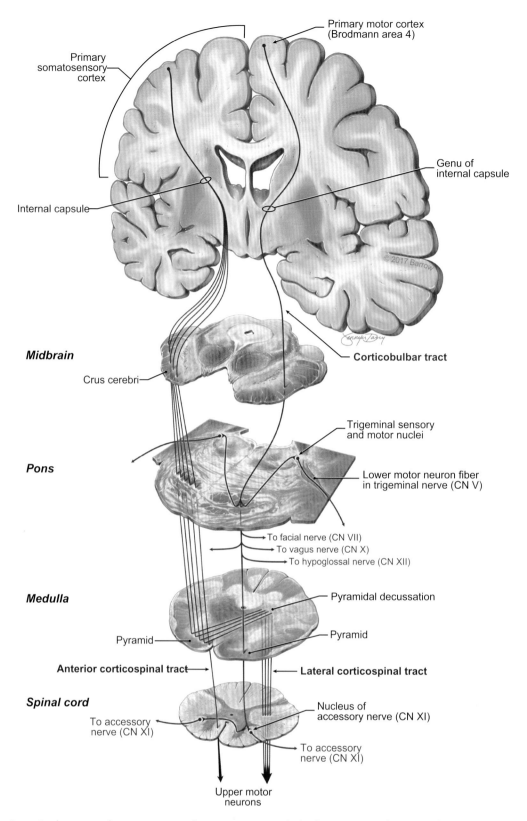

Primary motor cortex
(Brodmann area 4)

Primary
somatosensory
cortex

Genu of
internal capsule

Internal capsule

© 2017 Barrow

Midbrain

Corticobulbar tract

Crus cerebri

Pons

Trigeminal sensory
and motor nuclei

Lower motor neuron fiber
in trigeminal nerve (CN V)

To facial nerve (CN VII)
To vagus nerve (CN X)
To hypoglossal nerve (CN XII)

Medulla

Pyramidal decussation

Pyramid

Pyramid

Anterior corticospinal tract→

←Lateral corticospinal tract

Spinal cord

Nucleus of
accessory nerve (CN XI)

To accessory
nerve (CN XI)

To accessory
nerve (CN XI)

Upper motor
neurons

Figure 1.18. Corticospinal tracts. The corticospinal tracts constitute the major motor pathways. Nerves of this tract originate in the pyramidal cells in layer V of the cerebral cortex. The axons of these nerves travel from the cortex via the posterior limb of the internal capsule, into the cerebral peduncle and the anterior medulla. At the pyramids of the medulla, most of the fibers (80%) cross over to the opposite side from which they originated and form the lateral corticospinal tract. Some axons remain ipsilateral and form the anterior corticospinal tract. The descending fibers constitute upper motor neurons that migrate caudally in the spinal cord to the level of the organs they innervate. Once there, they form synapses with lower motor neurons or interneurons that ultimately form synapses with lower motor neurons in the anterior horn of the spinal cord. The corticobulbar tract is also known as the corticonuclear tract, and it is responsible for relaying motor information of the non-oculomotor cranial nerves between the cerebral cortex and the brainstem. The cranial nerves innervated by this tract include the trigeminal nerve (CN V), the facial nerve (CN VII), the vagus nerve (CN X), the accessory nerve (CN XI), and the hypoglossal nerve (CN XII). This tract originates in the primary motor cortex in Brodmann area 4. The tract descends through the corona radiata and the genu of the internal capsule to the midbrain. The internal capsule transitions to become the cerebral peduncles in the brainstem. White matter tracts migrate in the ventral portion of the peduncles in the crus cerebri. The corticospinal and corticobulbar fibers travel within the middle three-fifths of the crus cerebri. The fibers of the corticobulbar tract migrate in the crus cerebri and synapse at the level of the appropriate lower motor neurons controlling the cranial nerve of interest. This tract innervates cranial motor nuclei bilaterally, except for the lower facial nuclei and the hypoglossal nerve (CN XII), both of which are innervated unilaterally.

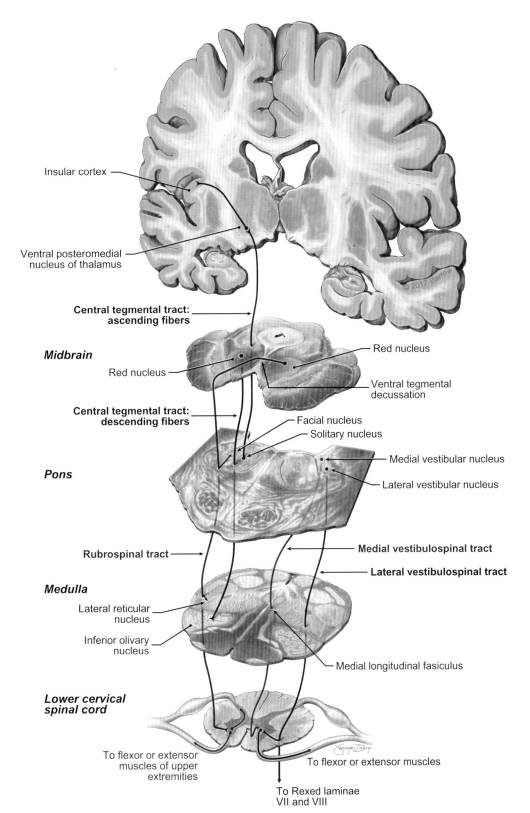

Insular cortex

Ventral posteromedial
nucleus of thalamus

Central tegmental tract:
ascending fibers

Midbrain

Red nucleus

Red nucleus

Ventral tegmental
decussation

Central tegmental tract:
descending fibers

Facial nucleus
Solitary nucleus

Pons

Medial vestibular nucleus

Lateral vestibular nucleus

Rubrospinal tract

Medial vestibulospinal tract

Lateral vestibulospinal tract

Medulla

Lateral reticular
nucleus

Inferior olivary
nucleus

Medial longitudinal fasiculus

Lower cervical
spinal cord

To flexor or extensor
muscles of upper
extremities

To flexor or extensor muscles

To Rexed laminae
VII and VIII

Figure 1.19. Rubrospinal, vestibulospinal, and central tegmental tracts. The rubrospinal tract constitutes one of the major motor pathways of voluntary movement. This pathway terminates in the upper cervical spinal cord and mediates flexion in the upper extremities. The fibers of this pathway originate in the midbrain at the magnocellular red nucleus and cross in the midbrain and descend in the lateral brainstem tegmentum. Once in the spinal cord, the rubrospinal tract travels through the lateral funiculus along with the lateral corticospinal tract. The vestibulospinal tract is a motor pathway responsible for maintaining posture and balance with head movement. It consists of a lateral tract and a medial tract. The lateral vestibulospinal tract originates in the lateral vestibular nucleus in the pons. These fibers descend ipsilaterally in the anterior lateral funiculus, ultimately terminating at the interneurons (or, in rare cases, at the alpha motor neurons) of Rexed laminae VII and VIII.

The medial vestibulospinal tract originates in the medial vestibular nucleus. These fibers unite with ipsilateral and contralateral medial longitudinal fasciculi and descend in the anterior funiculus into the spinal cord, where they terminate on neurons in Rexed laminae VII and VIII. The medial vestibulospinal tract predominantly innervates muscles of the head and terminates in the cervical spinal cord. The central tegmental tract is an axon tract that connects the subthalamus and the reticular formation with the inferior olivary nucleus. The central tegmental tract contains ascending and descending fibers. The ascending fibers arise from the rostral solitary nucleus and terminate in the ventral posteromedial nucleus of the thalamus. Information about taste is relayed from the thalamus to the insular cortex. The descending fibers arise from the red nucleus and project to the inferior olivary nucleus. The rubro-olivary tract connects to the contralateral cerebellum.

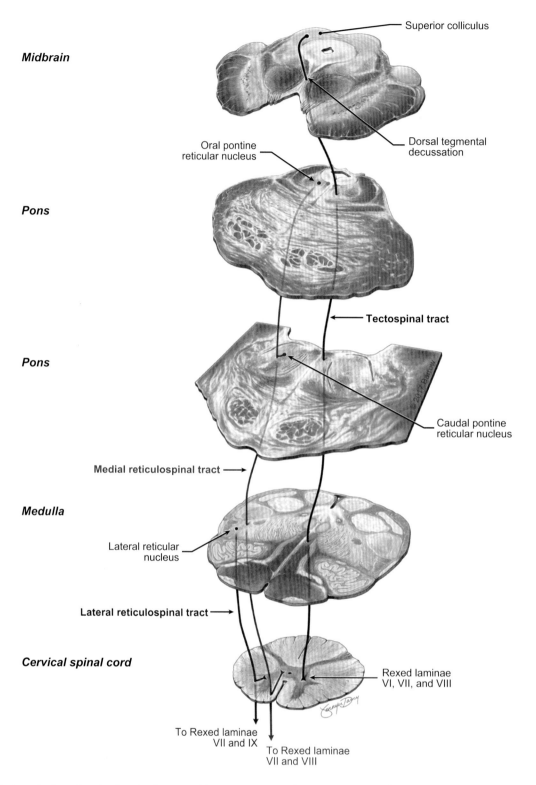

Midbrain

Superior colliculus

Oral pontine reticular nucleus

Dorsal tegmental decussation

Pons

Tectospinal tract

Pons

Caudal pontine reticular nucleus

Medial reticulospinal tract →

Medulla

Lateral reticular nucleus

Lateral reticulospinal tract →

Cervical spinal cord

Rexed laminae VI, VII, and VIII

To Rexed laminae VII and IX

To Rexed laminae VII and VIII

Figure 1.20. Tectospinal and reticulospinal tracts. The tectospinal tract connects the midbrain tectum to the spinal cord and is responsible for mediating reflex postural movements of the head to auditory and visual input. This tract originates in the superior colliculus, which has afferents from the oculomotor nuclei and projects to the contralateral and ipsilateral domains of the cervical neuromeres and the oculomotor, trochlear, and abducens nuclei. This tract descends in the spinal cord to terminate in Rexed laminae VI, VII, and VIII. The reticulospinal tract consists of the medial and lateral parts. The medial reticulospinal tract provides excitatory input to the antigravity extensor muscles. The fibers of this tract originate in the caudal pontine reticular nucleus and the oral pontine reticular nucleus, and they project to Rexed laminae VII and VIII of the spinal cord. The lateral reticulospinal tract exerts inhibitory control over excitatory axial extensor muscles. The fibers of this tract arise from the medullary reticular formation and descend in the anterior spinal cord in the lateral column to terminate in Rexed laminae VII and IX of the spinal cord.

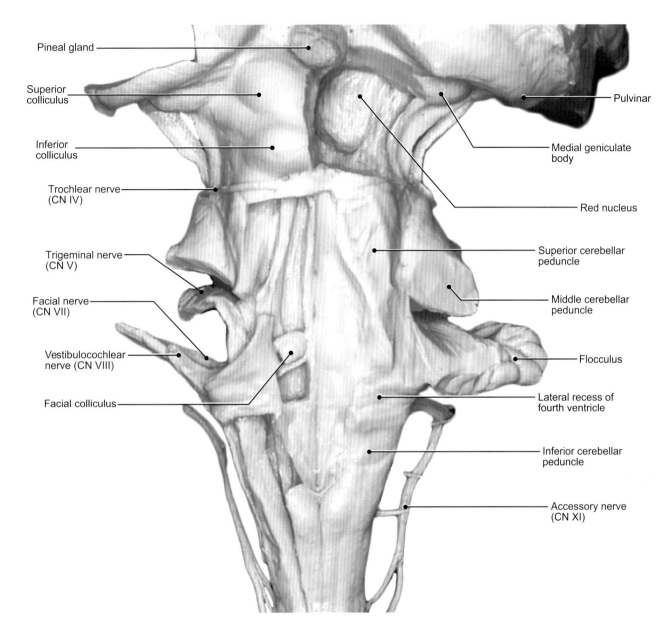

Pineal gland

Superior colliculus

Inferior colliculus

Trochlear nerve (CN IV)

Trigeminal nerve (CN V)

Facial nerve (CN VII)

Vestibulocochlear nerve (CN VIII)

Facial colliculus

Pulvinar

Medial geniculate body

Red nucleus

Superior cerebellar peduncle

Middle cerebellar peduncle

Flocculus

Lateral recess of fourth ventricle

Inferior cerebellar peduncle

Accessory nerve (CN XI)

Figure 1.21. Dorsal view of a cadaveric dissection showing the surface and internal structures of the brainstem. The midbrain has superior and inferior colliculi. The brachium of the inferior colliculus runs from the inferior colliculus to the medial geniculate body. The floor of the fourth ventricle has a rhomboid shape. The upper two-thirds of the floor of the fourth ventricle are on the dorsal surface of the pons, and the lower one-third is on the dorsal surface of the medulla. The floor of the fourth ventricle can be divided into a superior or a pontine part, an intermediate or a junctional part, and an inferior or a medullary part. The superior part of the floor of the fourth ventricle has a triangular shape. Its apex is at the cerebral aqueduct, its base is formed by an imaginary line connecting the lower margin of the cerebellar peduncles, and its lateral margins are the medial edge of the superior cerebellar peduncles. The intermediate or junctional part is at the same level as the lateral recesses. The medullary part has a triangular shape limited laterally by the inferolateral margin of the floor, along which the tela choroidea is attached, and its apex is at the obex. The medullary part contains the hypoglossal and vagal trigones and the area postrema, which is shaped like a pen nib and is thus called the calamus scriptorius.

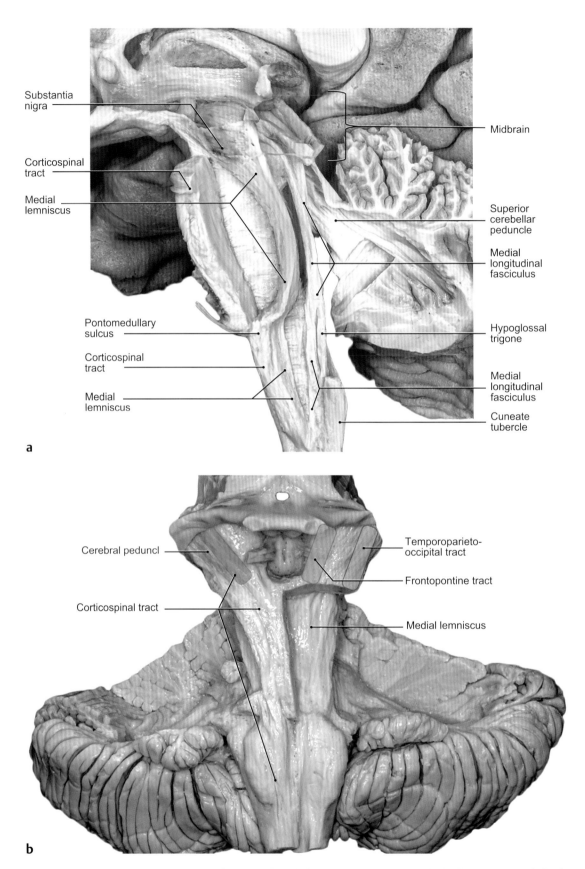

Substantia nigra

Corticospinal tract

Medial lemniscus

Midbrain

Superior cerebellar peduncle

Medial longitudinal fasciculus

Pontomedullary sulcus

Corticospinal tract

Medial lemniscus

Hypoglossal trigone

Medial longitudinal fasciculus

Cuneate tubercle

a

Cerebral peduncl

Corticospinal tract

Temporoparieto-occipital tract

Frontopontine tract

Medial lemniscus

b

Figure 1.22. Cadaveric dissections showing **(a)** the lateral and **(b)** the ventral views of the long tracts of the brainstem. The colored areas denote the various tracts within the bilateral cerebral peduncles.

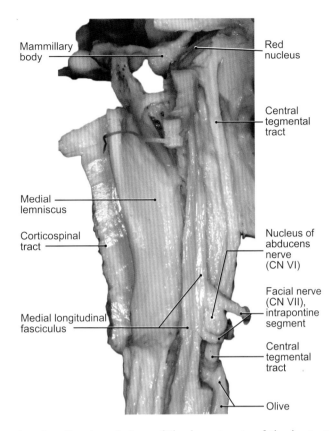

Figure 1.23. Cadaveric dissection showing the dorsal view of the long tracts of the brainstem.

Vascular Anatomy of the Brainstem

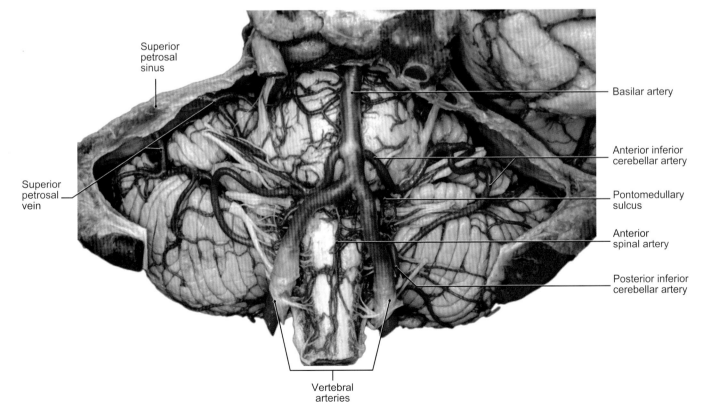

Figure 1.24. Ventral view of a cadaveric dissection of the vascular anatomy of the brainstem. At the level of the pontomedullary sulcus, the vertebral arteries come together to form the basilar artery, which ascends superiorly along the ventral surface of the pons to terminate as the two posterior cerebral arteries. This termination usually occurs at the level of the pontomesencephalic junction.

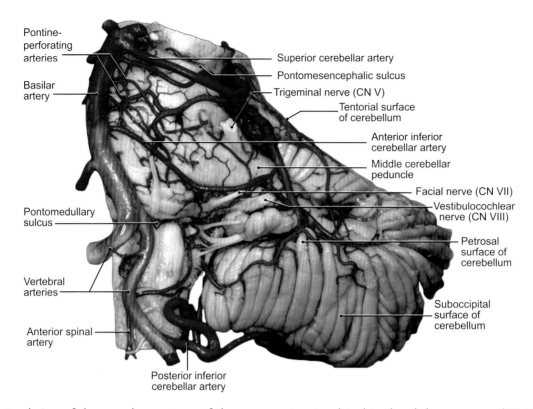

Labels (clockwise from top left):
- Pontine-perforating arteries
- Basilar artery
- Pontomedullary sulcus
- Vertebral arteries
- Anterior spinal artery
- Posterior inferior cerebellar artery
- Superior cerebellar artery
- Pontomesencephalic sulcus
- Trigeminal nerve (CN V)
- Tentorial surface of cerebellum
- Anterior inferior cerebellar artery
- Middle cerebellar peduncle
- Facial nerve (CN VII)
- Vestibulocochlear nerve (CN VIII)
- Petrosal surface of cerebellum
- Suboccipital surface of cerebellum

Figure 1.25. Lateral view of the vascular anatomy of the brainstem. The posterior inferior cerebellar artery arises from the vertebral arteries and supplies the medulla, the glossopharyngeal nerve (CN IX), the vagus nerve (CN X), the accessory nerve (CN XI), the inferior cerebellar peduncle, and the suboccipital surface of the cerebellum. The basilar artery gives rise to the pontine-perforating arteries and the anterior inferior cerebellar artery. The anterior inferior cerebellar artery is related to the abducens nerve (CN VI), the facial nerve (CN VII), the vestibulocochlear nerve (CN VIII), the middle cerebellar peduncle, and the petrosal surface of the cerebellum. The superior cerebellar artery arises from the basilar artery at the level of the pontomesencephalic sulcus and is related to the midbrain, superior cerebellar peduncle, and tentorial surface of the cerebellum.

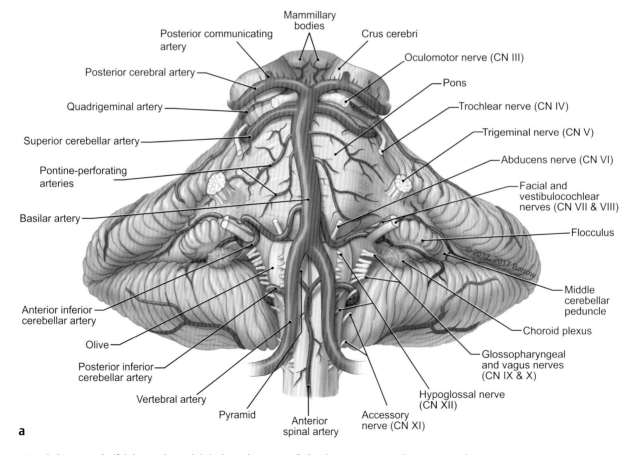

Labels (clockwise from top):
- Mammillary bodies
- Posterior communicating artery
- Posterior cerebral artery
- Quadrigeminal artery
- Superior cerebellar artery
- Pontine-perforating arteries
- Basilar artery
- Anterior inferior cerebellar artery
- Olive
- Posterior inferior cerebellar artery
- Vertebral artery
- Pyramid
- Anterior spinal artery
- Accessory nerve (CN XI)
- Hypoglossal nerve (CN XII)
- Glossopharyngeal and vagus nerves (CN IX & X)
- Choroid plexus
- Middle cerebellar peduncle
- Flocculus
- Facial and vestibulocochlear nerves (CN VII & VIII)
- Abducens nerve (CN VI)
- Trigeminal nerve (CN V)
- Trochlear nerve (CN IV)
- Pons
- Oculomotor nerve (CN III)
- Crus cerebri

© 2012–2017 Barrow

a

Figure 1.26. **(a)** Ventral, **(b)** lateral, and **(c)** dorsal views of the brainstem and associated arteries.

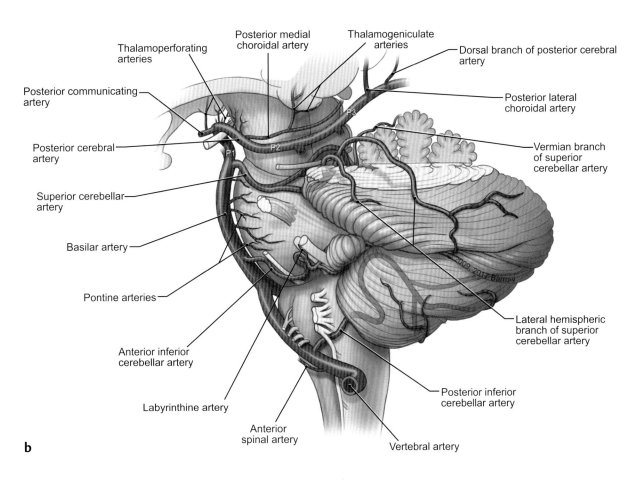

Thalamoperforating arteries

Posterior medial choroidal artery

Thalamogeniculate arteries

Dorsal branch of posterior cerebral artery

Posterior communicating artery

Posterior cerebral artery

Posterior lateral choroidal artery

Superior cerebellar artery

Vermian branch of superior cerebellar artery

Basilar artery

Pontine arteries

Anterior inferior cerebellar artery

Lateral hemispheric branch of superior cerebellar artery

Labyrinthine artery

Posterior inferior cerebellar artery

Anterior spinal artery

Vertebral artery

b

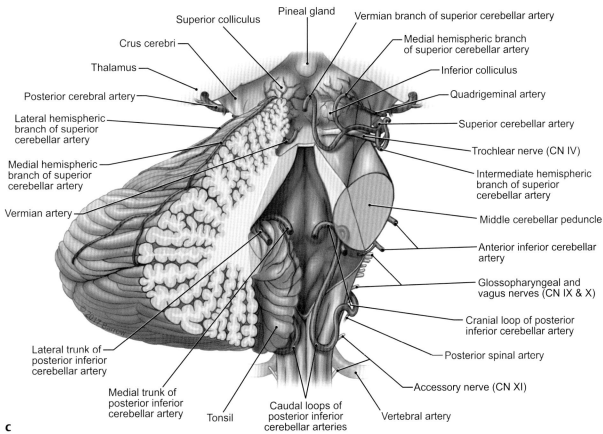

Superior colliculus

Pineal gland

Vermian branch of superior cerebellar artery

Crus cerebri

Medial hemispheric branch of superior cerebellar artery

Thalamus

Inferior colliculus

Posterior cerebral artery

Quadrigeminal artery

Lateral hemispheric branch of superior cerebellar artery

Superior cerebellar artery

Trochlear nerve (CN IV)

Medial hemispheric branch of superior cerebellar artery

Intermediate hemispheric branch of superior cerebellar artery

Vermian artery

Middle cerebellar peduncle

Anterior inferior cerebellar artery

Glossopharyngeal and vagus nerves (CN IX & X)

Cranial loop of posterior inferior cerebellar artery

Posterior spinal artery

Lateral trunk of posterior inferior cerebellar artery

Medial trunk of posterior inferior cerebellar artery

Tonsil

Caudal loops of posterior inferior cerebellar arteries

Vertebral artery

Accessory nerve (CN XI)

c

Figure 1.26. (Continued)

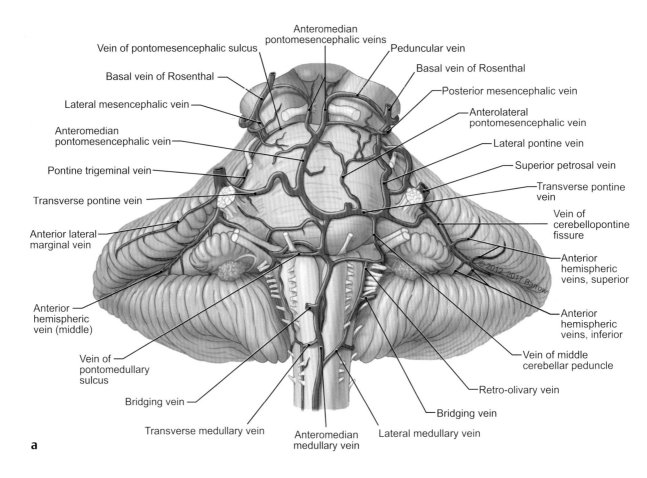

Anteromedian
pontomesencephalic veins

Vein of pontomesencephalic sulcus

Peduncular vein

Basal vein of Rosenthal

Basal vein of Rosenthal

Posterior mesencephalic vein

Lateral mesencephalic vein

Anterolateral
pontomesencephalic vein

Anteromedian
pontomesencephalic vein

Lateral pontine vein

Pontine trigeminal vein

Superior petrosal vein

Transverse pontine
vein

Transverse pontine vein

Vein of
cerebellopontine
fissure

Anterior lateral
marginal vein

Anterior
hemispheric
veins, superior

Anterior
hemispheric
vein (middle)

Anterior
hemispheric
veins, inferior

Vein of middle
cerebellar peduncle

Vein of
pontomedullary
sulcus

Retro-olivary vein

Bridging vein

Bridging vein

Transverse medullary vein

Anteromedian
medullary vein

Lateral medullary vein

a

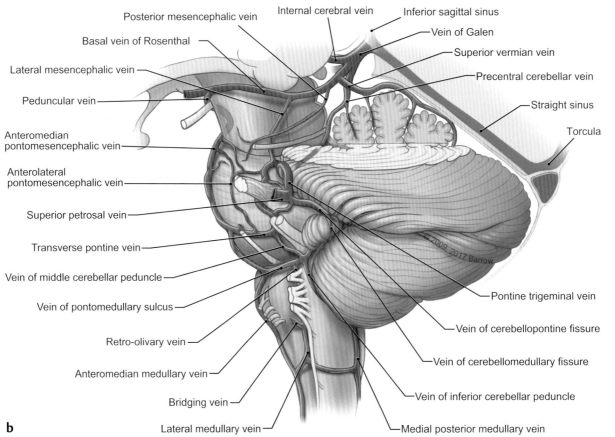

Posterior mesencephalic vein

Internal cerebral vein

Inferior sagittal sinus

Basal vein of Rosenthal

Vein of Galen

Superior vermian vein

Lateral mesencephalic vein

Precentral cerebellar vein

Peduncular vein

Straight sinus

Anteromedian
pontomesencephalic vein

Torcula

Anterolateral
pontomesencephalic vein

Superior petrosal vein

Transverse pontine vein

Vein of middle cerebellar peduncle

Vein of pontomedullary sulcus

Pontine trigeminal vein

Retro-olivary vein

Vein of cerebellopontine fissure

Vein of cerebellomedullary fissure

Anteromedian medullary vein

Vein of inferior cerebellar peduncle

Bridging vein

Medial posterior medullary vein

Lateral medullary vein

b

Figure 1.27. **(a)** Ventral, **(b)** lateral, and **(c)** dorsal views of the brainstem and associated veins.

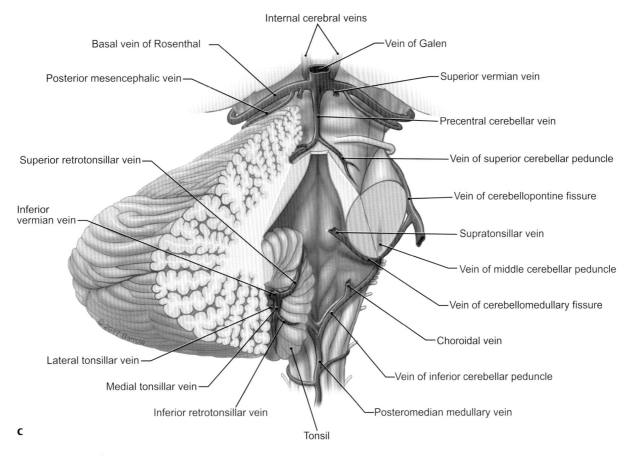

c

Figure 1.27. (*Continued*)

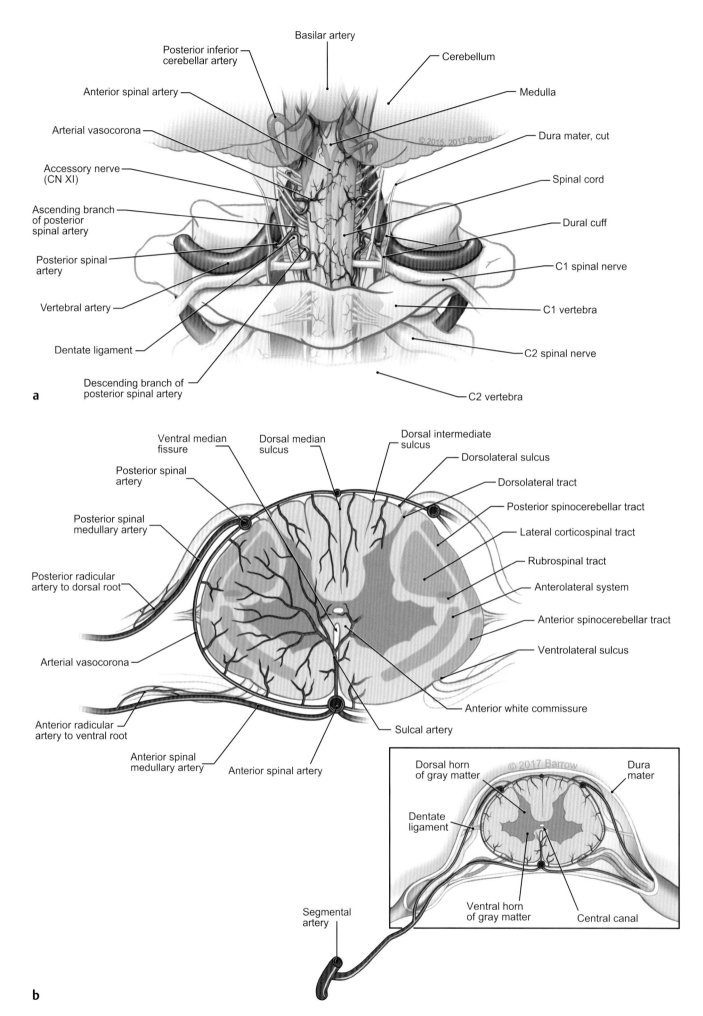

Figure 1.28. **(a)** Dorsal view of the spinal cord arteries at the level of the cervicomedullary junction, and **(b)** axial view of the medullary arterial system supplying the spinal cord.

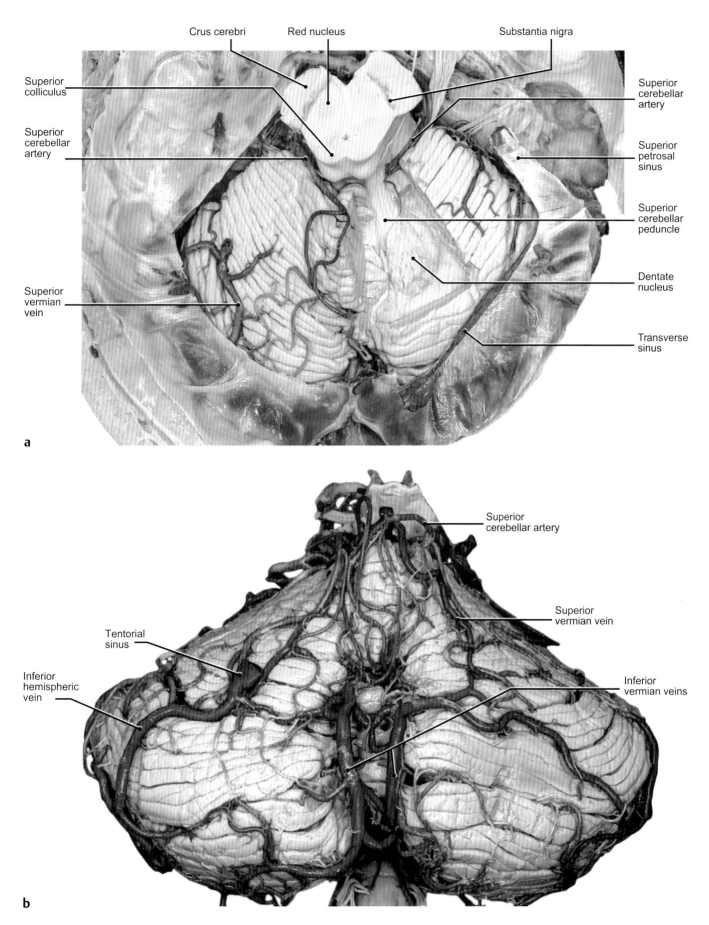

Figure 1.29. Cadaveric dissections showing **(a)** the superior view and **(b)** the dorsal view of the vasculature of the cerebellum.

Midbrain

Axial Sections of the Midbrain

Figure 1.30. (a–d) Sequential axial slices of the midbrain.

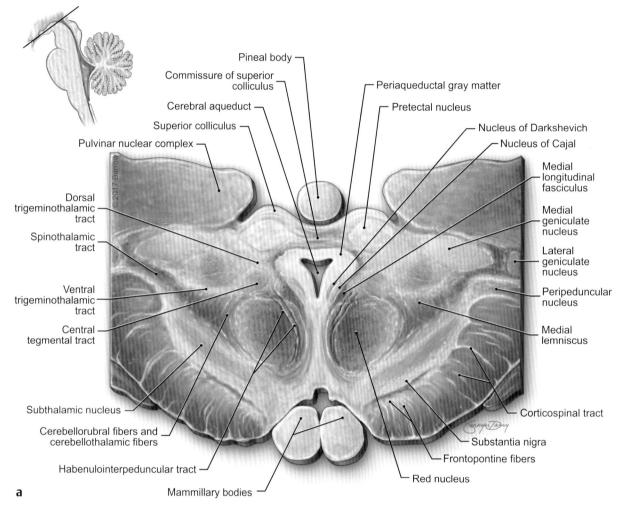

Pineal body

Commissure of superior colliculus

Cerebral aqueduct

Superior colliculus

Pulvinar nuclear complex

Periaqueductal gray matter

Pretectal nucleus

Nucleus of Darkshevich

Nucleus of Cajal

Medial longitudinal fasciculus

Medial geniculate nucleus

Lateral geniculate nucleus

Peripeduncular nucleus

Medial lemniscus

Dorsal trigeminothalamic tract

Spinothalamic tract

Ventral trigeminothalamic tract

Central tegmental tract

Subthalamic nucleus

Cerebellorubral fibers and cerebellothalamic fibers

Habenulointerpeduncular tract

Corticospinal tract

Substantia nigra

Frontopontine fibers

Red nucleus

a   Mammillary bodies

Figure 1.30. (a) Slightly oblique section through the midbrain–diencephalon junction. The section passes through the posterior commissure and the rostral end of the red nucleus, the pulvinar nuclear complex, and the lateral and medial geniculate bodies of the thalamus to end dorsal to the mammillary bodies. The medial longitudinal fasciculus ends at the nucleus of Cajal, which is located ventrolateral to the cerebral aqueduct and dorsomedial to the red nucleus. The central tegmental tract travels dorsal to the red nucleus to terminate at the capsule of the red nucleus. The subthalamic nucleus is located ventral to the red nucleus.

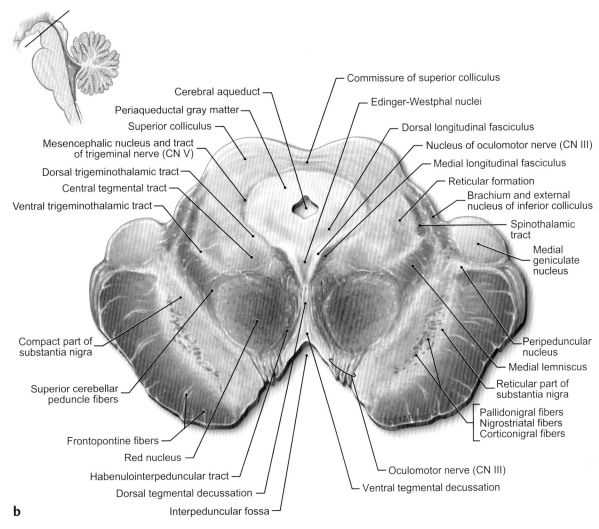

Commissure of superior colliculus

Edinger-Westphal nuclei

Cerebral aqueduct

Periaqueductal gray matter

Dorsal longitudinal fasciculus

Superior colliculus

Nucleus of oculomotor nerve (CN III)

Mesencephalic nucleus and tract
of trigeminal nerve (CN V)

Medial longitudinal fasciculus

Dorsal trigeminothalamic tract

Reticular formation

Central tegmental tract

Brachium and external
nucleus of inferior colliculus

Ventral trigeminothalamic tract

Spinothalamic
tract

Medial
geniculate
nucleus

Compact part of
substantia nigra

Peripeduncular
nucleus

Medial lemniscus

Superior cerebellar
peduncle fibers

Reticular part of
substantia nigra

Pallidonigral fibers
Nigrostriatal fibers
Corticonigral fibers

Frontopontine fibers

Red nucleus

Habenulointerpeduncular tract

Oculomotor nerve (CN III)

Dorsal tegmental decussation

Ventral tegmental decussation

b

Interpeduncular fossa

Figure 1.30. (b) Transverse section of the midbrain through the upper half of the superior colliculus, rostral portion of the oculomotor nucleus, including the Edinger-Westphal nuclei and the intramesencephalic segment of the oculomotor nerve (CN III). The superior cerebellar peduncle fibers form the dorsolateral capsule of the red nucleus. The oculomotor nucleus sits ventral to the cerebral aqueduct and comes together with the Edinger-Westphal nuclei in the midline.

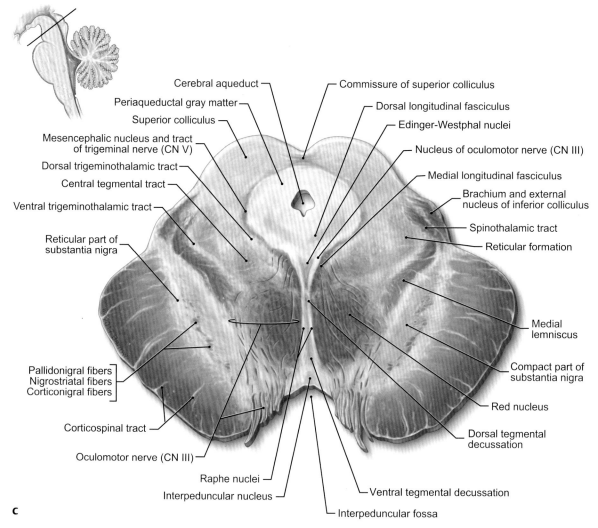

Cerebral aqueduct

Periaqueductal gray matter

Superior colliculus

Mesencephalic nucleus and tract
of trigeminal nerve (CN V)

Dorsal trigeminothalamic tract

Central tegmental tract

Ventral trigeminothalamic tract

Reticular part of
substantia nigra

Pallidonigral fibers
Nigrostriatal fibers
Corticonigral fibers

Corticospinal tract

Oculomotor nerve (CN III)

Raphe nuclei

Interpeduncular nucleus

Commissure of superior colliculus

Dorsal longitudinal fasciculus

Edinger-Westphal nuclei

Nucleus of oculomotor nerve (CN III)

Medial longitudinal fasciculus

Brachium and external
nucleus of inferior colliculus

Spinothalamic tract

Reticular formation

Medial
lemniscus

Compact part of
substantia nigra

Red nucleus

Dorsal tegmental
decussation

Ventral tegmental decussation

Interpeduncular fossa

c

Figure 1.30. (c) Transverse section of the midbrain through the red nucleus and the inferior half of the superior colliculus. The plane of the section is caudal to the Edinger-Westphal nuclei but includes rostral portions of the decussation of the superior peduncle. The decussating fibers pass through the red nucleus at this level. The intramesencephalic segment of the oculomotor nerve arising from the oculomotor nucleus passes through and is medial to the red nucleus. The corticospinal tract travels through the middle three-fifths of the crus cerebri.

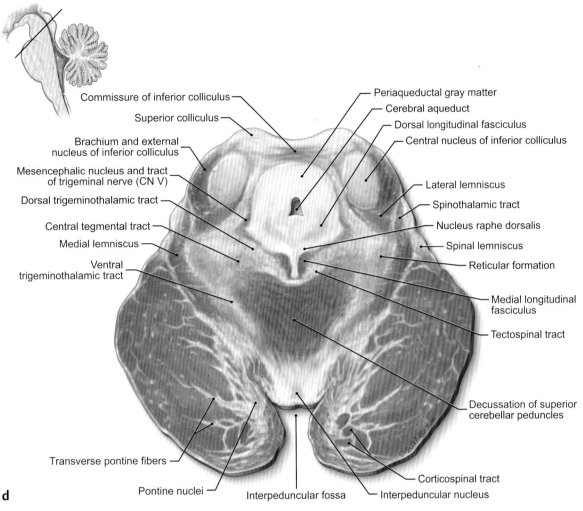

Commissure of inferior colliculus

Superior colliculus

Brachium and external nucleus of inferior colliculus

Mesencephalic nucleus and tract of trigeminal nerve (CN V)

Dorsal trigeminothalamic tract

Central tegmental tract

Medial lemniscus

Ventral trigeminothalamic tract

Periaqueductal gray matter

Cerebral aqueduct

Dorsal longitudinal fasciculus

Central nucleus of inferior colliculus

Lateral lemniscus

Spinothalamic tract

Nucleus raphe dorsalis

Spinal lemniscus

Reticular formation

Medial longitudinal fasciculus

Tectospinal tract

Decussation of superior cerebellar peduncles

Transverse pontine fibers

Pontine nuclei

Interpeduncular fossa

Interpeduncular nucleus

Corticospinal tract

d

Figure 1.30. (d) The transverse section of the midbrain through the junction of the superior and inferior colliculi and the ventral part of the pontomesencephalic sulcus. The section includes the rostral tip of the basilar pons, with the corticospinal tract located anteromedially. The superior cerebellar peduncle fibers (except the most laterally located fibers) decussate in the midline.

Surface Anatomy, Internal Structures, and Safe Entry Zones of the Midbrain

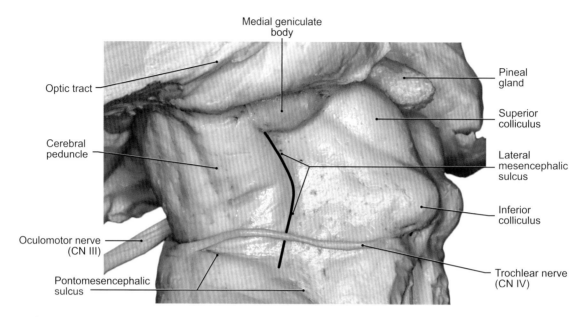

Figure 1.31. Cadaveric dissection showing the lateral surface of the midbrain. The lateral mesencephalic sulcus extends from the pontomesencephalic sulcus inferiorly to the medial geniculate body superiorly, and it forms the border between the cerebral peduncle and the tectum of the midbrain. The tectum contains the superior and inferior colliculi.

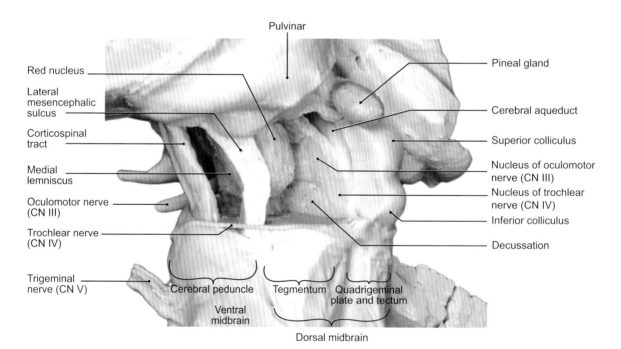

Figure 1.32. Lateral view of internal structures of the midbrain. The midbrain has a ventral part, which includes the crus cerebri, and a dorsal part, which includes the tegmentum and quadrigeminal plate (oculomotor, trochlear, and red nuclei) and the tectum (superior and inferior colliculi). The tegmentum of the midbrain is situated ventral to the cerebral aqueduct and the tectum of the midbrain is situated dorsal to the aqueduct. The lateral mesencephalic sulcus is positioned immediately lateral to the medial lemniscus at the border between the ventral and dorsal midbrain.

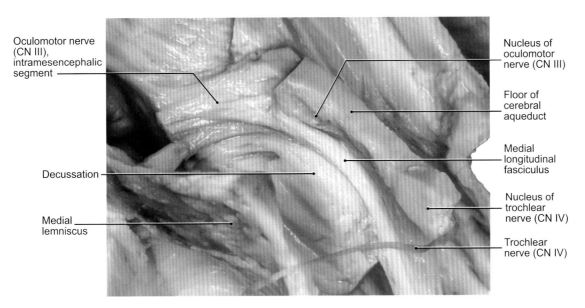

Oculomotor nerve (CN III), intramesencephalic segment

Nucleus of oculomotor nerve (CN III)

Floor of cerebral aqueduct

Medial longitudinal fasciculus

Decussation

Medial lemniscus

Nucleus of trochlear nerve (CN IV)

Trochlear nerve (CN IV)

Figure 1.33. Dissection showing a lateral view of the midbrain. The oculomotor and trochlear nuclei are situated ventral to the cerebral aqueduct. The medial longitudinal fasciculus connects with the oculomotor and trochlear nuclei.

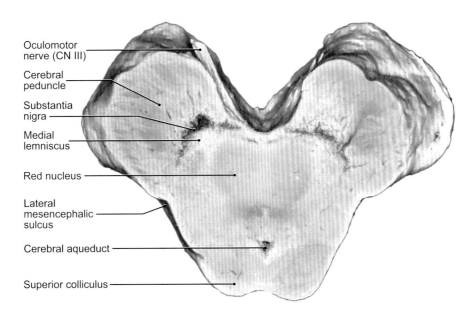

Oculomotor nerve (CN III)

Cerebral peduncle

Substantia nigra

Medial lemniscus

Red nucleus

Lateral mesencephalic sulcus

Cerebral aqueduct

Superior colliculus

Figure 1.34. Dissection showing the axial section of the midbrain at the level of the oculomotor nerve (CN III). This section demonstrates the location of various nuclei and tracts, and provides a rationale for safe entry zones in this area. For example, the location of the corticospinal tract in the middle three-fifths of the crus cerebri enables the surgeon to enter the ventral brainstem lateral to the oculomotor nerve between the posterior cerebral artery and the superior cerebellar artery at the anterior mesencephalic (alternatively called the perioculomotor) safe entry zone.

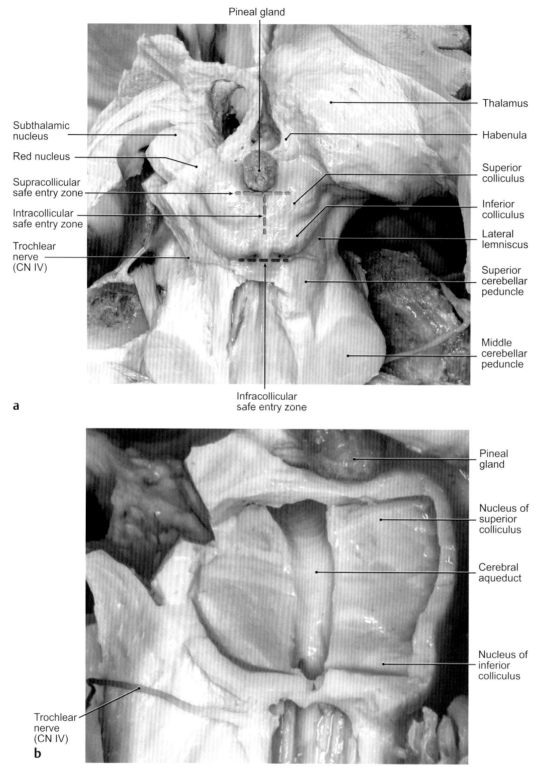

Figure 1.35. (a) Dorsal surface, safe entry zones, and internal structures of the midbrain. Three dorsally located safe entry zones can be used to resect deep-seated lesions in the midbrain. The supracollicular safe entry zone (*green dashed line*) is made above the superior colliculus, and the infracollicular safe entry zone (*blue dashed line*) is made below the inferior colliculus and above the trochlear nerve (CN IV). Both of these safe zones can be used for resection of lesions at the level of the colliculi. Alternatively, the intracollicular safe entry zone (*orange dashed line*) can be used with a vertical incision to resect extensive lesions in this area. **(b)** Stepwise dissection from the tectal (quadrigeminal) plate to the tegmentum. The cerebral aqueduct is the ventral limit of the intracollicular safe entry zones.

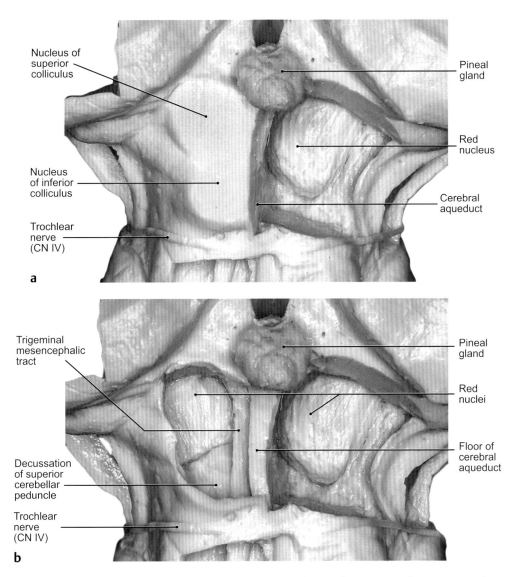

Nucleus of superior colliculus

Pineal gland

Red nucleus

Nucleus of inferior colliculus

Cerebral aqueduct

Trochlear nerve (CN IV)

a

Trigeminal mesencephalic tract

Pineal gland

Red nuclei

Decussation of superior cerebellar peduncle

Floor of cerebral aqueduct

Trochlear nerve (CN IV)

b

Figure 1.36. Dorsal view of the internal structures of the midbrain shown after ventrally passing the cerebral aqueduct. **(a)** The red nucleus is located at the tegmentum of the midbrain, which is situated ventral to the cerebral aqueduct. **(b)** The removal of the superior and inferior collicular nuclei exposes the tegmental part of the midbrain, which includes the red nuclei, decussation of the superior cerebellar peduncle, trigeminal mesencephalic tract dorsally, and central tegmental tract ventrally (not shown).

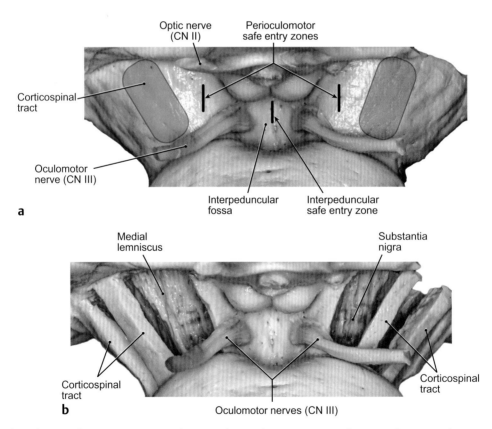

Figure 1.37. Dorsal view of the internal structures of the midbrain. The red nucleus extends from the midlevel of the inferior colliculus to the lateral wall of the third ventricle. The decussation of the superior cerebellar peduncle is situated at the level of the inferior colliculus. In the midbrain–diencephalic junction, the subthalamic nucleus is located ventrolateral to the red nucleus and dorsomedial to the internal capsule.

Figure 1.38. Ventral surface, safe entry zones, and internal structures of the midbrain. **(a)** The corticospinal tract is situated in the middle three-fifths of the crus cerebri. The anterior mesencephalic zone (perioculomotor zone) is directed through the frontopontine fibers and between the exit point of the oculomotor nucleus and the medial edge of the corticospinal tract. Alternatively, a second ventral safe entry zone, the interpeduncular safe entry zone, is located medial to the exit point of the oculomotor nerves (CN III) and directed through the interpeduncular fossa. **(b)** The removal of the frontopontine fibers exposes the medial lemniscus and substantia nigra.

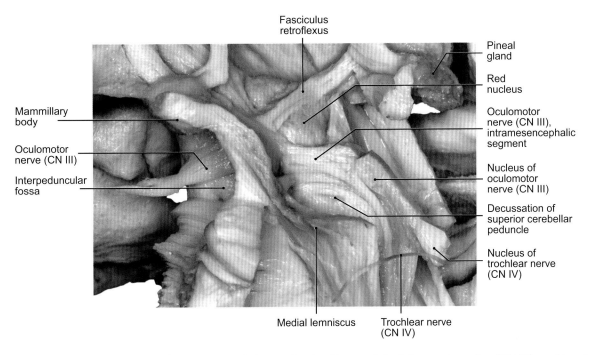

Figure 1.39. Lateral view of the internal structures of the midbrain. The nuclei of the oculomotor (CN III) and trochlear (CN IV) nerves are positioned in the midbrain just ventral to the cerebral aqueduct. The intramesencephalic segment of the oculomotor nerve arises from the oculomotor nucleus and passes medially and inside the red nucleus to exit through the interpeduncular fossa. The anterior mesencephalic (perioculomotor) safe entry zone can be seen.

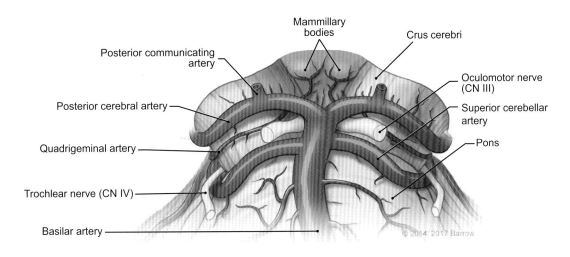

a

Figure 1.40. (a) Ventral view of the brainstem depicting the relationship of the posterior cerebral arteries, basilar artery, and their associated branches to midbrain structures and cranial nerves. **(b)** Axial view of the arteries of the midbrain. **(c)** Axial view of the veins of the midbrain.

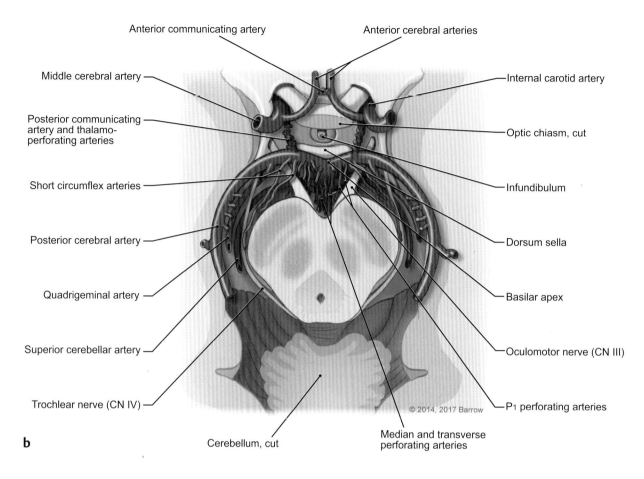

Anterior communicating artery

Anterior cerebral arteries

Middle cerebral artery

Internal carotid artery

Posterior communicating artery and thalamo-perforating arteries

Optic chiasm, cut

Short circumflex arteries

Infundibulum

Posterior cerebral artery

Dorsum sella

Quadrigeminal artery

Basilar apex

Superior cerebellar artery

Oculomotor nerve (CN III)

Trochlear nerve (CN IV)

P1 perforating arteries

© 2014, 2017 Barrow

b

Cerebellum, cut

Median and transverse perforating arteries

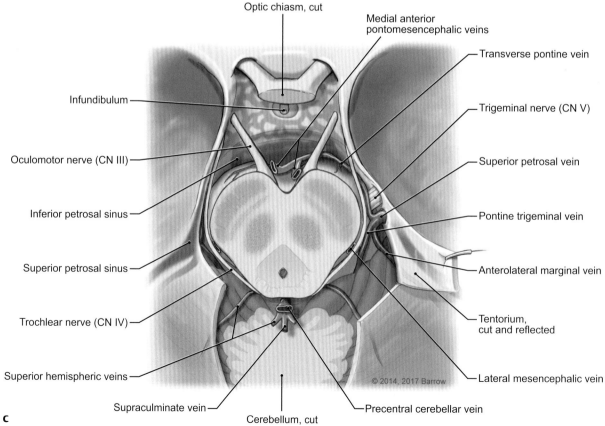

Optic chiasm, cut

Medial anterior pontomesencephalic veins

Transverse pontine vein

Infundibulum

Trigeminal nerve (CN V)

Oculomotor nerve (CN III)

Superior petrosal vein

Inferior petrosal sinus

Pontine trigeminal vein

Superior petrosal sinus

Anterolateral marginal vein

Trochlear nerve (CN IV)

Tentorium, cut and reflected

Superior hemispheric veins

Lateral mesencephalic vein

© 2014, 2017 Barrow

c

Supraculminate vein

Precentral cerebellar vein

Cerebellum, cut

Figure 1.40. (*Continued*)

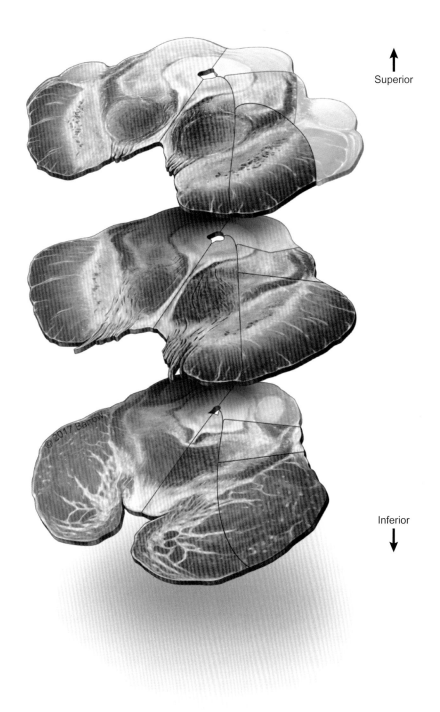

Superior

Inferior

Figure 1.41. Sequential slices of the midbrain depicting critical nuclei and vasculature supplying these nuclei. Pink denotes area supplied by the paramedian branches of the basilar bifurcation and the P1 segment of the posterior cerebral arteries. Purple denotes area supplied by the short circumferential branches of the quadrigeminal and the medial posterior choroidal arteries. Blue denotes region supplied by the lateral branches of the quadrigeminal artery (at the level of the inferior colliculus) and by the quadrigeminal and the posterior medial choroidal arteries (at the level of the superior colliculus). Teal denotes area supplied by the quadrigeminal artery and the superior cerebellar artery (at the level of the inferior colliculus) or the quadrigeminal and the posterior medial choroidal arteries (at the level of the superior colliculus). Green denotes region supplied by the thalamogeniculate artery.

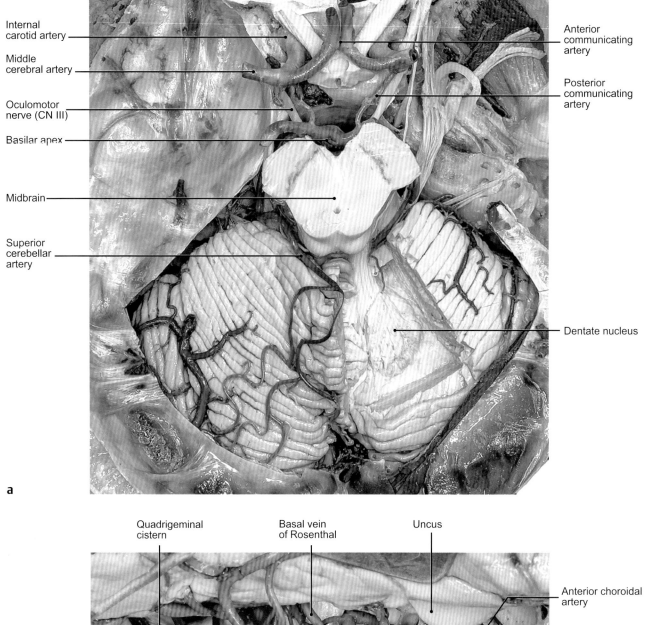

Internal carotid artery

Middle cerebral artery

Oculomotor nerve (CN III)

Basilar apex

Midbrain

Superior cerebellar artery

Anterior communicating artery

Posterior communicating artery

Dentate nucleus

a

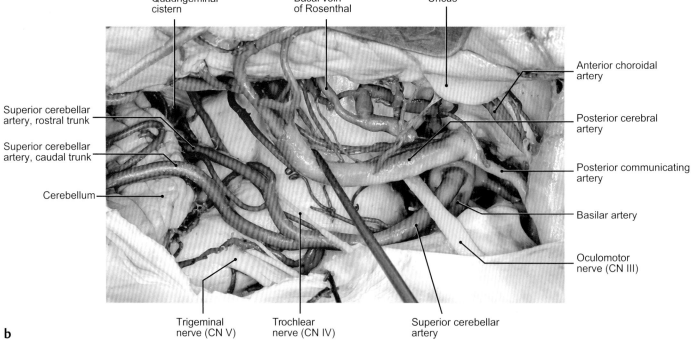

Quadrigeminal cistern

Basal vein of Rosenthal

Uncus

Superior cerebellar artery, rostral trunk

Superior cerebellar artery, caudal trunk

Cerebellum

Anterior choroidal artery

Posterior cerebral artery

Posterior communicating artery

Basilar artery

Oculomotor nerve (CN III)

Trigeminal nerve (CN V)

Trochlear nerve (CN IV)

Superior cerebellar artery

b

Figure 1.42. Cadaveric dissection showing the vascular anatomy of the midbrain and cerebellum. **(a)** Superior view of the midbrain and cerebellum. The superior cerebellar artery courses within the cerebellomesencephalic fissure and supplies the tentorial surface of the cerebellum and the dentate nucleus. **(b)** Lateral view of the midbrain. The superior cerebellar artery arises from the basilar artery and passes backward within the cerebellomesencephalic fissure to divide into the rostral and caudal trunks. The posterior cerebral artery and basal vein of Rosenthal course around the midbrain.

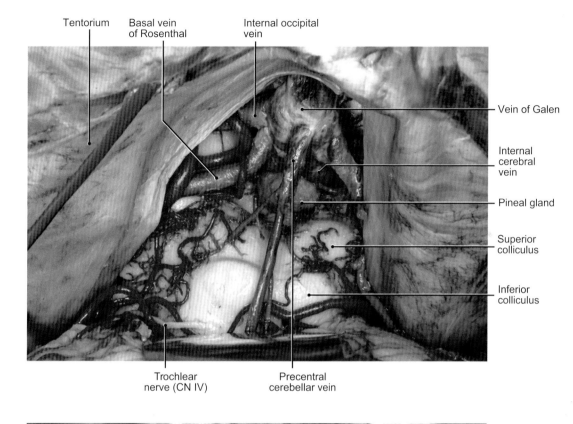

Tentorium Basal vein of Rosenthal Internal occipital vein

Vein of Galen

Internal cerebral vein

Pineal gland

Superior colliculus

Inferior colliculus

Trochlear nerve (CN IV) Precentral cerebellar vein

a

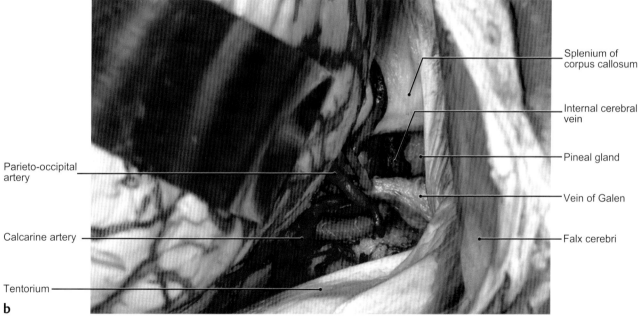

Splenium of corpus callosum

Internal cerebral vein

Pineal gland

Parieto-occipital artery

Vein of Galen

Calcarine artery

Falx cerebri

Tentorium

b

Figure 1.43. (a) Infratentorial dorsal and **(b)** supratentorial dorsal views of the arteries and veins of the midbrain and pineal region.

Pons

Axial Sections of the Pons

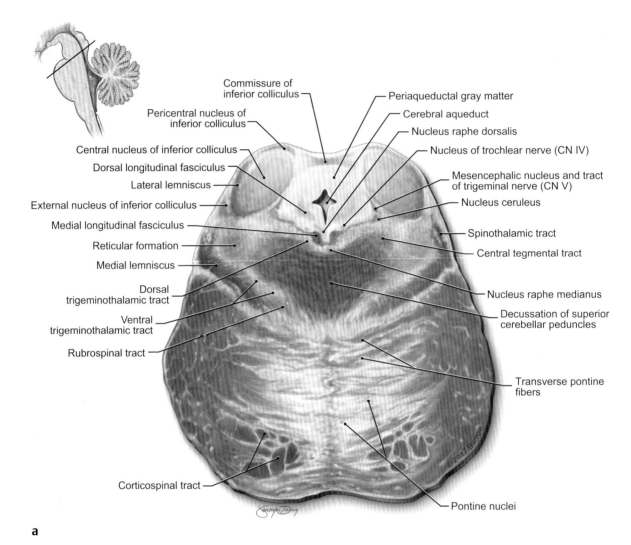

Commissure of inferior colliculus
Periaqueductal gray matter
Cerebral aqueduct
Pericentral nucleus of inferior colliculus
Nucleus raphe dorsalis
Central nucleus of inferior colliculus
Nucleus of trochlear nerve (CN IV)
Dorsal longitudinal fasciculus
Lateral lemniscus
Mesencephalic nucleus and tract of trigeminal nerve (CN V)
External nucleus of inferior colliculus
Nucleus ceruleus
Medial longitudinal fasciculus
Spinothalamic tract
Reticular formation
Central tegmental tract
Medial lemniscus
Dorsal trigeminothalamic tract
Nucleus raphe medianus
Ventral trigeminothalamic tract
Decussation of superior cerebellar peduncles
Rubrospinal tract
Transverse pontine fibers
Corticospinal tract
Pontine nuclei

a

Figure 1.44. Sequential axial slices through the pons depicting the critical nuclei and tracts. **(a)** Transverse section of the brainstem at the pontomesencephalic junction just caudal to the trochlear nerve (CN IV), through the inferior colliculus, caudal portions of the decussation of the superior cerebellar peduncle, and rostral parts of the basilar pons. The corticospinal tracts travel in the anteromedial part of the ventral pons. **(b)** Transverse section of the upper pons at the level of the exit of the trochlear nerve to the level of the exit of the trigeminal nerve (CN V). The medial lemniscus divides the brainstem into the ventral and dorsal pons. **(c)** Transverse section of the pons through the principal sensory motor nuclei of the trigeminal nerve. The dorsal longitudinal fasciculus, medial longitudinal fasciculus, and reticular formation are located bilateral to the midline, in order from dorsal to ventral. The trigeminal motor and main sensory nuclei are located ventral to the superior cerebellar peduncle. The rubrospinal tract travels just lateral to the medial lemniscus. **(d)** Transverse section of the pons through the rostral pole of the facial nucleus and the genu of the facial nerve (CN VII) and rostral portions of the abducens nucleus. **(e)** Transverse section of the caudal pons through the facial colliculus.

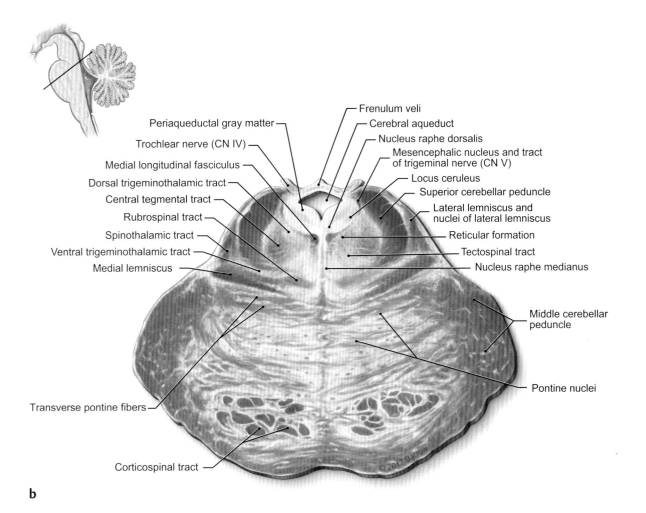

Frenulum veli
Periaqueductal gray matter
Cerebral aqueduct
Trochlear nerve (CN IV)
Nucleus raphe dorsalis
Medial longitudinal fasciculus
Mesencephalic nucleus and tract of trigeminal nerve (CN V)
Dorsal trigeminothalamic tract
Locus ceruleus
Central tegmental tract
Superior cerebellar peduncle
Rubrospinal tract
Lateral lemniscus and nuclei of lateral lemniscus
Spinothalamic tract
Reticular formation
Ventral trigeminothalamic tract
Tectospinal tract
Medial lemniscus
Nucleus raphe medianus
Middle cerebellar peduncle
Pontine nuclei
Transverse pontine fibers
Corticospinal tract

b

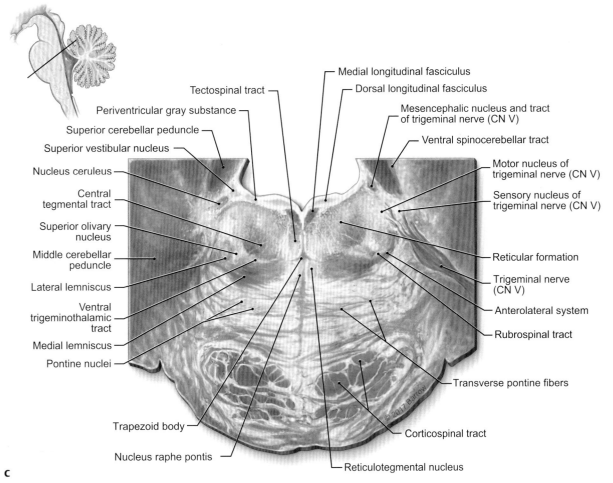

Medial longitudinal fasciculus
Tectospinal tract
Dorsal longitudinal fasciculus
Periventricular gray substance
Mesencephalic nucleus and tract of trigeminal nerve (CN V)
Superior cerebellar peduncle
Ventral spinocerebellar tract
Superior vestibular nucleus
Nucleus ceruleus
Motor nucleus of trigeminal nerve (CN V)
Central tegmental tract
Sensory nucleus of trigeminal nerve (CN V)
Superior olivary nucleus
Middle cerebellar peduncle
Reticular formation
Lateral lemniscus
Trigeminal nerve (CN V)
Ventral trigeminothalamic tract
Anterolateral system
Medial lemniscus
Rubrospinal tract
Pontine nuclei
Transverse pontine fibers
Trapezoid body
Corticospinal tract
Nucleus raphe pontis
Reticulotegmental nucleus

c

Figure 1.44. (*Continued*)

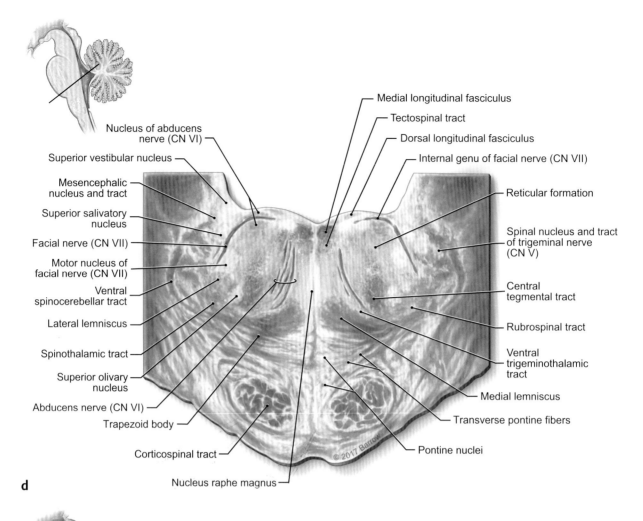

Nucleus of abducens nerve (CN VI)
Superior vestibular nucleus
Mesencephalic nucleus and tract
Superior salivatory nucleus
Facial nerve (CN VII)
Motor nucleus of facial nerve (CN VII)
Ventral spinocerebellar tract
Lateral lemniscus
Spinothalamic tract
Superior olivary nucleus
Abducens nerve (CN VI)
Trapezoid body
Corticospinal tract
Nucleus raphe magnus

Medial longitudinal fasciculus
Tectospinal tract
Dorsal longitudinal fasciculus
Internal genu of facial nerve (CN VII)
Reticular formation
Spinal nucleus and tract of trigeminal nerve (CN V)
Central tegmental tract
Rubrospinal tract
Ventral trigeminothalamic tract
Medial lemniscus
Transverse pontine fibers
Pontine nuclei

© 2017 Barrow

d

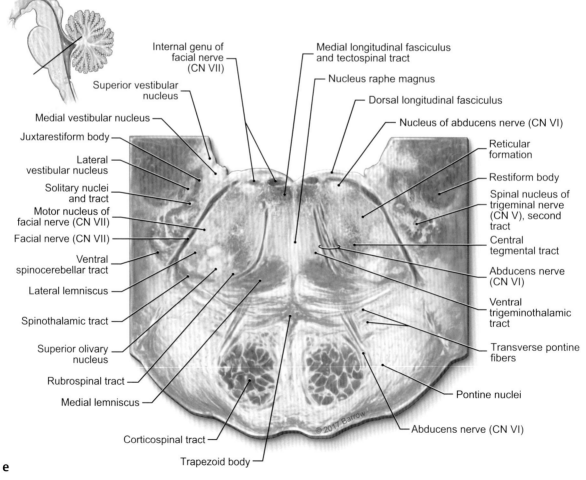

Internal genu of facial nerve (CN VII)
Superior vestibular nucleus
Medial vestibular nucleus
Juxtarestiform body
Lateral vestibular nucleus
Solitary nuclei and tract
Motor nucleus of facial nerve (CN VII)
Facial nerve (CN VII)
Ventral spinocerebellar tract
Lateral lemniscus
Spinothalamic tract
Superior olivary nucleus
Rubrospinal tract
Medial lemniscus
Corticospinal tract
Trapezoid body

Medial longitudinal fasciculus and tectospinal tract
Nucleus raphe magnus
Dorsal longitudinal fasciculus
Nucleus of abducens nerve (CN VI)
Reticular formation
Restiform body
Spinal nucleus of trigeminal nerve (CN V), second tract
Central tegmental tract
Abducens nerve (CN VI)
Ventral trigeminothalamic tract
Transverse pontine fibers
Pontine nuclei
Abducens nerve (CN VI)

© 2017 Barrow

e

Figure 1.44. (*Continued*)

Surface Anatomy, Internal Structures, and Safe Entry Zones of the Pons

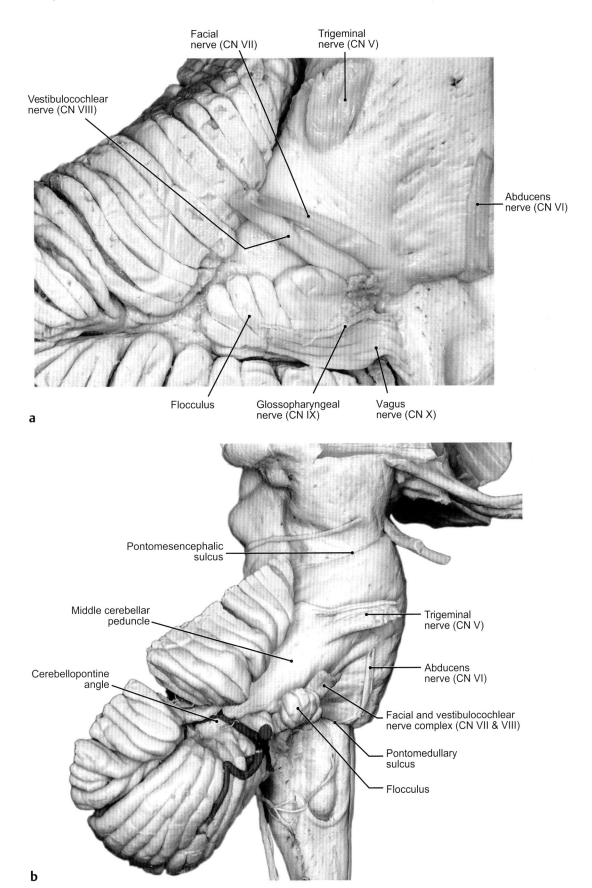

Figure 1.45. (a) Anterior and **(b)** lateral surfaces of the pons.

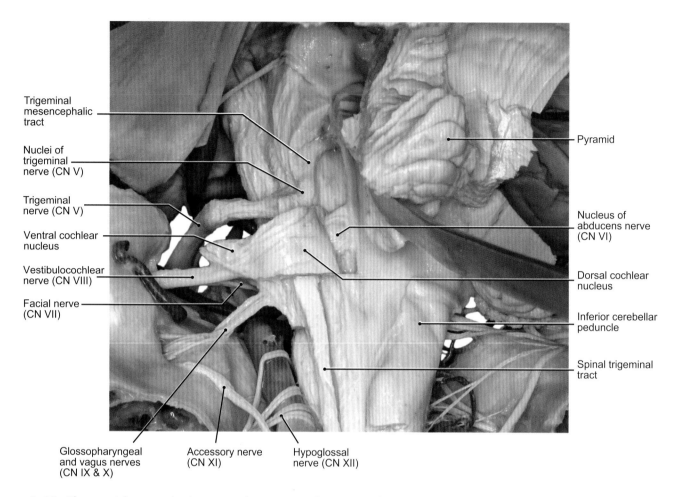

Trigeminal mesencephalic tract

Nuclei of trigeminal nerve (CN V)

Trigeminal nerve (CN V)

Ventral cochlear nucleus

Vestibulocochlear nerve (CN VIII)

Facial nerve (CN VII)

Pyramid

Nucleus of abducens nerve (CN VI)

Dorsal cochlear nucleus

Inferior cerebellar peduncle

Spinal trigeminal tract

Glossopharyngeal and vagus nerves (CN IX & X)

Accessory nerve (CN XI)

Hypoglossal nerve (CN XII)

Figure 1.46. The cranial nerves in the pons: the trigeminal (CN V), abducens (CN VI), facial (CN VII), and vestibulocochlear (CN VIII) nerves. A dorsal view of the floor of the fourth ventricle. The trigeminal motor and main sensory nuclei are located at the midpontine level and deep to the lateral edge of the floor of the fourth ventricle. The trigeminal mesencephalic tract ascends deep to the superior half of the floor of the fourth ventricle to reach the midbrain. The spinal trigeminal tract descends between the intrapontine segment and dorsal cochlear nucleus of the vestibulocochlear nerve dorsally and the intrapontine segment of the facial nerve and glossopharyngeal (CN IX), vagus (CN X), accessory (XI), and hypoglossal (CN XII) nerves ventrally to reach the upper spinal cord. The dorsal cochlear nucleus sits on the floor of the lateral recess of the fourth ventricle, where it forms a smooth prominence called the auditory tubercle.

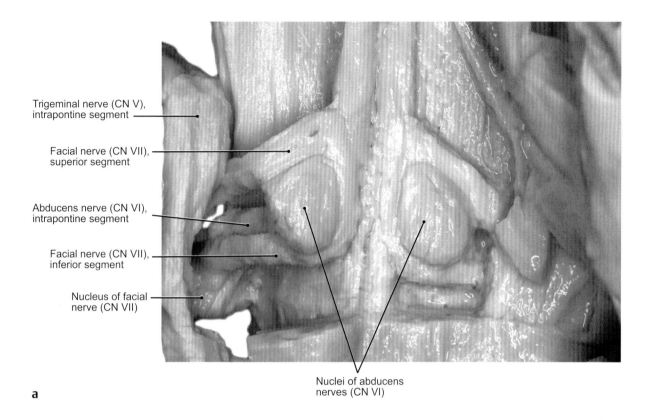

Trigeminal nerve (CN V), intrapontine segment

Facial nerve (CN VII), superior segment

Abducens nerve (CN VI), intrapontine segment

Facial nerve (CN VII), inferior segment

Nucleus of facial nerve (CN VII)

Nuclei of abducens nerves (CN VI)

a

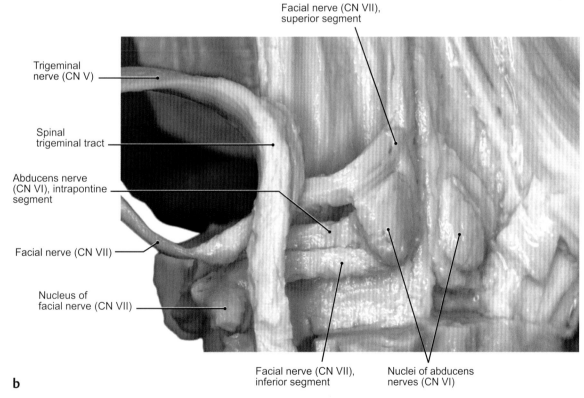

Facial nerve (CN VII), superior segment

Trigeminal nerve (CN V)

Spinal trigeminal tract

Abducens nerve (CN VI), intrapontine segment

Facial nerve (CN VII)

Nucleus of facial nerve (CN VII)

Facial nerve (CN VII), inferior segment

Nuclei of abducens nerves (CN VI)

b

Figure 1.47. Cranial nerves in the pons: the trigeminal (CN V), abducens (CN VI), and facial (CN VII) nerves. **(a)** The abducens nucleus and intrapontine segment of the facial nerve form the facial colliculus, which in most cases creates a prominence on the floor of the fourth ventricle. **(b)** Dorsolateral view of the abducens and facial nerves at the level of the facial colliculus. The intrapontine segment of the facial nerve arises from the facial nucleus and courses backward to circle the abducens nucleus. After it circles the abducens nucleus, it courses forward to exit the brainstem. The intrapontine segment of the abducens nerve arises from the abducens nucleus and travels forward to exit the brainstem. The nuclei and intrapontine segments of the abducens and facial nerves are situated medial to the trigeminal nerve.

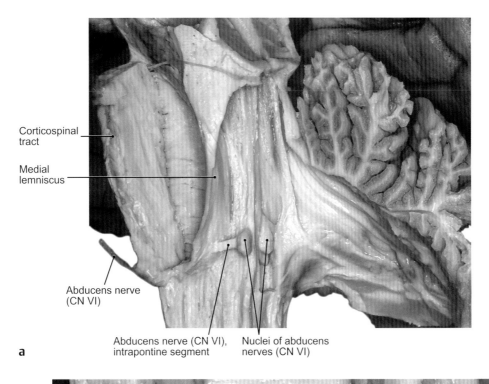

Corticospinal tract

Medial lemniscus

Abducens nerve (CN VI)

Abducens nerve (CN VI), intrapontine segment

Nuclei of abducens nerves (CN VI)

a

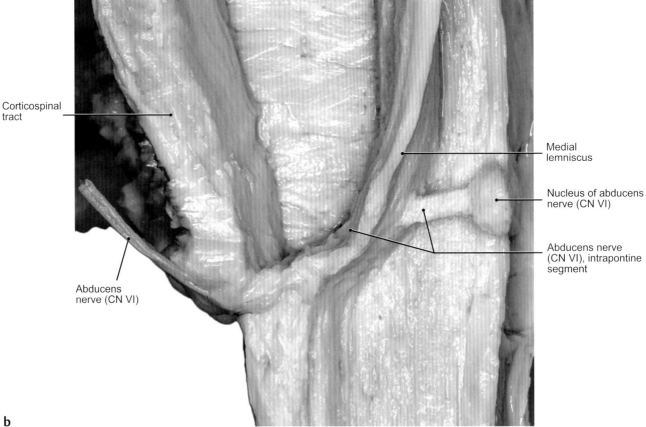

Corticospinal tract

Medial lemniscus

Nucleus of abducens nerve (CN VI)

Abducens nerve (CN VI), intrapontine segment

Abducens nerve (CN VI)

b

Figure 1.48. Cranial nerves in the pons: the abducens nerve (CN VI). **(a)** Dorsolateral view of the abducens nerve (after removal of the facial nerve [CN VII]). The intrapontine segment of the abducens nerve arises from the abducens nucleus, which is located underneath the floor of the fourth ventricle, and passes lateral to the corticospinal tract to exit the brainstem. **(b)** Lateral view of the nucleus and course of the abducens nerve, which runs through the medial lemniscus.

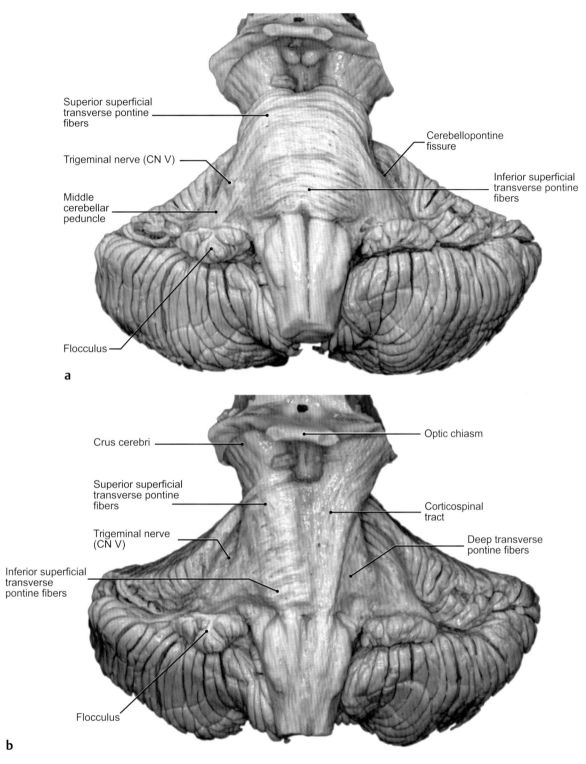

Figure 1.49. Ventral pons and internal structures. **(a)** The transverse pontine fibers are called the middle cerebellar peduncle at the point lateral to the level of the exit zone of the trigeminal nerve (CN V) from the pons. The transverse pontine fibers located ventral to the corticospinal tract are called the superficial transverse pontine fibers, which are divided into a superior and an inferior part according to their positions relative to the exit zone of the trigeminal nerve from the pons. **(b)** The transverse pontine fibers located dorsal to the corticospinal tract are referred to as the deep transverse pontine fibers. The corticospinal tract courses in the pons anteromedially.

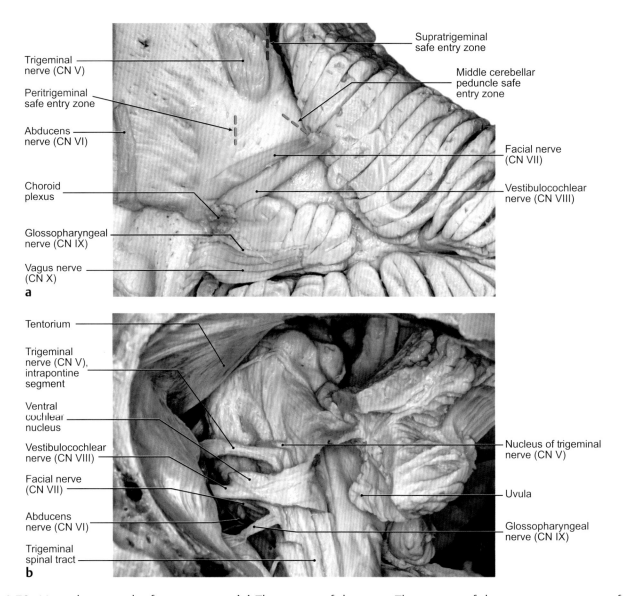

Trigeminal nerve (CN V)

Supratrigeminal safe entry zone

Peritrigeminal safe entry zone

Middle cerebellar peduncle safe entry zone

Abducens nerve (CN VI)

Facial nerve (CN VII)

Choroid plexus

Vestibulocochlear nerve (CN VIII)

Glossopharyngeal nerve (CN IX)

Vagus nerve (CN X)

a

Tentorium

Trigeminal nerve (CN V), intrapontine segment

Ventral cochlear nucleus

Nucleus of trigeminal nerve (CN V)

Vestibulocochlear nerve (CN VIII)

Facial nerve (CN VII)

Uvula

Abducens nerve (CN VI)

Glossopharyngeal nerve (CN IX)

Trigeminal spinal tract

b

Figure 1.50. Ventral pons and safe entry zones. **(a)** The middle cerebellar peduncle, peritrigeminal, and supratrigeminal safe entry zones. The peritrigeminal safe entry zone (*green dashed line*) is located medially between the trigeminal nerve (CN V) and the facial nerve (CN VII). Alternatively, the pons may be entered using the middle cerebellar peduncle safe entry zone (*orange dashed line*), which is located lateral to the trigeminal and facial nerves. The supratrigeminal safe entry zone (*blue dashed line*) is located just above and lateral to the trigeminal nerve. **(b)** The retrosigmoid view depicting the internal structures of the pons. The courses of the tracts create areas of sparse fiber tract density or areas with a scarcity of perforating arteries that may be used to traverse the brainstem. **(c)** The critical neurologic structures in the peritrigeminal safe entry zone (*green dashed line*) are the intrapontine fibers of the trigeminal nerve superiorly; the intrapontine fibers of the abducens nerve (CN VI) inferiorly; the spinal tract of the trigeminal nerve, the motor nucleus of the trigeminal nerve, and the intrapontine segment of the facial nerve posteromedially; and the corticospinal tract anteromedially.

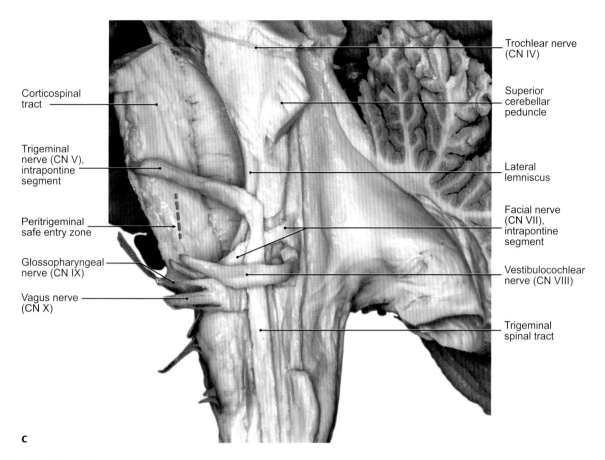

Trochlear nerve (CN IV)

Corticospinal tract

Superior cerebellar peduncle

Trigeminal nerve (CN V), intrapontine segment

Lateral lemniscus

Peritrigeminal safe entry zone

Facial nerve (CN VII), intrapontine segment

Glossopharyngeal nerve (CN IX)

Vestibulocochlear nerve (CN VIII)

Vagus nerve (CN X)

Trigeminal spinal tract

c

Figure 1.50. (*Continued*)

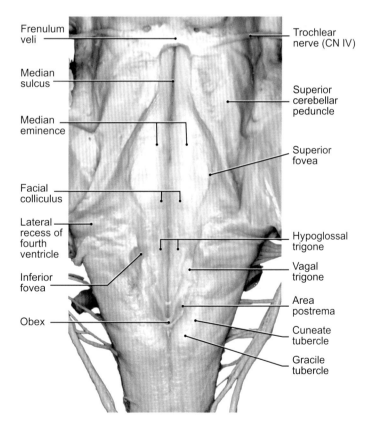

Frenulum veli

Trochlear nerve (CN IV)

Median sulcus

Superior cerebellar peduncle

Median eminence

Superior fovea

Facial colliculus

Lateral recess of fourth ventricle

Hypoglossal trigone

Inferior fovea

Vagal trigone

Area postrema

Obex

Cuneate tubercle

Gracile tubercle

Figure 1.51. Dorsal pontine surface. The floor of the fourth ventricle is divided in the midline by the median sulcus. The sulcus limitans extends along the floor lateral to the median sulcus. The floor is divided into three parts: the superior or pontine, intermediate or junctional, and inferior or medullary parts. The superior fovea is positioned lateral to the facial colliculus, and the inferior fovea is lateral to the hypoglossal trigone. The median eminence is the longitudinal prominence between the median sulcus and the sulcus limitans. It is the site of the facial colliculus, prominences overlying the hypoglossal and vagal nuclei, and the area postrema. These three paired triangular areas overlying the hypoglossal and vagal nuclei and area postrema in the medullary part of the floor give this area a pen nib–shaped appearance, and consequently, the name *calamus scriptorius*.

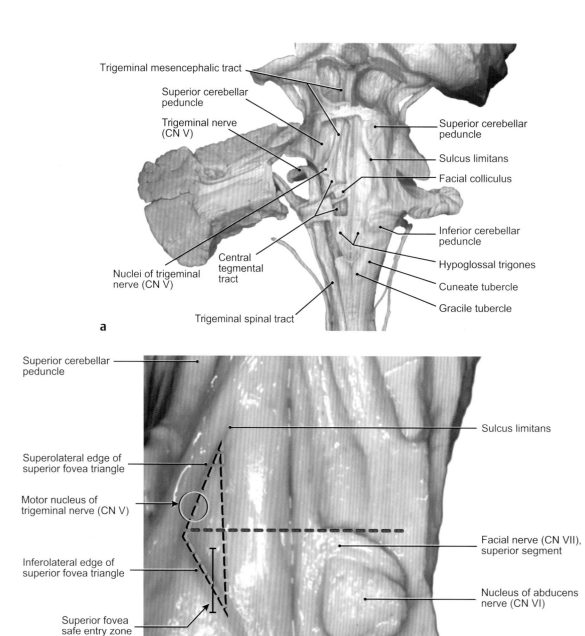

Trigeminal mesencephalic tract

Superior cerebellar peduncle

Trigeminal nerve (CN V)

Nuclei of trigeminal nerve (CN V)

Central tegmental tract

Trigeminal spinal tract

Superior cerebellar peduncle

Sulcus limitans

Facial colliculus

Inferior cerebellar peduncle

Hypoglossal trigones

Cuneate tubercle

Gracile tubercle

a

Superior cerebellar peduncle

Superolateral edge of superior fovea triangle

Motor nucleus of trigeminal nerve (CN V)

Inferolateral edge of superior fovea triangle

Superior fovea safe entry zone

Vestibular area

Sulcus limitans

Facial nerve (CN VII), superior segment

Nucleus of abducens nerve (CN VI)

Facial nerve (CN VII), inferior segment

b

Figure 1.52. Surface anatomy and internal structures of the dorsal pons. **(a)** The medial longitudinal fasciculus courses adjacent to the midline near the floor of the fourth ventricle and interconnects with the nuclei of the oculomotor (CN III), trochlear (CN IV), and abducens (CN VI) nerves. The medial longitudinal fasciculus passes medial to the nucleus of the abducens nerve and the intrapontine segment of the facial nerve (CN VII). The trigeminal nerve (CN V), after reaching its motor and main sensory nuclei, divides into the rostrally directed trigeminal mesencephalic tract and the caudally directed spinal tract. The central tegmental tract connects the red nucleus to the inferior olivary nucleus. The trigeminal mesencephalic tract and central tegmental tract course deep between the sulcus limitans medially and the superior cerebellar peduncle laterally. **(b)** Dorsal view of the superior fovea triangle and safe entry zone. The superior fovea triangle (*green dashed line*) is bordered superolaterally by the superior cerebellar peduncle, inferolaterally by the vestibular area, and medially by the sulcus limitans. The lateral apex of the triangle is located at the same axial level as the upper edge of the facial colliculus (*blue dashed line*). The motor nucleus of the trigeminal nerve (*circle*) sits deep to the superolateral edge of the superior fovea triangle. The inferior half of the superior fovea triangle is used as a safe entry zone (*black line*) for lesions located at the level of the facial colliculus.

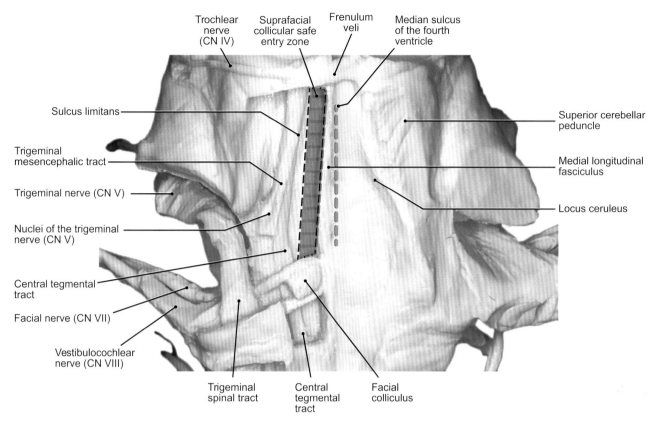

Figure 1.53. The suprafacial collicular safe entry zone (*shaded area inside green dashed lines*) is bordered medially by the medial longitudinal fasciculus, laterally by the sulcus limitans, superiorly by the frenulum veli, and inferiorly by the facial colliculus. Alternatively, the median sulcus of the fourth ventricle (*orange dashed line*) can be opened between the frenulum veli and the lowermost level of the facial colliculus.

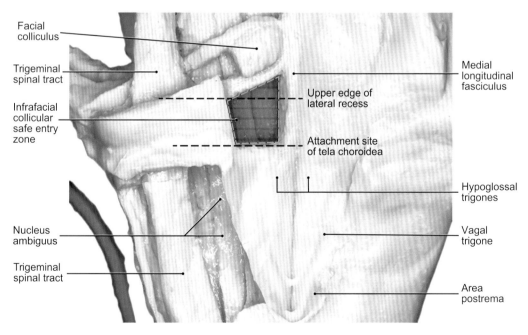

Figure 1.54. The infrafacial collicular safe entry zone (*shaded area inside green dashed lines*) is limited medially by the medial longitudinal fasciculus, laterally by the nucleus ambiguus, superiorly by the facial colliculus, and inferiorly by the hypoglossal trigone. Thus, the lateral border of the infrafacial collicular safe entry zone corresponds to the most medial point of attachment of the tela choroidea along the lower margin of the lateral recess, whereas the rostral and caudal borders are the same as the upper and lower edges of the lateral recess.

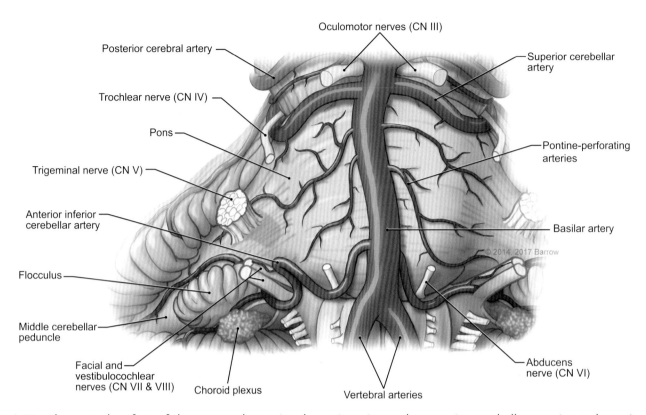

Figure 1.55. The ventral surface of the pons and associated cranial nerves and arteries. The basilar artery gives rise to the anterior inferior cerebellar artery, which courses around the abducens nerve (CN VI), the facial nerve (CN VII), and the vestibulocochlear nerve (CN VIII). The basilar artery then gives rise to the superior cerebellar arteries and terminates after giving rise to the posterior cerebral arteries. The basilar artery also gives off the pontine-perforating arteries, which supply the ventral pons.

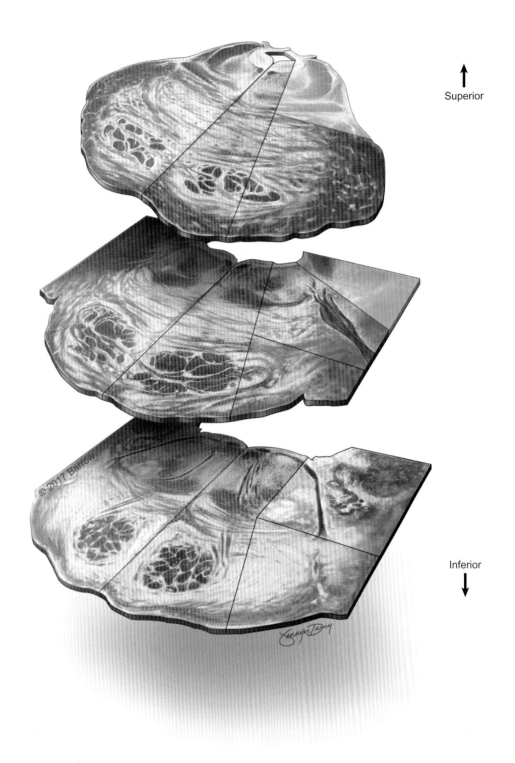

Superior

Inferior

Figure 1.56. Sequential axial slices of the pons depicting critical nuclei and the vasculature supplying these nuclei. Pink denotes region of the pons supplied by the paramedian branches of the basilar artery. Purple denotes area supplied by the short circumferential branches of the basilar artery. Blue denotes region supplied by the long circumferential branches of the basilar artery and the branches of the anterior inferior cerebellar artery. Teal denotes area supplied by the long circumferential branches of the basilar artery and the branches of the superior cerebellar artery.

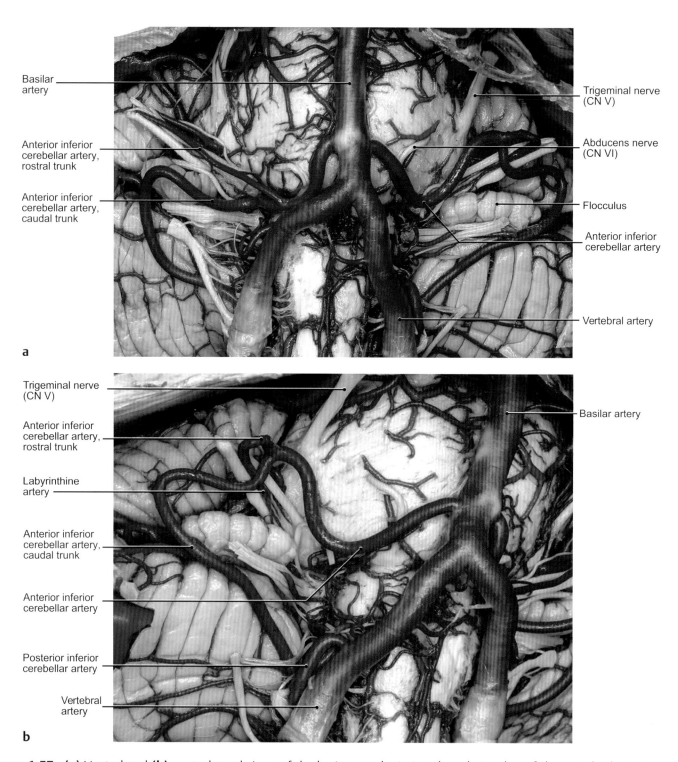

Basilar artery

Anterior inferior cerebellar artery, rostral trunk

Anterior inferior cerebellar artery, caudal trunk

Trigeminal nerve (CN V)

Abducens nerve (CN VI)

Flocculus

Anterior inferior cerebellar artery

Vertebral artery

a

Trigeminal nerve (CN V)

Anterior inferior cerebellar artery, rostral trunk

Labyrinthine artery

Anterior inferior cerebellar artery, caudal trunk

Anterior inferior cerebellar artery

Posterior inferior cerebellar artery

Vertebral artery

Basilar artery

b

Figure 1.57. (a) Ventral and **(b)** ventrolateral views of the brainstem depicting the relationship of the vertebral arteries, basilar artery, and associated branches to the pons, cerebellum, and cranial nerves.

Medulla

Axial Sections of the Medulla and Cervicomedullary Junction

Figure 1.58. (a–f) Sequential axial slices of the medulla extending to the cervicomedullary junction.

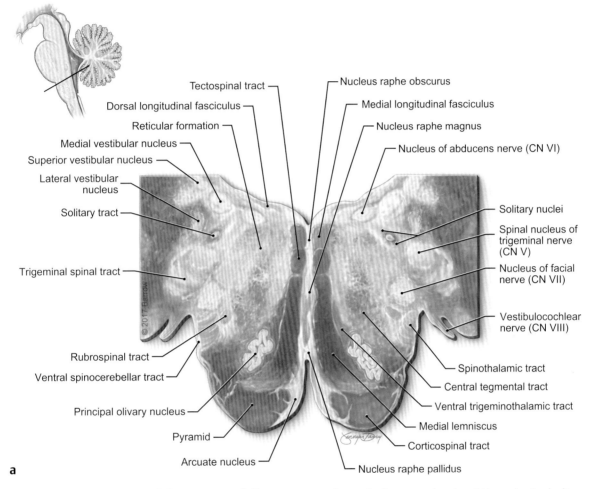

a

Figure 1.58. (a) Transverse section of the pontomedullary junction through the rostral pole of the principal olivary nucleus and through the motor nucleus of the facial nerve (CN VII). This plane is just caudal to the main portion of the nucleus of the abducens nerve (CN VI). The pontine nuclei are also called the arcuate nuclei at this level.

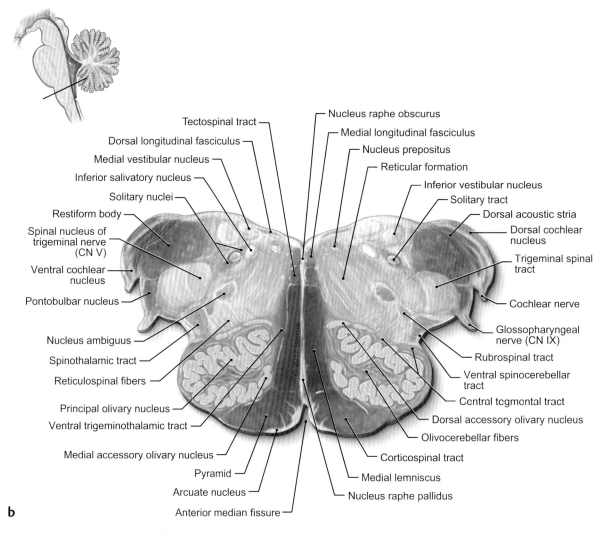

Tectospinal tract
Dorsal longitudinal fasciculus
Medial vestibular nucleus
Inferior salivatory nucleus
Solitary nuclei
Restiform body
Spinal nucleus of trigeminal nerve (CN V)
Ventral cochlear nucleus
Pontobulbar nucleus
Nucleus ambiguus
Spinothalamic tract
Reticulospinal fibers
Principal olivary nucleus
Ventral trigeminothalamic tract
Medial accessory olivary nucleus
Pyramid
Arcuate nucleus
Anterior median fissure

Nucleus raphe obscurus
Medial longitudinal fasciculus
Nucleus prepositus
Reticular formation
Inferior vestibular nucleus
Solitary tract
Dorsal acoustic stria
Dorsal cochlear nucleus
Trigeminal spinal tract
Cochlear nerve
Glossopharyngeal nerve (CN IX)
Rubrospinal tract
Ventral spinocerebellar tract
Central tegmental tract
Dorsal accessory olivary nucleus
Olivocerebellar fibers
Corticospinal tract
Medial lemniscus
Nucleus raphe pallidus

b

Figure 1.58. (b) Transverse section of the medulla through the upper half of the principal olivary nucleus and through the lateral recess of the fourth ventricle.

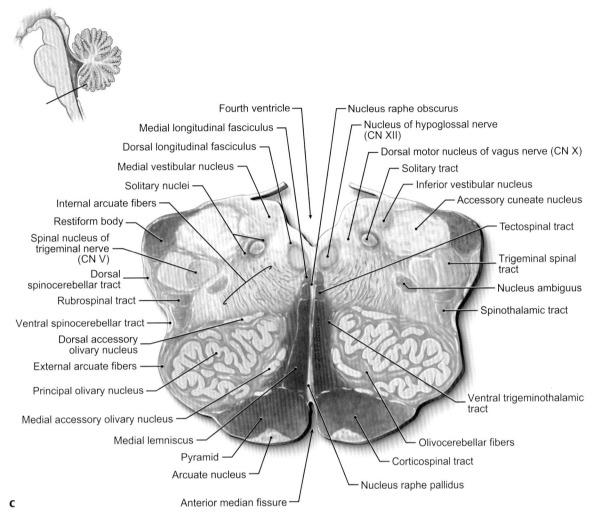

Figure 1.58. (c) Transverse section of the medulla through the midpoint of the principal olivary nucleus and the root of the glossopharyngeal nerve (CN IX). This level also corresponds to the level of the nucleus of the hypoglossal nerve (CN XII) and the dorsal motor nucleus of the vagus nerve (CN X). The internal arcuate fibers are the second-order neurons of the posterior column–medial lemniscus pathway.

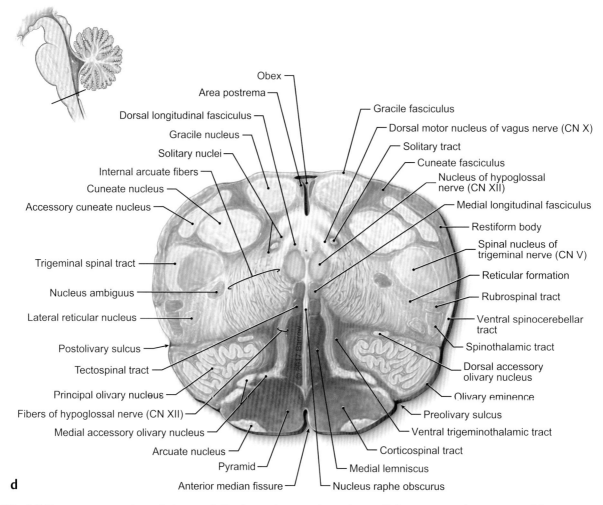

Obex
Area postrema
Dorsal longitudinal fasciculus
Gracile nucleus
Solitary nuclei
Internal arcuate fibers
Cuneate nucleus
Accessory cuneate nucleus
Trigeminal spinal tract
Nucleus ambiguus
Lateral reticular nucleus
Postolivary sulcus
Tectospinal tract
Principal olivary nucleus
Fibers of hypoglossal nerve (CN XII)
Medial accessory olivary nucleus
Arcuate nucleus
Pyramid
Anterior median fissure

Gracile fasciculus
Dorsal motor nucleus of vagus nerve (CN X)
Solitary tract
Cuneate fasciculus
Nucleus of hypoglossal nerve (CN XII)
Medial longitudinal fasciculus
Restiform body
Spinal nucleus of trigeminal nerve (CN V)
Reticular formation
Rubrospinal tract
Ventral spinocerebellar tract
Spinothalamic tract
Dorsal accessory olivary nucleus
Olivary eminence
Preolivary sulcus
Ventral trigeminothalamic tract
Corticospinal tract
Medial lemniscus
Nucleus raphe obscurus

d

Figure 1.58. (d) Transverse section of the medulla through rostral portions of the sensory decussation (the crossing of the internal arcuate fibers), the obex, and the caudal one-third of the nucleus of the hypoglossal nerve and the principal olivary nucleus.

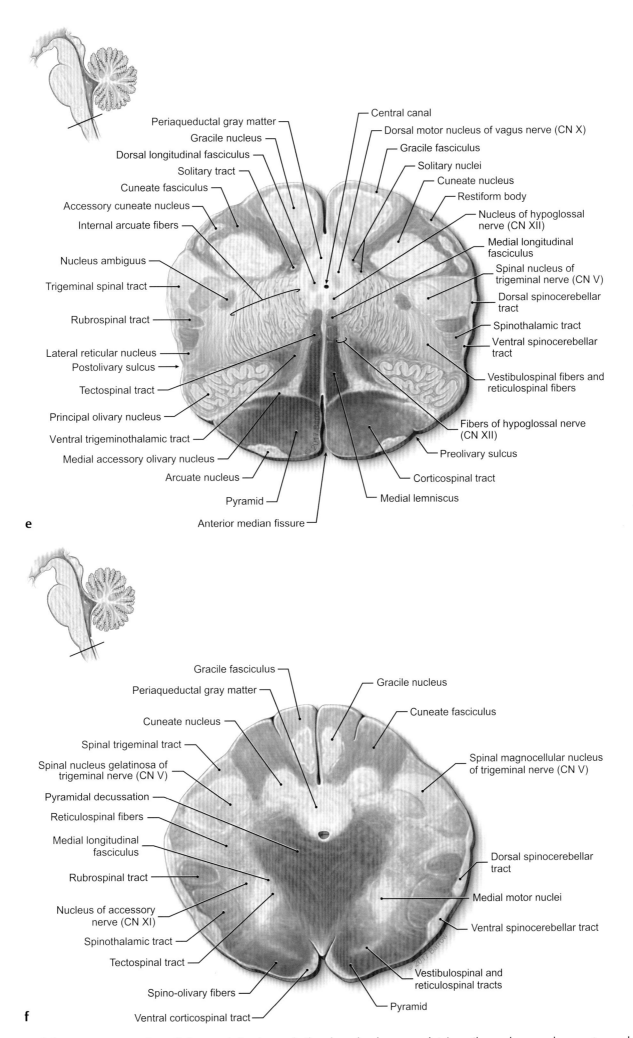

Figure 1.58. (e) Transverse section of the medulla through the dorsal column nuclei (gracile nucleus and cuneate nucleus), caudal portions of the nucleus of the hypoglossal nerve, caudal end of the principal olivary nucleus, and middle portions of the sensory decussation. **(f)** Transverse section of the medulla through the pyramidal decussation of the corticospinal tract.

Surface Anatomy of the Medulla

Figure 1.59. Surface anatomy of the ventral medulla.

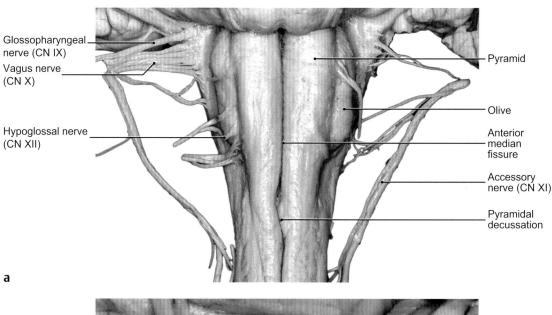

Glossopharyngeal nerve (CN IX)

Vagus nerve (CN X)

Hypoglossal nerve (CN XII)

Pyramid

Olive

Anterior median fissure

Accessory nerve (CN XI)

Pyramidal decussation

a

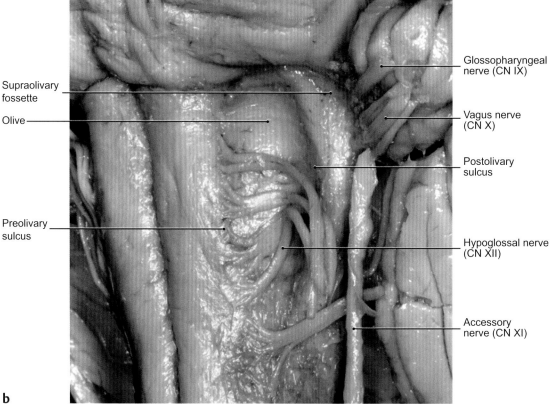

Supraolivary fossette

Olive

Preolivary sulcus

Glossopharyngeal nerve (CN IX)

Vagus nerve (CN X)

Postolivary sulcus

Hypoglossal nerve (CN XII)

Accessory nerve (CN XI)

b

Figure 1.59. (a) The medulla contains the glossopharyngeal (CN IX), vagus (CN X), accessory (CN XI), and hypoglossal (CN XII) nerves. The medulla is divided in the midline by the anterior median fissure. The corticospinal tract runs within the pyramid. **(b)** Lateral view of the medulla. The preolivary sulcus is located between the pyramid and olive, and the postolivary sulcus is located behind the olive. The hypoglossal nerve exits from the preolivary sulcus, and the accessory nerve exits from the postolivary sulcus. The depression rostral to the olive, the supraolivary fossette, is just below the junction of the facial nerve (CN VII) and the vestibulocochlear nerve (CN VIII) with the brainstem. The glossopharyngeal, vagus, and accessory nerves exit the medulla just dorsal to the postolivary sulcus, which is located between the olive and the inferior cerebellar peduncle.

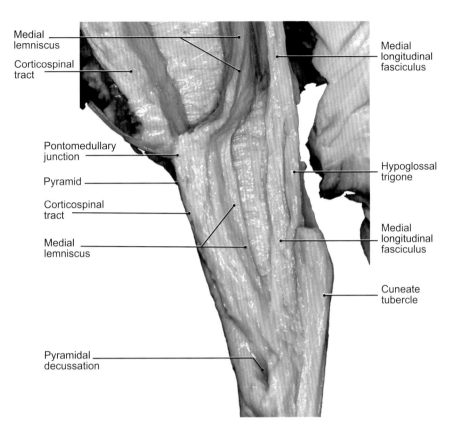

Figure 1.60. Internal structures of the ventral medulla. Lateral view after removal of the olive. In the medulla, the medial lemniscus is located just behind the pyramids formed by the corticospinal tracts that descend in the ventral medulla. The medial lemniscus is located medial to the olive and ventral to the hypoglossal trigone. The medial longitudinal fasciculus crosses the medial lemniscus at the level of the gracile and cuneate tubercles and descends in the ventral funiculus of the spinal cord.

Safe Entry Zones of the Ventral Medulla

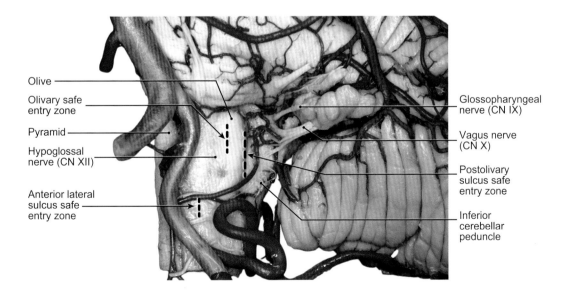

Figure 1.61. The anterior lateral sulcus (preolivary sulcus) safe entry zone is located between the caudal roots of the hypoglossal nerve (CN XII) and the rostral C1 rootlets. The postolivary sulcus safe entry zone is entered between the olive and the inferior cerebellar peduncle and is ventral to the glossopharyngeal and vagus rootlets. Alternatively, the medulla may be entered directly through the olive.

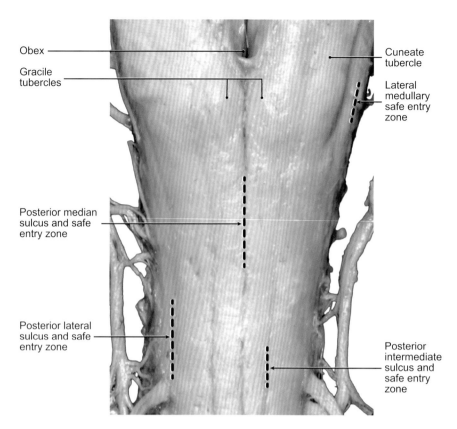

Figure 1.62. The surface anatomy and safe entry zones of the dorsal medulla. There are three dorsal medullary sulci, which have been used to gain entry to the dorsal medulla and have been described as safe entry zones. These include the posterior median sulcus below the obex in the midline, the posterior intermediate sulcus between the gracile tubercle and the cuneate tubercle, and the posterior lateral sulcus along the lateral margin of the cuneate tubercle. An additional safe entry zone, the lateral medullary zone, through the inferior cerebellar peduncle has been proposed.

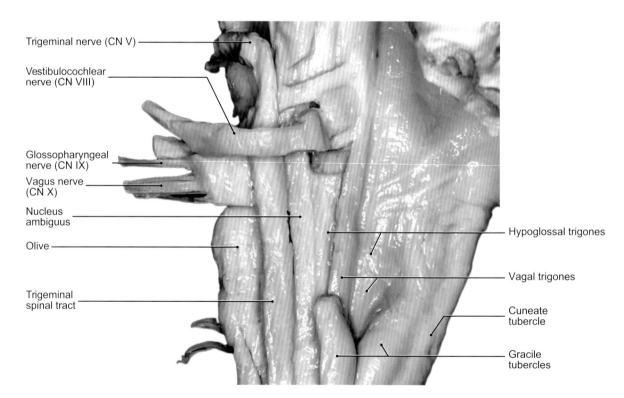

Figure 1.63. Internal structures of the dorsal medulla. Dorsal view of the medulla. The nucleus ambiguus is located ventrolateral to the vagal trigone, ventromedial to the trigeminal spinal tract, ventral to the cuneate tubercle, dorsal to the olive, and caudal to the facial motor nucleus. The intramedullary segments of the glossopharyngeal (CN IX), vagus (CN X), and accessory (CN XI) nerves exit the nucleus ambiguus to travel laterally, ventral to the trigeminal spinal tract, to exit the medulla along the retro-olivary sulcus.

Vascular Anatomy of the Medulla

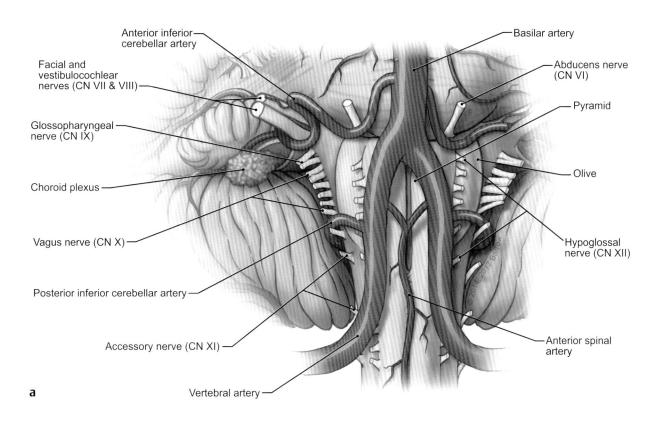

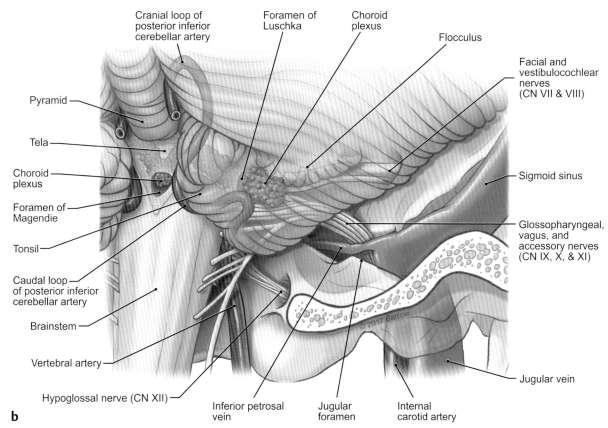

Figure 1.64. (a) Ventral and **(b)** dorsal views of the medulla with associated vasculature.

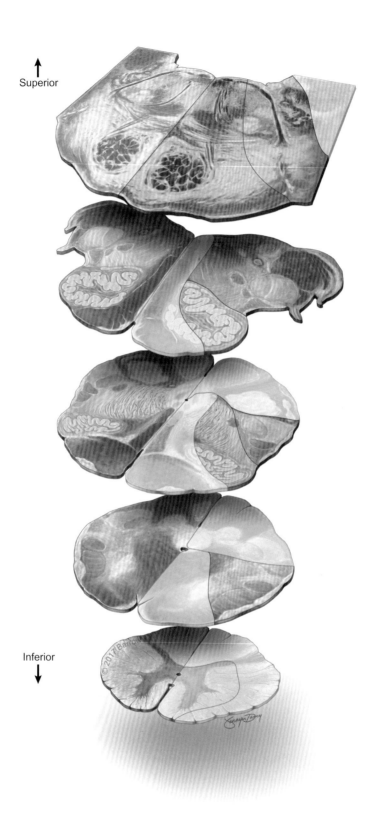

Superior

Inferior

Figure 1.65. Sequential axial slices of the cervicomedullary junction depicting critical nuclei and vasculature supplying these nuclei. Yellow denotes area supplied by the anterior inferior cerebellar artery. Pink denotes region supplied by the vertebral artery plus the paramedian branches of the caudal portions of the basilar artery. Purple denotes area supplied by the posterior inferior cerebellar artery. Blue denotes region supplied by the vertebral artery. Teal denotes area supplied by the anterior spinal artery. Green denotes region supplied by the posterior spinal artery and arterial vasocorona in the spinal cord.

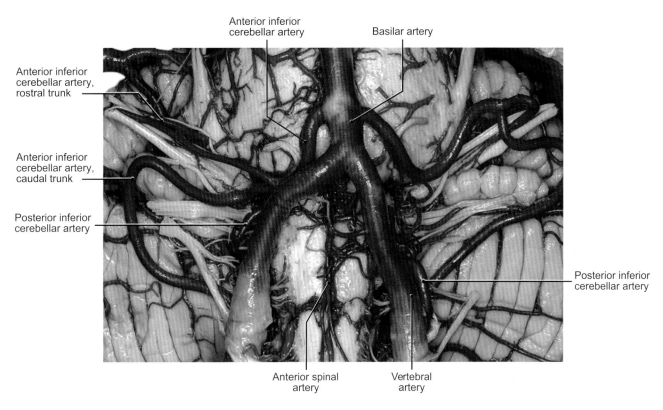

Anterior inferior
cerebellar artery

Basilar artery

Anterior inferior
cerebellar artery,
rostral trunk

Anterior inferior
cerebellar artery,
caudal trunk

Posterior inferior
cerebellar artery

Posterior inferior
cerebellar artery

Anterior spinal
artery

Vertebral
artery

Figure 1.66. Ventral surface of the dissected medulla and associated vasculature and nerves. The vertebral arteries give rise to the posterior inferior cerebellar arteries. The anterior spinal artery usually arises more rostrally from the vertebral arteries or from the vertebrobasilar junction. The posterior inferior cerebellar artery runs in close proximity to the lower cranial nerves.

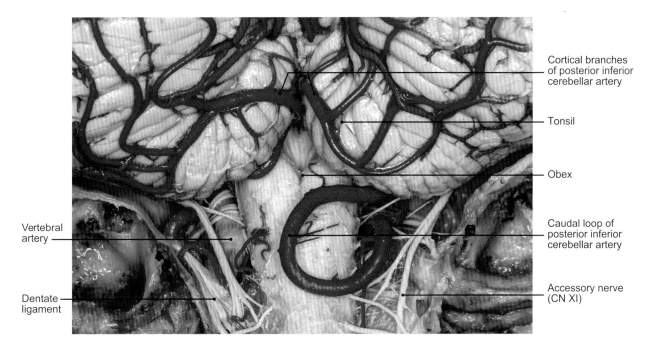

Cortical branches
of posterior inferior
cerebellar artery

Tonsil

Obex

Caudal loop of
posterior inferior
cerebellar artery

Accessory nerve
(CN XI)

Vertebral
artery

Dentate
ligament

Figure 1.67. Dorsal view of the medulla. This dorsal view of the suboccipital surface and the cerebellomedullary fissure demonstrates the relationship of the medullary blood supply to the lower cranial nerves.

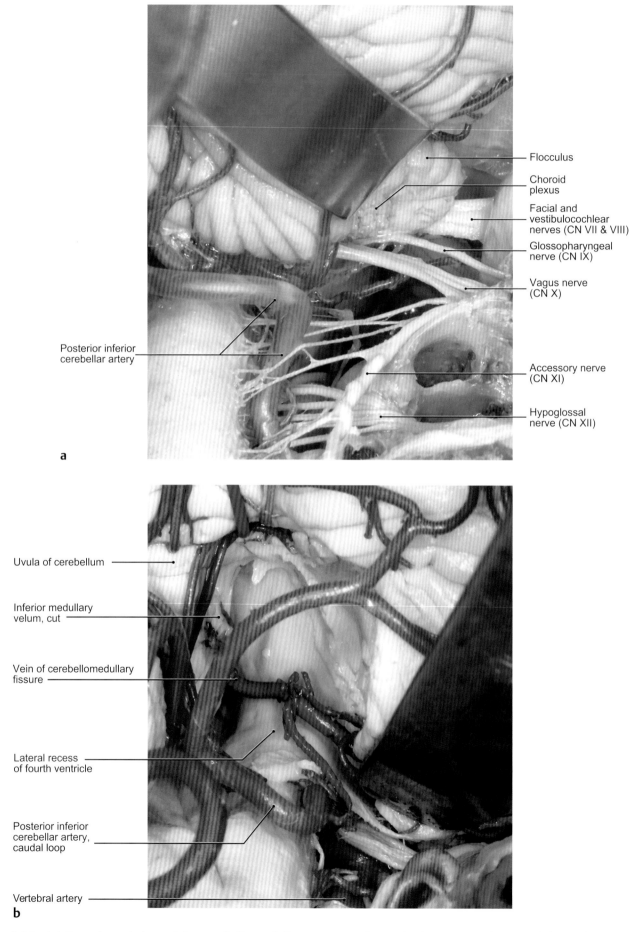

Flocculus

Choroid
plexus

Facial and
vestibulocochlear
nerves (CN VII & VIII)

Glossopharyngeal
nerve (CN IX)

Vagus nerve
(CN X)

Posterior inferior
cerebellar artery

Accessory nerve
(CN XI)

Hypoglossal
nerve (CN XII)

a

Uvula of cerebellum

Inferior medullary
velum, cut

Vein of cerebellomedullary
fissure

Lateral recess
of fourth ventricle

Posterior inferior
cerebellar artery,
caudal loop

Vertebral artery

b

Figure 1.68. **(a)** Dorsolateral view of the cerebellomedullary junction shows the lower cranial nerves (glossopharyngeal [CN IX], vagus [CN X], accessory [CN XI], and hypoglossal [CN XII] nerves) and their relationship to the vertebral artery and its branches. **(b)** Dorsal view of the telovelar junction and associated vessels.

Dentate Nucleus and Cerebellar Peduncles

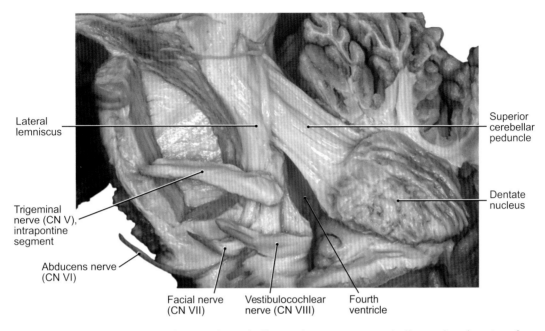

Lateral lemniscus

Trigeminal nerve (CN V), intrapontine segment

Abducens nerve (CN VI)

Facial nerve (CN VII)

Vestibulocochlear nerve (CN VIII)

Fourth ventricle

Superior cerebellar peduncle

Dentate nucleus

Figure 1.69. Lateral view of the dentate nucleus and cerebellum. The superior cerebellar peduncle arises from the dentate nucleus and ascends via the midbrain to the thalamus. It also forms the superior half of the lateral wall of the fourth ventricle.

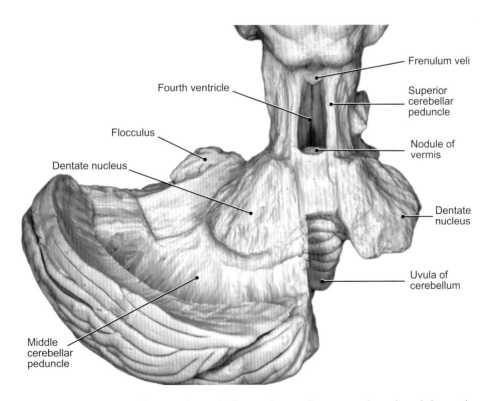

Fourth ventricle

Flocculus

Dentate nucleus

Middle cerebellar peduncle

Frenulum veli

Superior cerebellar peduncle

Nodule of vermis

Dentate nucleus

Uvula of cerebellum

Figure 1.70. Dorsal view of the dentate nucleus and cerebellum. The uvula, pyramid, and nodule are located at the midline, and the bilateral dentate nuclei are located paramedially. The dentate nucleus is the major outflow of the cerebellum.

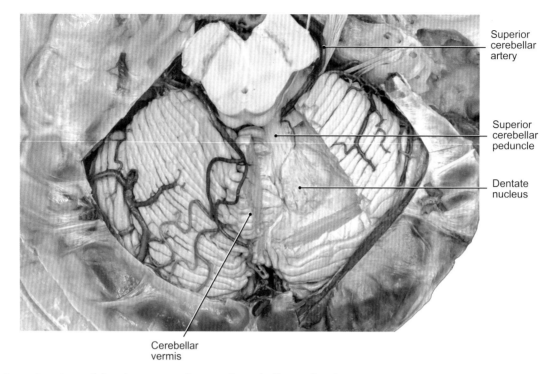

Superior cerebellar artery

Superior cerebellar peduncle

Dentate nucleus

Cerebellar vermis

Figure 1.71. Superior view of the dentate nucleus and cerebellum. The dentate nucleus sits in the quadrangular lobule and is supplied by the superior cerebellar artery.

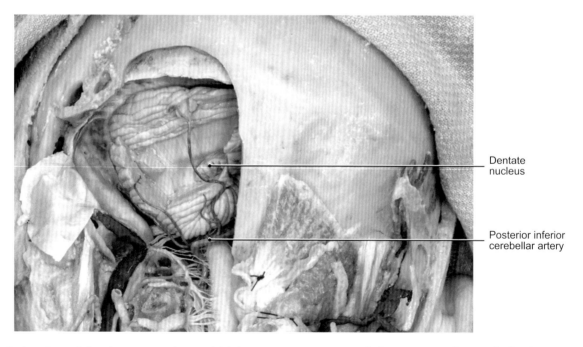

Dentate nucleus

Posterior inferior cerebellar artery

Figure 1.72. Inferior view of the dentate nucleus, which has a centrosuperomedial position in the cerebellar hemisphere.

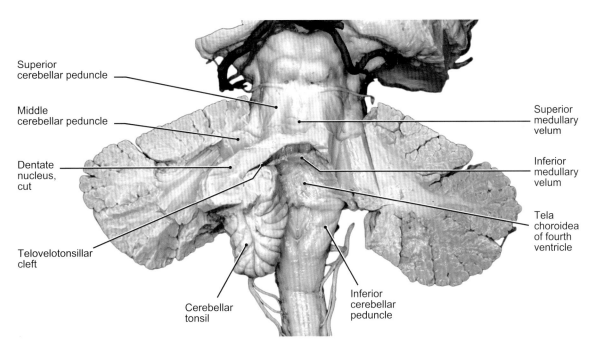

Superior
cerebellar peduncle

Middle
cerebellar peduncle

Dentate
nucleus,
cut

Telovelotonsillar
cleft

Cerebellar
tonsil

Superior
medullary
velum

Inferior
medullary
velum

Tela
choroidea
of fourth
ventricle

Inferior
cerebellar
peduncle

Figure 1.73. Posterior view of the telovelotonsillar cleft, which can be used as a landmark for the superior limit of the cerebellar tonsillectomy.

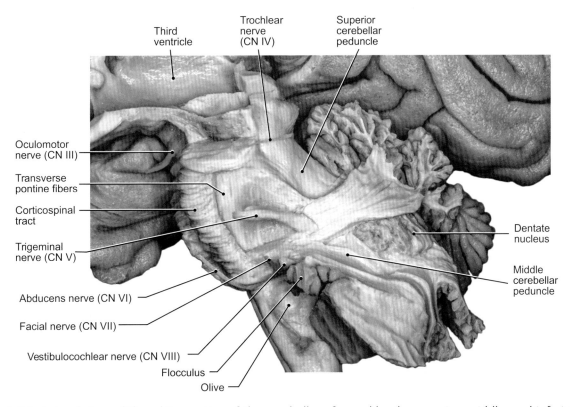

Third
ventricle

Trochlear
nerve
(CN IV)

Superior
cerebellar
peduncle

Oculomotor
nerve (CN III)

Transverse
pontine fibers

Corticospinal
tract

Trigeminal
nerve (CN V)

Abducens nerve (CN VI)

Facial nerve (CN VII)

Vestibulocochlear nerve (CN VIII)

Flocculus

Olive

Dentate
nucleus

Middle
cerebellar
peduncle

Figure 1.74. Lateral view of the white matter of the cerebellum formed by the superior, middle, and inferior cerebellar peduncles. The superior cerebellar peduncle connects the cerebellum to the midbrain, the middle cerebellar peduncle connects the pons to the cerebellum, and the inferior cerebellar peduncle connects the medulla and spinal cord to the cerebellum.

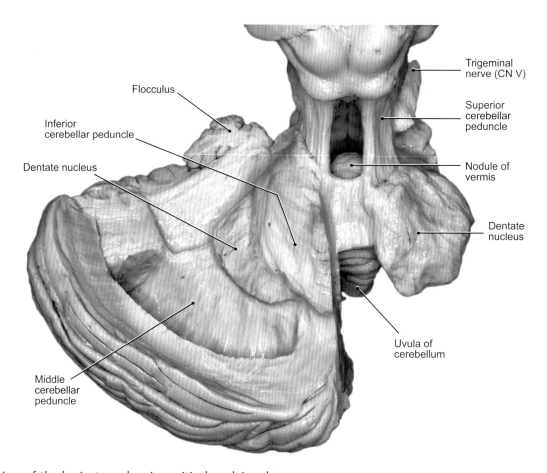

Figure 1.75. Dorsal view of the brainstem showing critical nuclei and tracts.

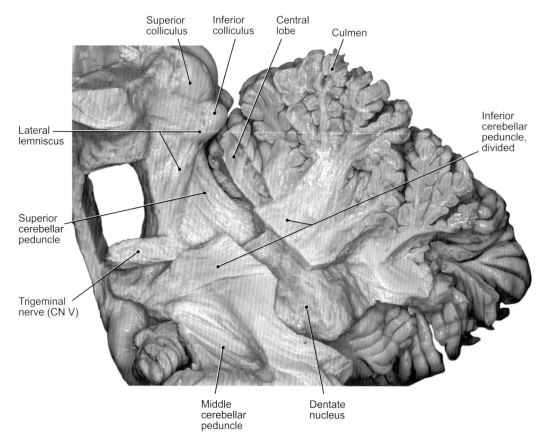

Figure 1.76. Lateral view of the brainstem showing critical nuclei and tracts.

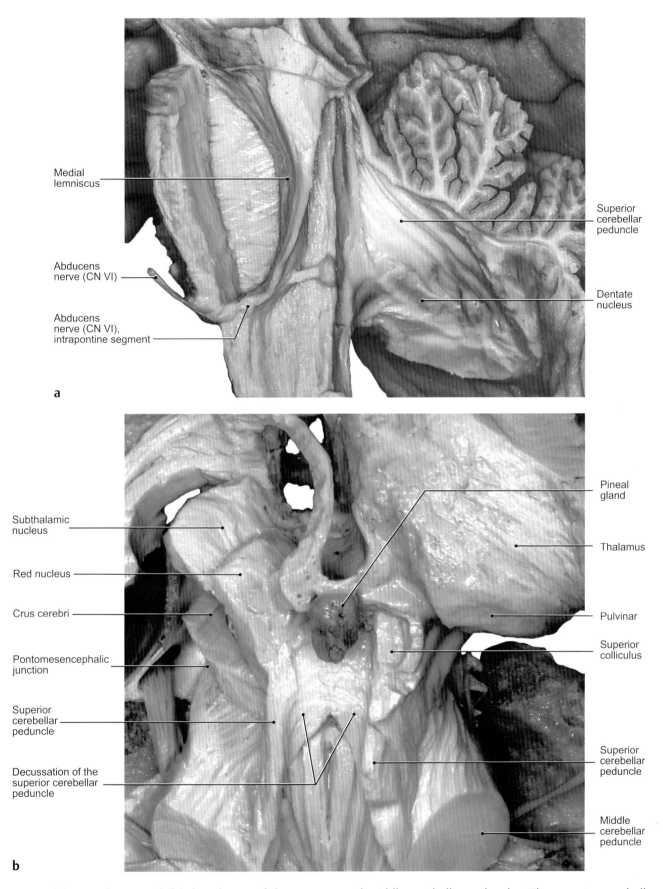

Figure 1.77. (a) Lateral view and **(b)** dorsal view of the superior and middle cerebellar peduncles. The superior cerebellar peduncle fibers decussate in the midbrain to form the capsule of the red nucleus. The middle cerebellar peduncle connects the cerebellum to the pons.

Cranial Nerves and Skull Base

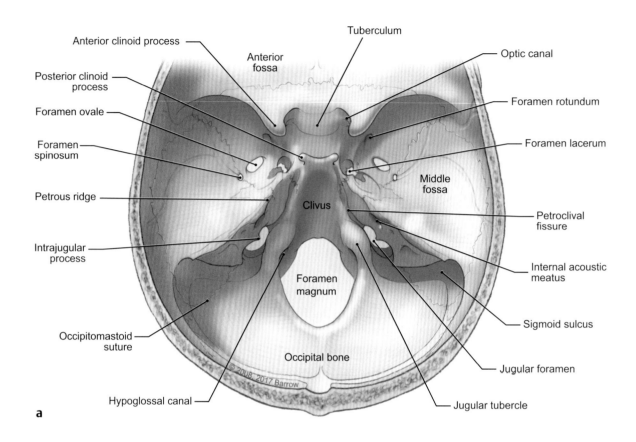

a

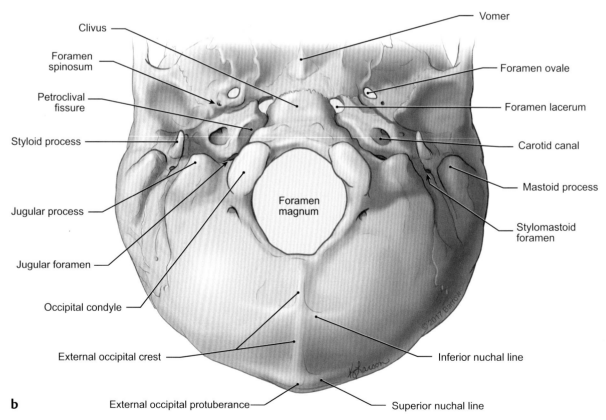

b

Figure 1.78. (a) The intracranial skull base and the foramina, which serve as the site of exit of the spinal cord, cranial nerves, and vasculature. **(b)** The extracranial view of the foramen magnum.

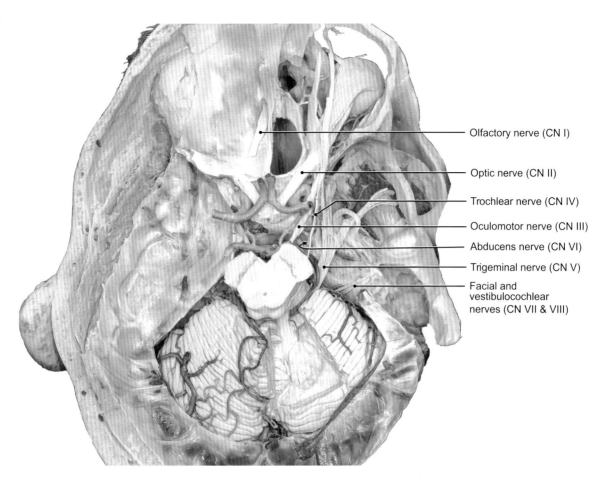

Olfactory nerve (CN I)

Optic nerve (CN II)

Trochlear nerve (CN IV)

Oculomotor nerve (CN III)

Abducens nerve (CN VI)

Trigeminal nerve (CN V)

Facial and vestibulocochlear nerves (CN VII & VIII)

Figure 1.79. Superior view of the olfactory (CN I), optic (CN II), oculomotor (CN III), trochlear (CN IV), trigeminal (CN V), abducens (CN VI), facial (CN VII), and vestibulocochlear (CN VIII) nerves and their courses.

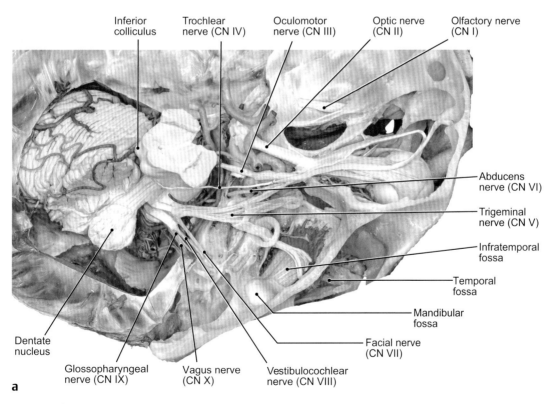

Inferior colliculus

Trochlear nerve (CN IV)

Oculomotor nerve (CN III)

Optic nerve (CN II)

Olfactory nerve (CN I)

Abducens nerve (CN VI)

Trigeminal nerve (CN V)

Infratemporal fossa

Temporal fossa

Mandibular fossa

Facial nerve (CN VII)

Vestibulocochlear nerve (CN VIII)

Vagus nerve (CN X)

Glossopharyngeal nerve (CN IX)

Dentate nucleus

a

Figure 1.80. (a) Superolateral view of the olfactory (CN I), optic (CN II), oculomotor (CN III), trochlear (CN IV), trigeminal (CN V), abducens (CN VI), facial (CN VII), vestibulocochlear (CN VIII), glossopharyngeal (CN IX), and vagus (CN X) nerves and their courses through the posterior to anterior fossae. **(b)** High-magnification lateral view of the brainstem and cranial nerves demonstrates the close proximity of the facial nerve and the glossopharyngeal nerve at the level of their root entry zone at the cerebellopontine angle cistern.

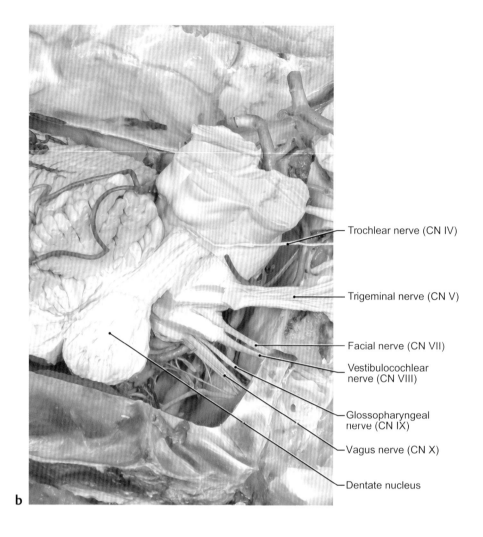

Trochlear nerve (CN IV)

Trigeminal nerve (CN V)

Facial nerve (CN VII)

Vestibulocochlear
nerve (CN VIII)

Glossopharyngeal
nerve (CN IX)

Vagus nerve (CN X)

Dentate nucleus

b

Figure 1.80. (*Continued*)

Trochlear
nerve
(CN IV)

Abducens
nerve
(CN VI)

Oculomotor
nerve
(CN III)

Optic
nerve
(CN II)

Olfactory
nerve
(CN I)

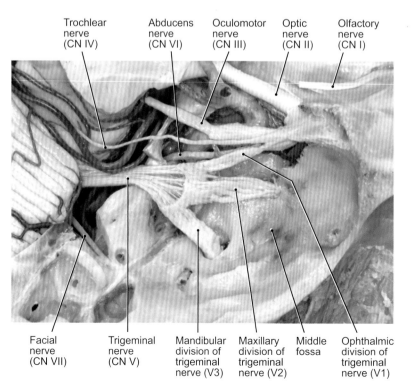

Facial
nerve
(CN VII)

Trigeminal
nerve
(CN V)

Mandibular
division of
trigeminal
nerve (V3)

Maxillary
division of
trigeminal
nerve (V2)

Middle
fossa

Ophthalmic
division of
trigeminal
nerve (V1)

Figure 1.81. Lateral view of the skull demonstrating the path of the olfactory (CN I), optic (CN II), oculomotor (CN III), trochlear (CN IV), trigeminal (CN V), abducens (CN VI), and facial (CN VII) nerves.

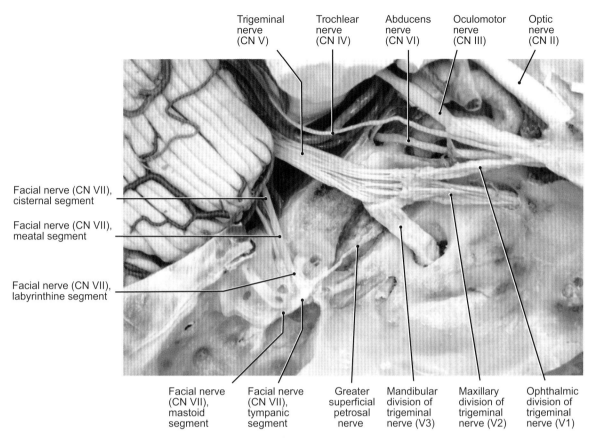

Trigeminal nerve (CN V)

Trochlear nerve (CN IV)

Abducens nerve (CN VI)

Oculomotor nerve (CN III)

Optic nerve (CN II)

Facial nerve (CN VII), cisternal segment

Facial nerve (CN VII), meatal segment

Facial nerve (CN VII), labyrinthine segment

Facial nerve (CN VII), mastoid segment

Facial nerve (CN VII), tympanic segment

Greater superficial petrosal nerve

Mandibular division of trigeminal nerve (V3)

Maxillary division of trigeminal nerve (V2)

Ophthalmic division of trigeminal nerve (V1)

Figure 1.82. Lateral view of the skull base demonstrating the relationship of the oculomotor (CN III), trochlear (CN IV), trigeminal (CN V), and abducens (CN VI) nerves as they migrate through the cavernous sinus (removed for clarity).

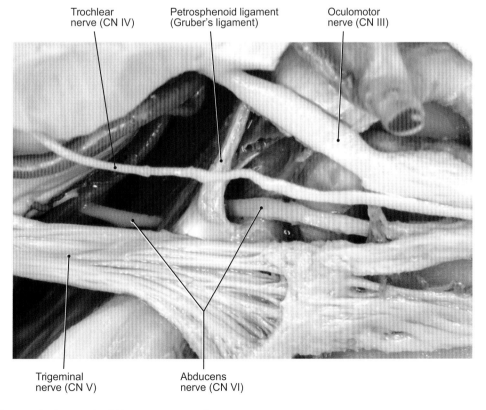

Trochlear nerve (CN IV)

Petrosphenoid ligament (Gruber's ligament)

Oculomotor nerve (CN III)

Trigeminal nerve (CN V)

Abducens nerve (CN VI)

Figure 1.83. Lateral view of the posterior part of the cavernous sinus.

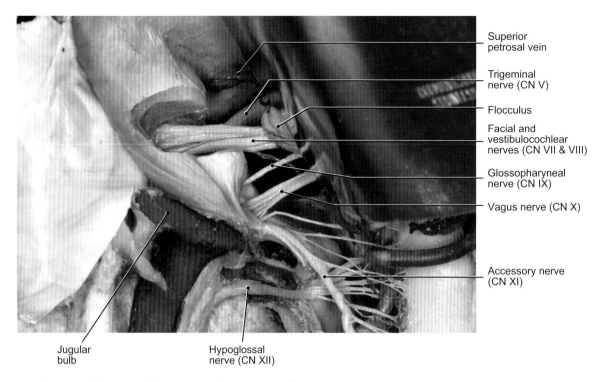

Superior
petrosal vein

Trigeminal
nerve (CN V)

Flocculus

Facial and
vestibulocochlear
nerves (CN VII & VIII)

Glossopharyneal
nerve (CN IX)

Vagus nerve (CN X)

Accessory nerve
(CN XI)

Jugular
bulb

Hypoglossal
nerve (CN XII)

Figure 1.84. Lateral view of the cranial nerves in the posterior fossa.

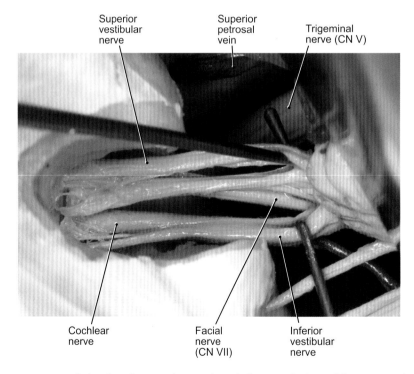

Superior
vestibular
nerve

Superior
petrosal
vein

Trigeminal
nerve (CN V)

Cochlear
nerve

Facial
nerve
(CN VII)

Inferior
vestibular
nerve

Figure 1.85. The relative orientation of the facial nerve (CN VII) and the vestibulocochlear nerve (CN VIII).

2 Safe Entry Zones

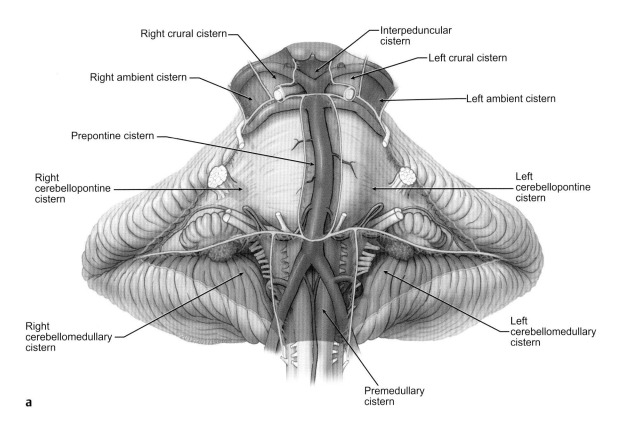

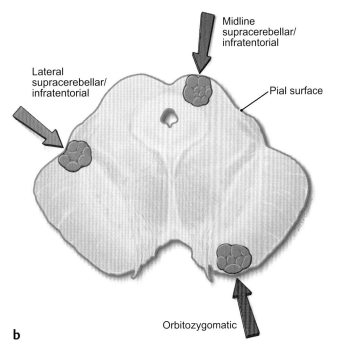

Figure 2.1. (a) Anterior view. The cerebrospinal cisterns provide natural pathways to the brainstem. **(b)** Axial view. These pathways can be reached using skull base approaches (*arrows*), judicious subarachnoid dissection, and release of cerebrospinal fluid. Lesions should be approached where they abut a pial or an ependymal surface to minimize injury to critical neurovascular bundles.

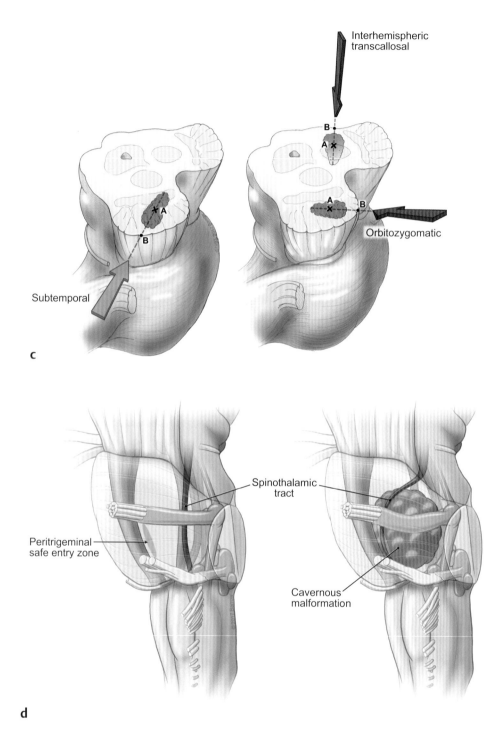

Figure 2.1. (c) Axial view. When a lesion does not abut a pial or an ependymal surface, the surgeon should use the path that is least likely to disturb eloquent neural structures. The two-point method can assist with selection of the approach both in cases of deep lesions and in cases where the lesion abuts a pial or an ependymal surface. To perform the two-point method, first place a mark (*point A*) at the center of the lesion, then place a second mark (*point B*) where the lesion is closest to a surface of the brainstem or at the least eloquent entry point. Next draw a line from point *A* to point *B* and ultimately to the surface of the skull. The approach is dictated by this line (*arrows*). **(d)** Anterolateral view. Pathology can displace critical nuclei and tracts, which could nullify safe entry into the surgical zones. For example, the peritrigeminal safe entry zone (*blue oval*) enables the surgeon to access lesions in the lateral pons, but a hemorrhage or tumor can displace tracts so that entry via this safe entry zone could compromise neurologic function.

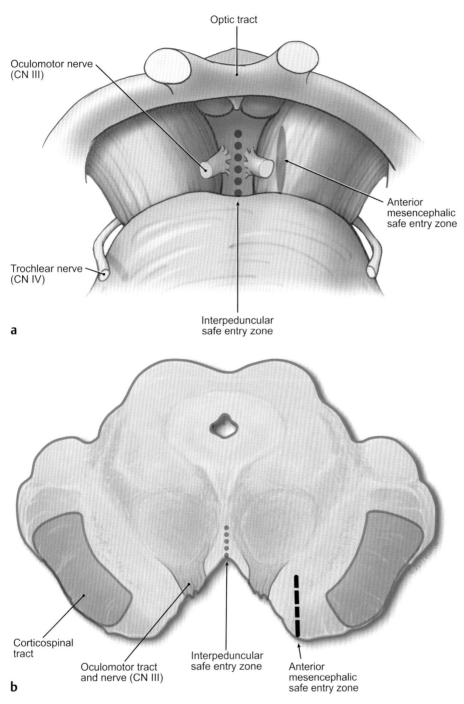

Optic tract

Oculomotor nerve
(CN III)

Anterior
mesencephalic
safe entry zone

Trochlear nerve
(CN IV)

Interpeduncular
safe entry zone

a

Corticospinal
tract

Oculomotor tract
and nerve (CN III)

Interpeduncular
safe entry zone

Anterior
mesencephalic
safe entry zone

b

Figure 2.2. **(a)** Anterior view. Ventral midbrain lesions can be accessed using any of the anterior or anterolateral approaches through the cerebral peduncle via the anterior mesencephalic (also known as the perioculomotor) safe entry zone (*blue oval*). This safe entry zone is located lateral to the oculomotor nerve (CN III) between the posterior cerebral artery and the superior cerebellar artery. An alternative ventral safe entry zone is the interpeduncular safe entry zone (*dotted line*). **(b)** Axial view. The anterior mesencephalic safe entry zone (*dashed line*) is bordered medially by the oculomotor tract and nerve, laterally by the corticospinal tract, superiorly by the posterior cerebral artery, and inferiorly by the superior cerebellar artery. The interpeduncular safe entry zone (*dotted line*) is bordered laterally by the oculomotor nerves.

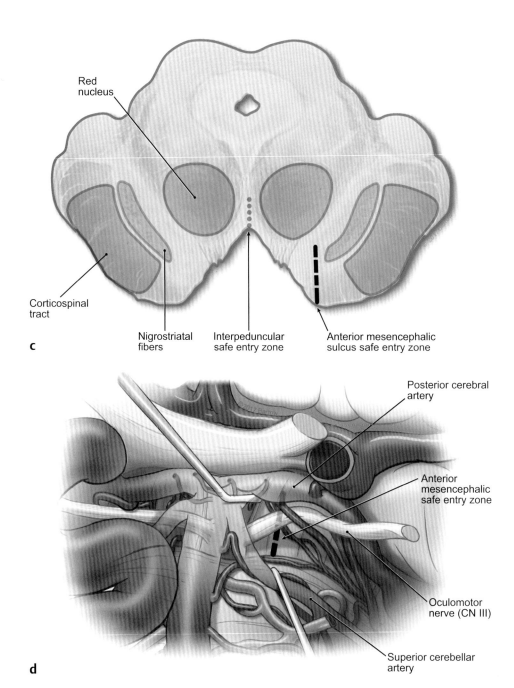

c

Red nucleus

Corticospinal tract

Nigrostriatal fibers

Interpeduncular safe entry zone

Anterior mesencephalic sulcus safe entry zone

d

Posterior cerebral artery

Anterior mesencephalic safe entry zone

Oculomotor nerve (CN III)

Superior cerebellar artery

Figure 2.2. (c) Axial view. The anterior mesencephalic safe entry zone (*dashed line*) makes use of the distribution of the corticospinal tract fibers in the middle three-fifths of the cerebral peduncle and the fact that the red nucleus and nigrostriatal circuit are in a deep location. The interpeduncular safe entry zone (*dotted line*) makes use of the sparse nature of critical fibers in this region, but the proximity to the basilar artery and the variability of distribution of the basilar perforators can make this safe entry zone challenging to use. **(d)** The anterior mesencephalic safe entry zone (*dashed line*) is bound superiorly by the posterior cerebral artery and inferiorly by the superior cerebellar artery.

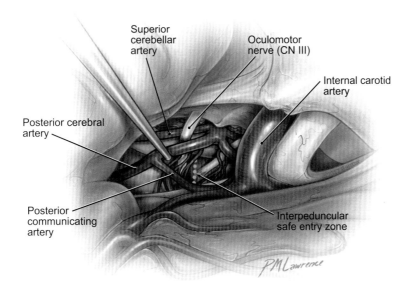

e

Figure 2.2. (e) The interpeduncular safe entry zone (*dotted line*) can be used for select lesions that are located ventrally and midline to the oculomotor nerve nucleus.

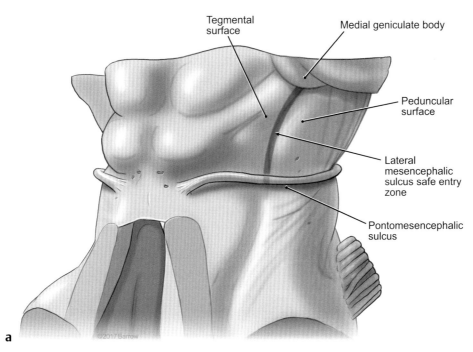

a

Figure 2.3. (a) Posterolateral view. Extending from the medial geniculate body to the pontomesencephalic sulcus, the lateral mesencephalic sulcus (*blue line*) is another safe entry zone into the midbrain. The lateral mesencephalic sulcus is often hidden by the lateral mesencephalic vein. The sulcus separates the peduncular and tegmental surfaces of the midbrain facing the middle incisural space.

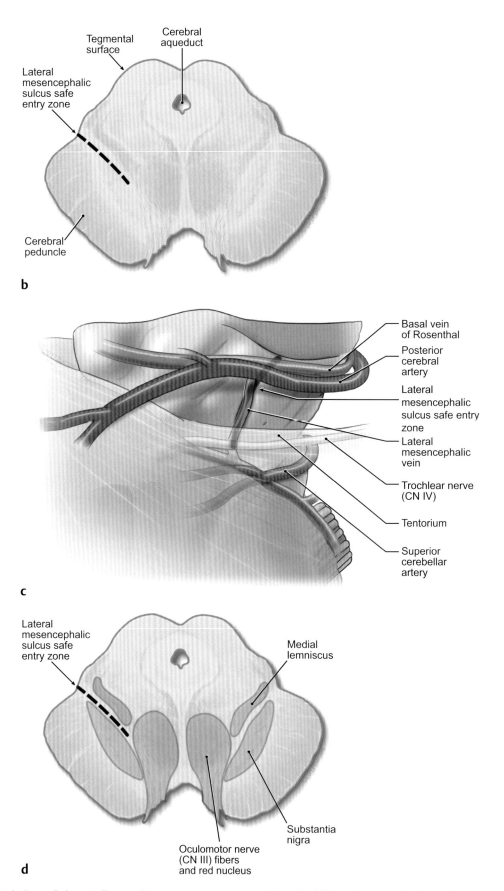

Figure 2.3. **(b)** Axial slice of the midbrain demonstrating the lateral mesencephalic sulcus safe entry zone (*dashed line*). **(c)** Posterolateral view. The posterior cerebral artery crosses the lateral mesencephalic sulcus safe entry zone (*blue line*) superiorly, whereas the cerebellomesencephalic segments of the superior cerebellar artery, the trochlear nerve (CN IV), and the tentorial edge cross the zone inferiorly. **(d)** Axial view. The lateral mesencephalic sulcus safe entry zone (*dashed line*) rests between the substantia nigra anterolaterally and the medial lemniscus posteriorly. The anteromedial limit of the safe entry zone is defined by the oculomotor fibers crossing from the red nucleus to the substantia nigra.

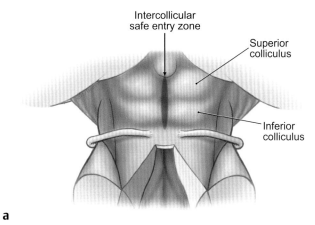

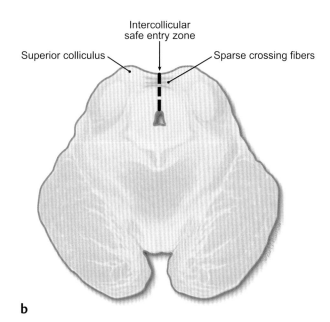

Figure 2.4. (a) Dorsal view. The superior and inferior colliculi constitute the dorsal surface of the midbrain. The intercollicular safe entry zone (*blue oval*) is bordered laterally by the colliculi. **(b)** Axial view of the intercollicular safe entry zone (*dashed line*). The intercollicular region has relatively sparse crossing fibers. The anterior limit of this safe entry zone is the cerebral aqueduct.

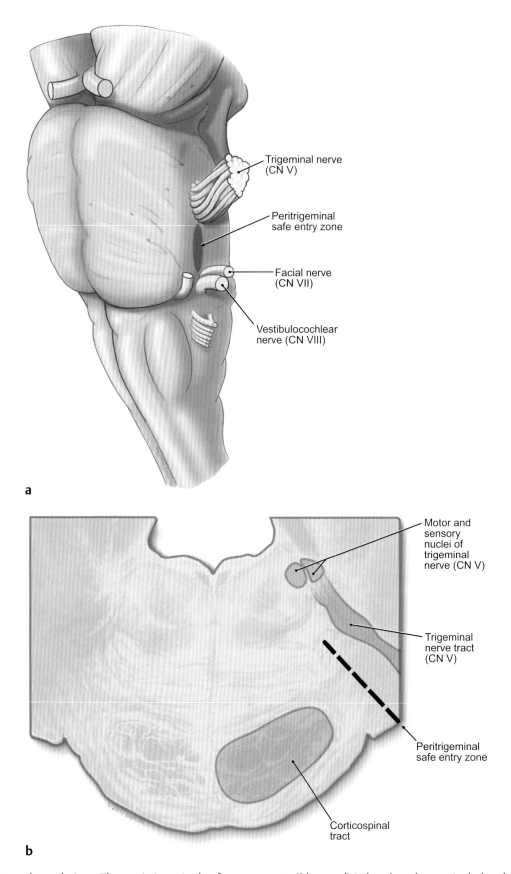

Trigeminal nerve (CN V)

Peritrigeminal safe entry zone

Facial nerve (CN VII)

Vestibulocochlear nerve (CN VIII)

a

Motor and sensory nuclei of trigeminal nerve (CN V)

Trigeminal nerve tract (CN V)

Peritrigeminal safe entry zone

Corticospinal tract

b

Figure 2.5. (a) Anterolateral view. The peritrigeminal safe entry zone (*blue oval*) is bordered superiorly by the trigeminal nerve (CN V) and inferiorly by the facial (CN VII) and vestibulocochlear nerve (CN VIII) complex. **(b)** Axial view. The peritrigeminal safe entry zone (*dashed line*) is anterior to the motor and sensory nuclei of the trigeminal nerve and lateral to the corticospinal tract.

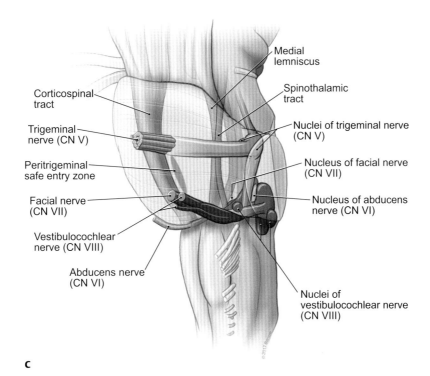

Corticospinal tract
Trigeminal nerve (CN V)
Peritrigeminal safe entry zone
Facial nerve (CN VII)
Vestibulocochlear nerve (CN VIII)
Abducens nerve (CN VI)
Medial lemniscus
Spinothalamic tract
Nuclei of trigeminal nerve (CN V)
Nucleus of facial nerve (CN VII)
Nucleus of abducens nerve (CN VI)
Nuclei of vestibulocochlear nerve (CN VIII)

c

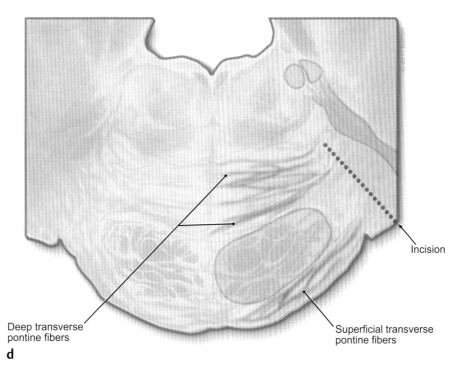

Deep transverse pontine fibers
Superficial transverse pontine fibers
Incision

d

Figure 2.5. **(c)** Anterolateral view. The fibers of the abducens (CN VI), facial, and vestibulocochlear nerves run caudally and pass posterior to the trigeminal nuclei; these fibers define the inferior border of the peritrigeminal safe entry zone (*blue oval*). Injury to these nuclei should be avoided by not proceeding too inferoposteriorly when using this safe entry zone. The fibers of the trigeminal nerve run rostrally and define the superior extent of the safe entry zone. **(d)** Axial view of the peritrigeminal safe entry zone. The incision is made longitudinally between the trigeminal and facial nerves. The incision (*dotted line*) crosses the superficial transverse pontine fibers. As the incision is deepened, it can reach the pontine nuclei and ultimately cross the deep transverse pontine fibers. Making an incision dorsal to the trigeminal nerve may injure the intrapontine segment of the nerve and the ventral cochlear nucleus.

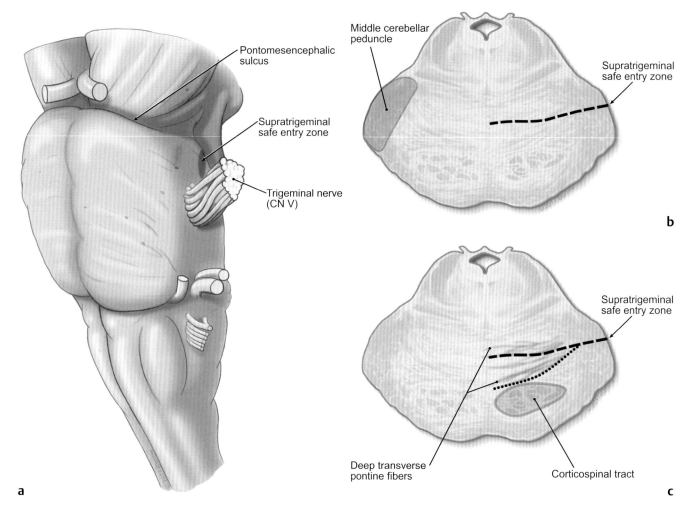

Figure 2.6. (a) Anterolateral view. Another possible point of entry into the pons is the supratrigeminal safe entry zone (*blue oval*), which rests above the trigeminal nerve (CN V) root on the middle cerebellar peduncle. **(b)** Axial view of the supratrigeminal safe entry zone (*dashed line*). **(c)** Axial view.

The posterolateral location of the middle cerebellar peduncle and of the pontine transverse fibers makes it possible to dissect along the fibers medially (*dashed line*) or anteromedially (*dotted line*), posterior to the corticospinal tract.

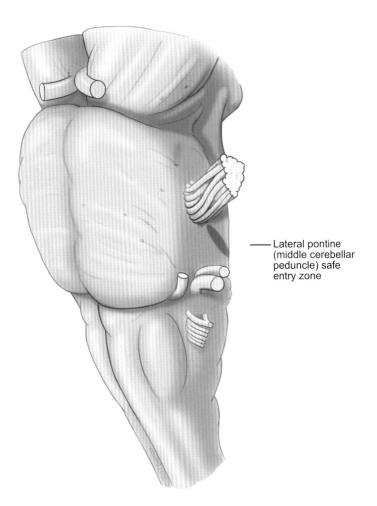

Lateral pontine (middle cerebellar peduncle) safe entry zone

Figure 2.7. Anterolateral view. The lateral pontine or middle cerebellar peduncle safe entry zone (*blue oval*) rests at the junction between the cerebellum and the pons.

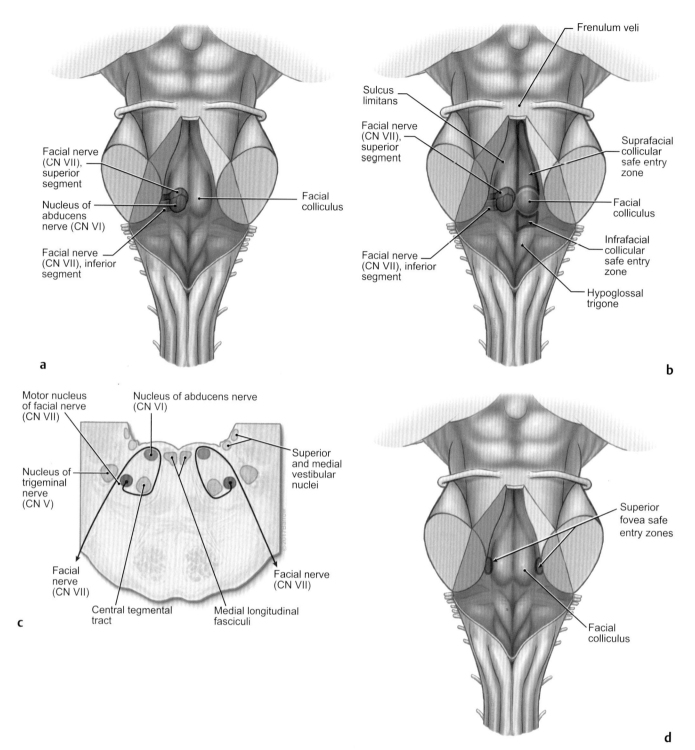

Figure 2.8. **(a)** Dorsal view. At the floor of the fourth ventricle, the facial nerve (CN VII) passes around the nucleus of the abducens nerve (CN VI), forming the facial colliculus. Two safe entry zones, the suprafacial collicular and infrafacial collicular safe entry zones, reside adjacent to this structure. **(b)** Dorsal view. The suprafacial collicular safe entry zone is defined as a triangle, delineated caudally by the facial nerve, laterally by the sulcus limitans, and medially by the medial longitudinal fasciculus (not shown). The superior limit is the frenulum veli. The infrafacial collicular zone is delineated by the hypoglossal trigone caudally, the facial nerve laterally, and the medial longitudinal fasciculus medially. The superior limit is the inferior segment of the facial nerve. **(c)** Axial view. The incision in the suprafacial collicular safe entry zone must be made with care so that it does not extend medially and deeply into the medial longitudinal fasciculus or laterally to the sulcus limitans. This approach avoids injury to the trigeminal mesencephalic and central tegmental tracts located deep to the locus ceruleus, and it limits injury to the trigeminal motor and main sensory nuclei, which are located deep to the superolateral edge of the superior fovea triangle. Transverse infracollicular incisions that extend laterally may injure the superior cerebellar peduncle and the lateral lemniscus. **(d)** Dorsal view. A third safe entry zone at the level of the facial colliculus is the superior fovea safe entry zone (*blue ovals*), which is located in the lower half of the superior fovea triangle lateral to the facial colliculus.

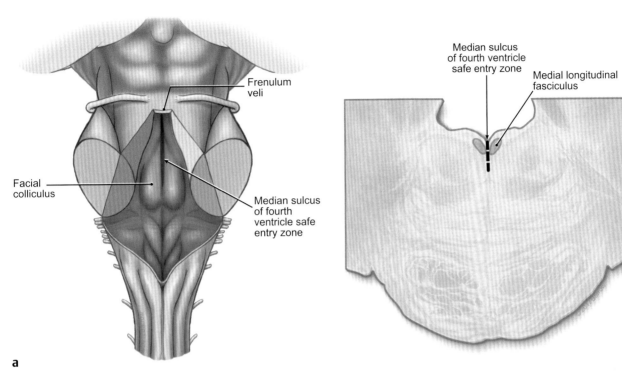

Figure 2.9. (a) Dorsal view. The median sulcus of the fourth ventricle is a safe entry zone (*narrow blue oval*). There are no crossing fibers at the midline between the frenulum veli and the facial colliculus. **(b)** Axial view. Extreme care must be taken because even the slightest retraction of the adjacent brainstem can cause extraocular movement paresis due to injury of the medial longitudinal fasciculi (*blue areas*), which are deep and lateral to the median sulcus of the fourth ventricle safe entry zone (*dashed line*).

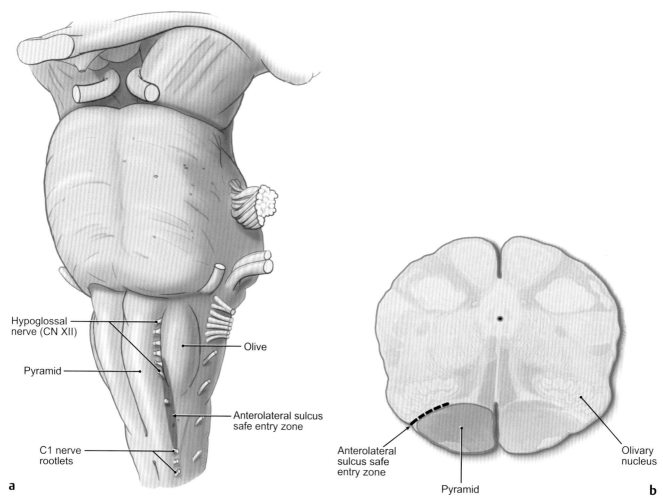

Hypoglossal
nerve (CN XII)

Pyramid

C1 nerve
rootlets

Olive

Anterolateral sulcus
safe entry zone

a

Anterolateral
sulcus safe
entry zone

Pyramid

Olivary
nucleus

b

Figure 2.10. **(a)** Anterolateral view. Lateral to the pyramid, the rootlets of the hypoglossal nerve (CN XII) leave the brainstem from the anterolateral sulcus. The space between the hypoglossal nerve rootlets and the C1 nerve rootlets delineate the anterolateral sulcus safe entry zone (*blue oval*), which coincides with the decussation of the corticospinal tract. Oblique paramedian dissection avoids the corticospinal tract. **(b)** Axial view. The anterolateral sulcus (*dashed line*) of the medulla is a safe entry zone.

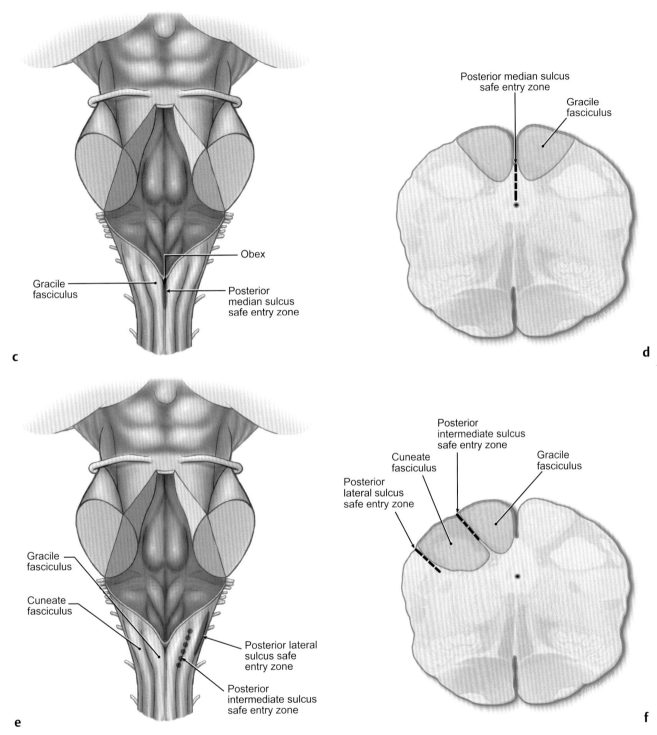

c

d

e

f

Figure 2.10. (c) Dorsal view. The posterior median sulcus safe entry zone (*blue oval*) is located below the obex and is restricted laterally by the clava, which covers the gracile fasciculus. This safe entry zone, which is similar to the dorsal midline raphe safe entry zone **(Figure 2.13)** of the cervical spine, enables the removal of lesions that are located in the posterior medulla. **(d)** Axial view. The posterior median sulcus (*dashed line*) is another safe entry zone. **(e)** Dorsal view. The posterior intermediate sulcus safe entry zone (*dotted line*) is located between the gracile and cuneate fasciculi, and the posterior lateral sulcus safe entry zone (*blue oval*) is located lateral to the cuneate fasciculus. **(f)** Axial view of the posterior intermediate sulcus and the posterior lateral sulcus safe entry zones (*dashed lines*).

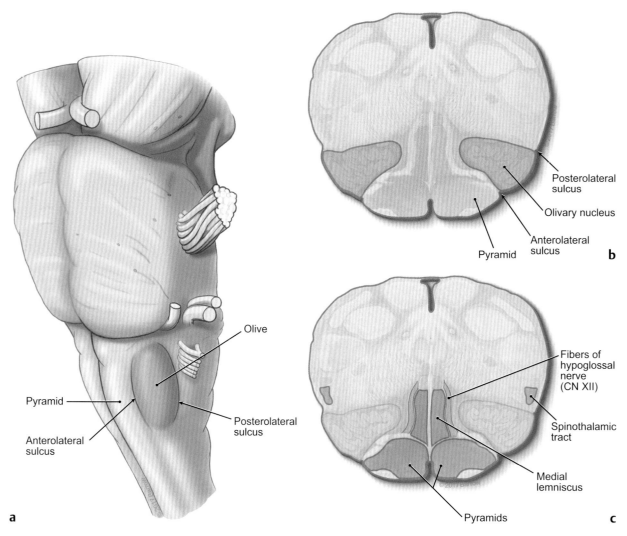

Figure 2.11. **(a)** Anterolateral view. The olives are oval prominences on the anterolateral surfaces of the medulla limited medially by the anterolateral sulcus and pyramids and posteriorly by the posterolateral sulcus. **(b)** Axial view through the bilateral olives (*blue area*), anterolateral sulcus, and posterolateral sulcus. **(c)** Axial view at the level of the inferior olivary nuclei (olives), where fibers of the hypoglossal nerves (CN XII) separate the olives from the corticospinal tracts. The olives are limited medially by the hypoglossal nerve fibers and the medial lemnisci and posteriorly by the spinothalamic tracts.

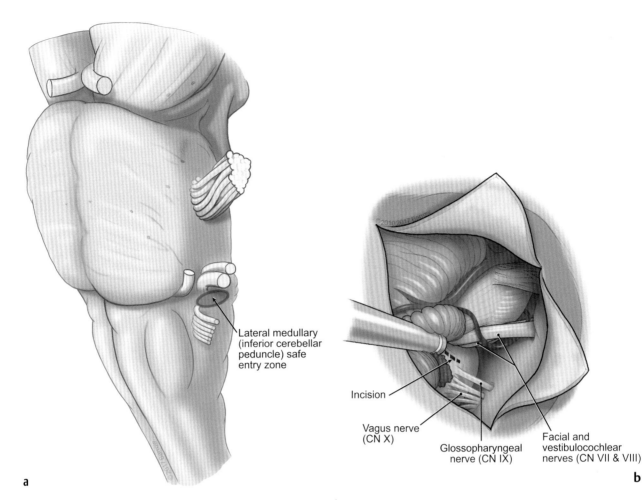

a

b

Figure 2.12. (a) Anterolateral view of the lateral medullary or inferior cerebellar peduncle safe entry zone (*blue area*). This zone can be approached via a retrosigmoid or far-lateral craniotomy through the inferior cerebellar peduncle. **(b)** The foramen of Luschka is opened, and the origins of the

glossopharyngeal (CN IX) and vagus (CN X) nerves are identified. A small transverse incision (*dashed line*) is made in the inferior cerebellar peduncle inferior to the cochlear nuclei and posterior to the origin of the glossopharyngeal and vagus nerves.

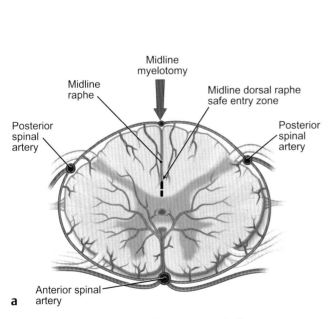

a

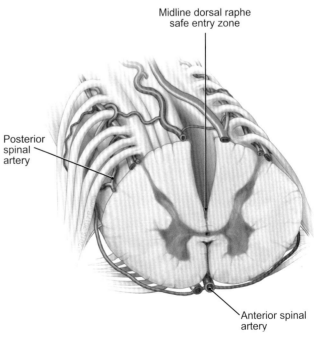

b

Figure 2.13. (a) Axial view of cervicomedullary junction. One approach to lesions within the cervicomedullary junction and the upper cervical spinal cord is through the dorsal raphe safe entry zone (*dashed line*) via a midline

myelotomy (*arrow*). **(b)** Axial view. The midline dorsal raphe (*arrow*) can be opened extensively in a rostrocaudal direction to minimize retraction and compression of the fibers in the cervicomedullary junction.

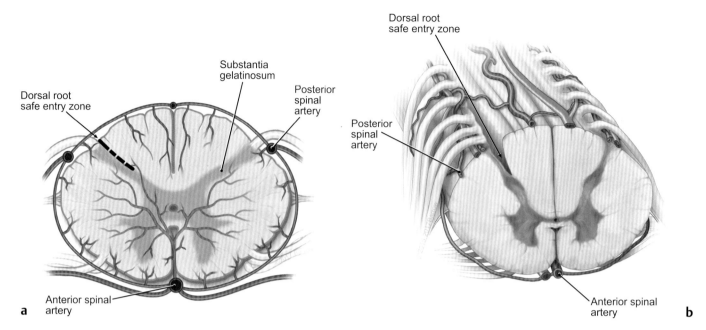

Figure 2.14. **(a)** Axial view of the cervicomedullary junction. The dorsal root safe entry zone (*dashed line*) can be used to remove lesions within the cervicomedullary junction and the upper cervical spinal cord via the substantia gelatinosum. **(b)** Axial view. The dorsal root safe entry zone (*arrow*) may be opened to access lesions in the posterolateral spinal cord.

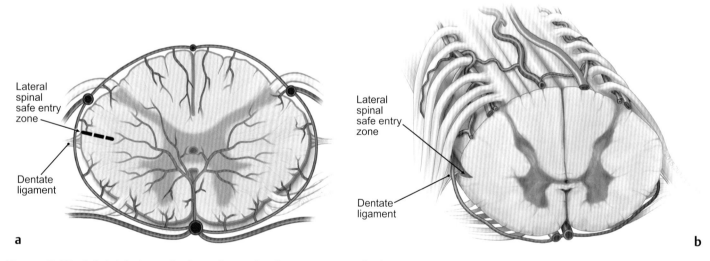

Figure 2.15. **(a)** Axial view. The lateral spinal safe entry zone, which is located between the nerve roots at the level of the dentate ligament (dashed line), can be used to remove lesions within the cervicomedullary junction and the spinal cord. **(b)** Axial view. The lateral spinal safe entry zone (*arrow*) may be opened by cutting the dentate ligament at multiple levels to gain access to lesions in the lateral spinal cord and to expose some ventral lesions.

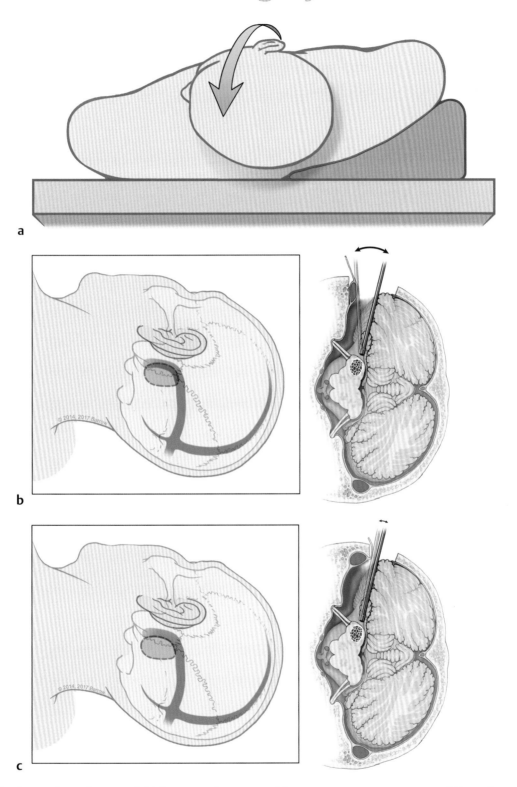

Figure 3.1. Positioning and craniotomy. **(a)** The operation begins with the proper positioning of the patient, so that the surgeon can perform the operation in a relaxed and comfortable manner. The patient should be placed in a position that minimizes pressure points, facilitates venous outflow to minimize congestion, and enables the surgeon to obtain many working trajectories by simply turning the bed. For an extreme-lateral supracerebellar infratentorial approach, for example, the patient is positioned with the head turned to the contralateral side, the chin tucked, and the neck slightly extended (*arrow*) toward the floor to enable gravity-dependent retraction of the cerebellar hemisphere and a more generous working space for the surgeon to perform the operation. **(b)** The proper placement of a craniotomy provides adequate exposure to deep structures without unnecessary exposure of the adjacent brain or vessels. For a retrosigmoid craniotomy, for example, the craniotomy should be placed to expose the transverse–sigmoid junction to enable the surgeon to obtain a flat view of the petrous ridge while being able to dynamically retract the exposed sinus edge. **(c)** Failure to expose the junction, such as by leaving bone over the sinus, hinders the approach to the cerebellopontine angle, resulting in the need for more cerebellar retraction to obtain similar exposure. Careful attention to craniotomy positioning significantly decreases morbidity without sacrificing the working space necessary to successfully perform an operation on the brainstem. Note that the contents of the cerebellopontine angle are well visualized using the craniotomy in **(b)**, where the transverse–sigmoid junction is mobilized.

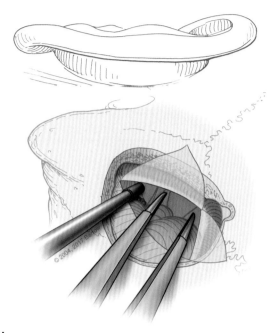

d

Figure 3.1. (d) The keyhole philosophy should be used whenever possible to optimize the craniotomy size, working trajectory, and visualization. A keyhole craniotomy is tailored but not necessarily small; rather, it is the smallest and most optimally placed craniotomy to enable the surgeon to perform the procedure without sacrificing quality or placing the patient at undue risk by minimizing visualization. The smallest permissible craniotomy is one that is large enough for bipolar forceps and a suction device to readily pass through.

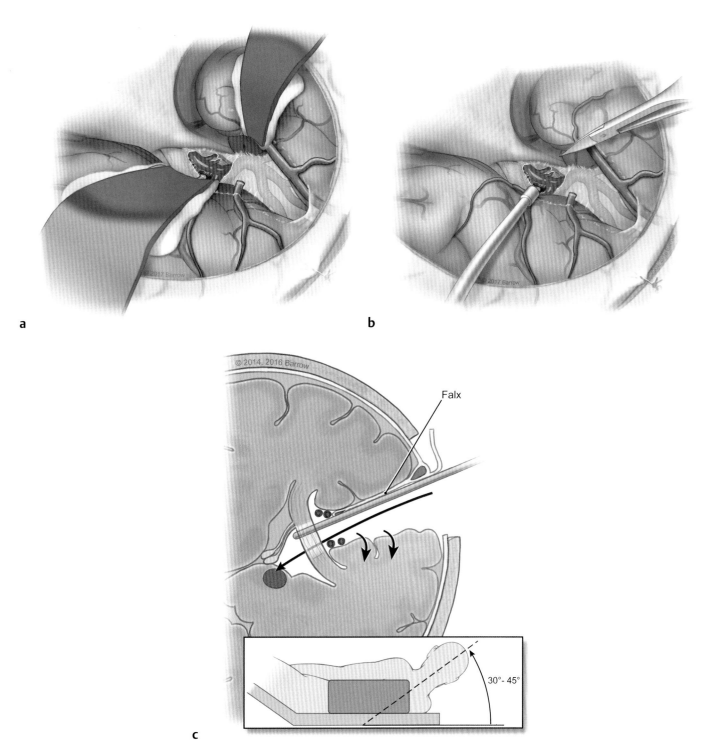

a

b

c

Figure 3.2. Dynamic and gravity retraction. **(a)** With properly placed craniotomies, it is rarely necessary to use the rigid retractor system to provide exposure. **(b)** The surgeon can obtain the same views with dynamic retraction using bipolar forceps, suction devices, or other microinstruments.

(c) Natural anatomic barriers, such as the falx, can be used in conjunction with gravity (*inset*) to perform the task of a rigid retractor. This point emphasizes the importance of patient positioning and proper planning of craniotomies to decrease the risk of patient morbidity.

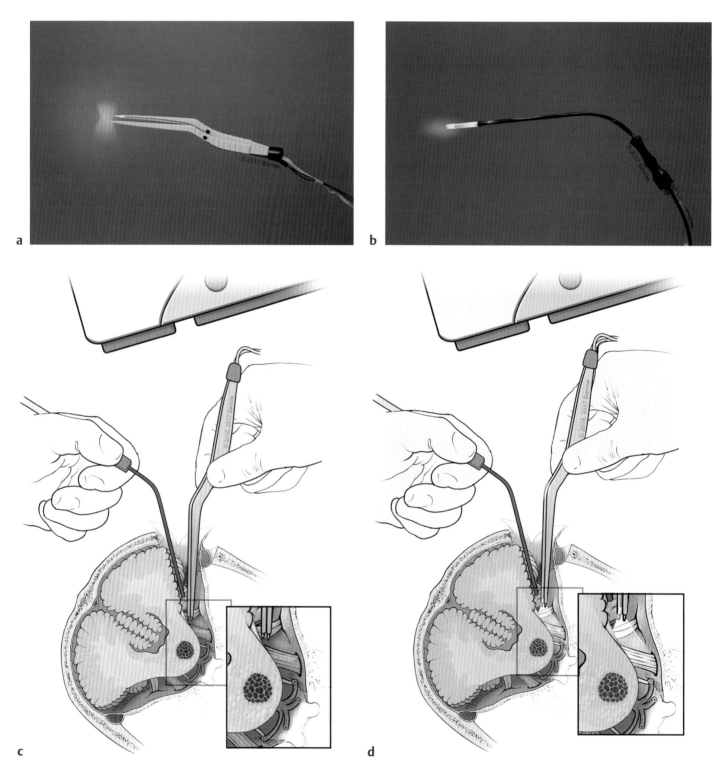

Figure 3.3. New tools and lighted instruments. Surgery for lesions of the brainstem and adjacent structures requires working through deep corridors. Flexible, bayonetted instruments enable the surgeon to work in tight, narrow corridors and still accomplish what previously required larger openings using less flexible instruments with a higher profile. Although the operative microscope has greatly aided the illumination of surgical fields, the considerable working depths necessary to approach lesions in the brainstem have required the invention of new surgical tools and instruments.

(a) Lighted bipolar forceps and **(b)** lighted suction devices provide enhanced illumination at the depth of the surgical field. **(c)** Illustration of the view obtained with the operative microscope. **(d)** Depiction of the same view as in **(c)** obtained with the addition of lighted bipolar forceps. Note the improved ability to visualize the cavity at the depth of the field. Specialized microinstruments enable improved surgical handling of pathology within the eloquent confines of the brainstem.

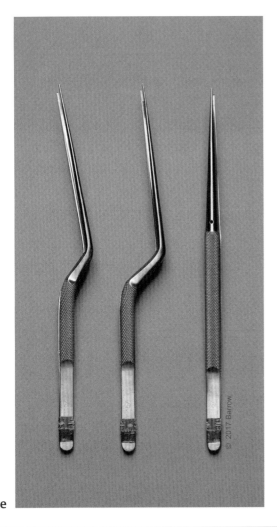

e

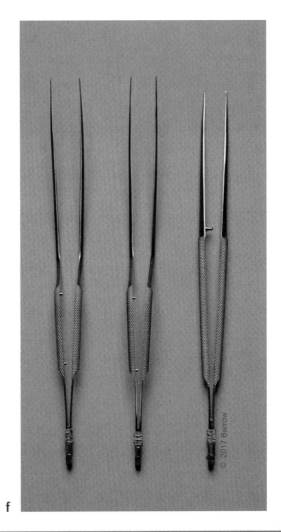

f

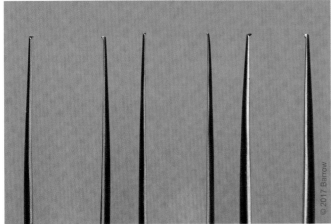
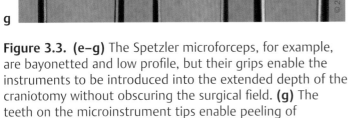

g

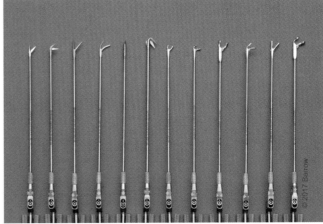

h

Figure 3.3. (e–g) The Spetzler microforceps, for example, are bayonetted and low profile, but their grips enable the instruments to be introduced into the extended depth of the craniotomy without obscuring the surgical field. **(g)** The teeth on the microinstrument tips enable peeling of cavernous malformation remnants from the surgical cavity. **(h)** Single-shaft instruments provide a low-profile means for operating at the depth of the surgical field with minimal hindrance.

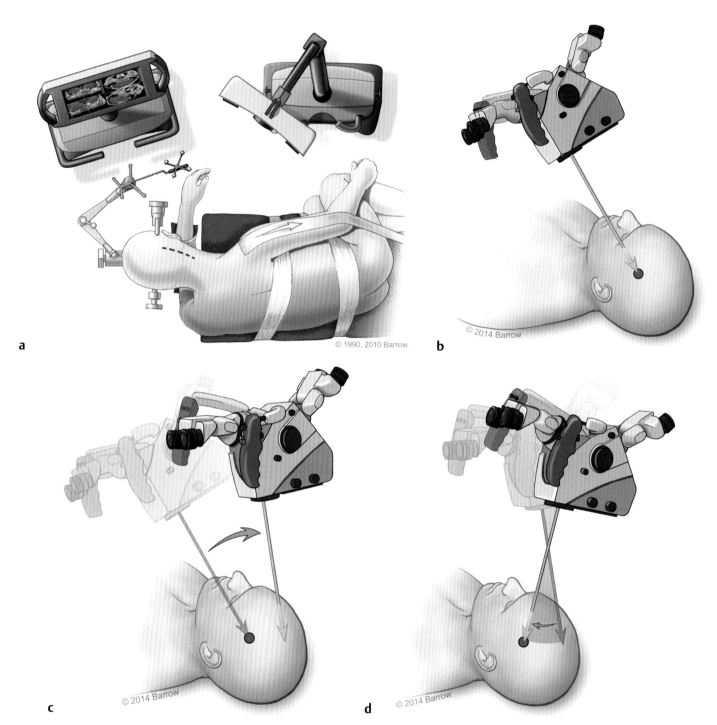

a

b

c

d

Figure 3.4. Stereotactic navigation has greatly facilitated planning and executing operations in eloquent regions. The neuronavigation system can assist in the optimal planning of a craniotomy and in identifying safe entry zones and sites where the pathology abuts pial or ependymal planes. The system also assists the surgeon in identifying the borders of the pathology. **(a)** The stereotactic navigation system can be integrated with the operative microscope to lock onto the pathology at the depth of the surgical field, giving the

surgeon the flexibility to maneuver to visualize adjacent anatomy while preserving the ability to return to the site of the pathology with the simple push of a button. **(b)** AutoLock Current Point feature. The microscope's focal point is used to set the target. **(c)** The microscope can be manually moved after the target is set. **(d)** With activation of the AutoLock Current Point feature, the focal point automatically returns to the designated target.

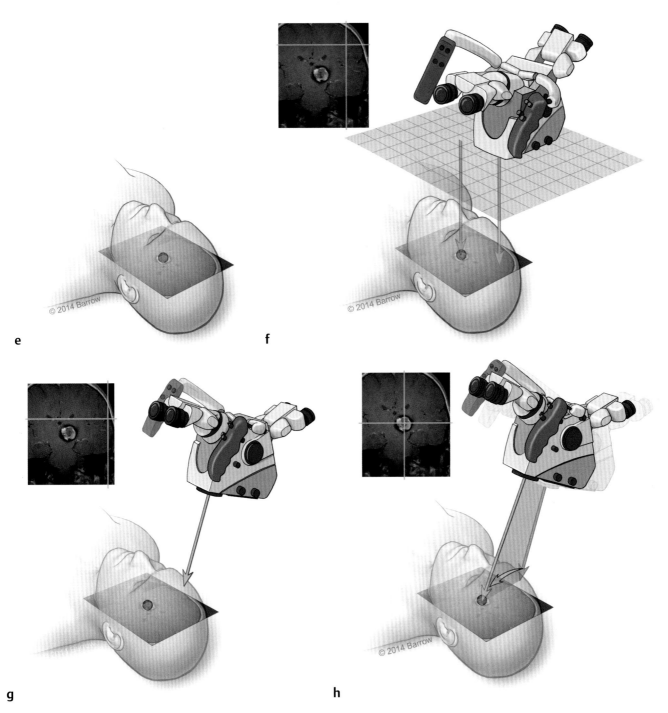

Figure 3.4. (e) Align Parallel to Plane feature. The target is identified, and a surgical plane is defined.
(f) With the Align Parallel to Plane feature activated, the microscope automatically aligns parallel to the selected plane and focuses on the plane that intersects the target point. **(g)** Point to Plane Target feature. The target is predefined. **(h)** With the Point to Plane Target feature activated, the microscope automatically rotates and focuses on the target point.

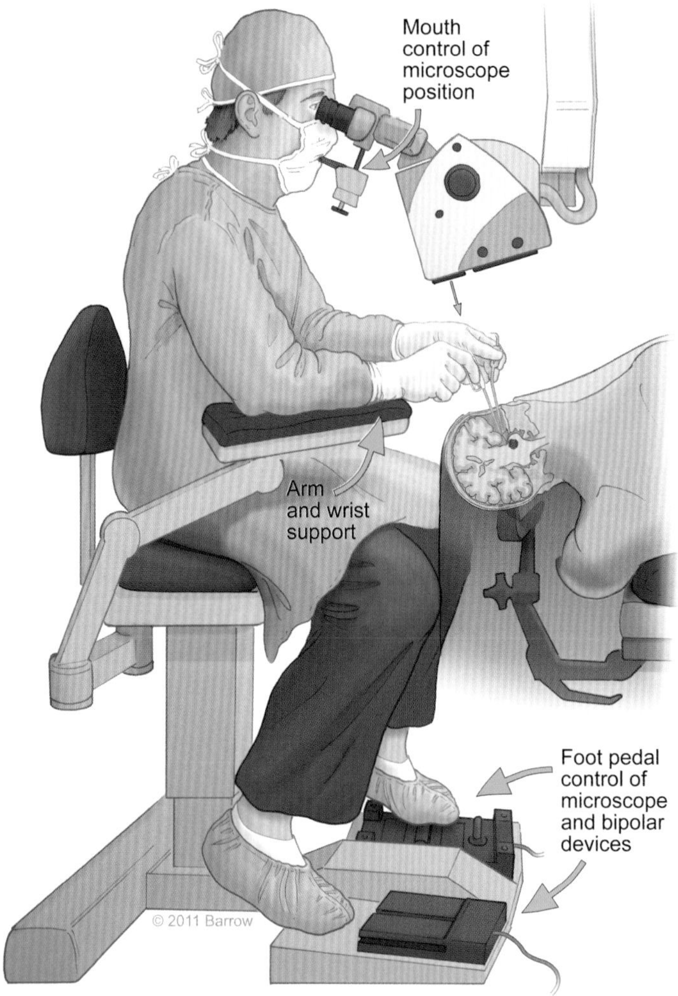

Mouth control of microscope position

Arm and wrist support

Foot pedal control of microscope and bipolar devices

© 2011 Barrow

Figure 3.5. Operative chair designed for surgeon comfort, with armrests, foot pedals, and microscope with mouth controls. The importance of surgeon comfort for the successful execution of an operation should not be underestimated. The operative chair with an armrest enables the surgeon to remain seated while carrying out intricate operations. The armrests help minimize fatigue while stabilizing the surgeon's forearms close to the patient and enabling the surgeon to operate in the same position for hours. The foot pedals attached to the operative chair enable hands-free manipulation of the microscope, greatly facilitating the operation by minimizing the time necessary for the surgeon to adjust the focus and light intensity. The mouthpiece controls enable hands-free, fine movement of the microscope.

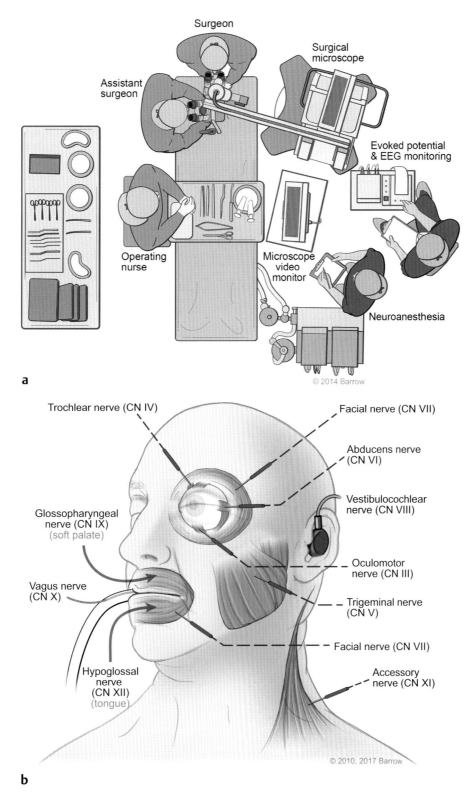

Figure 3.6. Neuroanesthesia and monitoring. **(a)** Successful execution of every operation requires that the team be well versed in the techniques of neurologic anesthesia and monitoring. An anesthesiologist familiar and comfortable with surgery in eloquent brain domains greatly facilitates the intraoperative care of patients. Brainstem operations often require the monitoring of somatosensory evoked potentials and motor evoked potentials, as well as cranial nerve-specific monitoring, and the neuroanesthesia team should be aware of and able to accommodate these monitoring modalities. **(b)** Neurologic monitoring of critical tracts and motor and sensory pathways is essential to decrease the likelihood of patient morbidity. At Barrow Neurological Institute, all patients with planned operations in the brainstem undergo monitoring of somatosensory evoked potentials, motor evoked potentials, and the appropriate cranial nerves.

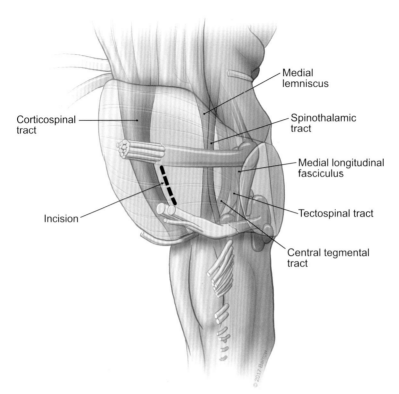

Figure 3.7. Method of entry into the brainstem (anterolateral view). Entry into the brainstem should be at points where the pathology abuts a pial or an ependymal plane, using a safe entry zone or an entry point that minimizes brain transgression and the likelihood of injury to critical tracts. The two-point method greatly assists with selection of the surgical approach and site of entry. When the brainstem is entered, the method of entry should be such that it disturbs the least number of tracts possible. Ideally, an opening parallel to the critical fiber tracts (*dashed line*) decreases the likelihood of morbidity to essential functions such as lower cranial nerves.

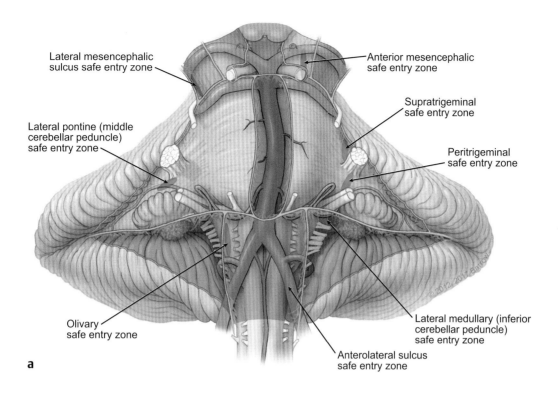

Lateral mesencephalic
sulcus safe entry zone

Anterior mesencephalic
safe entry zone

Supratrigeminal
safe entry zone

Lateral pontine (middle
cerebellar peduncle)
safe entry zone

Peritrigeminal
safe entry zone

Olivary
safe entry zone

Lateral medullary (inferior
cerebellar peduncle)
safe entry zone

Anterolateral sulcus
safe entry zone

a

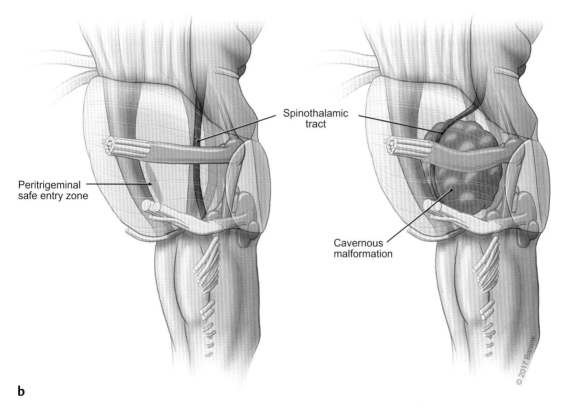

Spinothalamic
tract

Peritrigeminal
safe entry zone

Cavernous
malformation

b

Figure 3.8. Safe entry zones and natural planes of entry (anterior view). **(a)** The importance of using safe entry zones (*blue ovals*) and cisterns to gain entry to pathologies in the thalamus and brainstem cannot be overstressed. The judicious use of cerebrospinal fluid cisterns facilitates brain relaxation and minimizes transgression of neural pathways while enabling the surgeon to arrive at points of safe entry into the brainstem. Akin to the opening of the interhemispheric or sylvian fissures, the opening of posterior fossa fissures minimizes the need to traverse structures such as the middle cerebellar peduncle. A thorough discussion of safe entry zones (*blue ovals*) can be found in Section 2. These safe entry zones traverse areas between tracts or are located in areas where perforating vessels are sparse. **(b)** It is important to remember that large lesions may distort surgical safe entry zones (*blue ovals*) and displace critical tracts (anterolateral view).

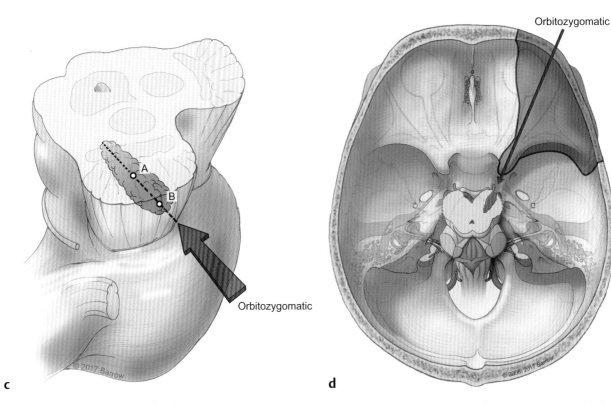

c

d

Figure 3.8. (c) The two-point method assists in selecting the approach to the intrinsic brainstem pathology and in determining the entry point that is least likely to cause morbidity. This method depends on identifying the longest axis of the lesion, noting the location where it comes closest to or abuts a pial or an ependymal plane, and transferring that trajectory onto the skull to identify the ideal point for the craniotomy. To perform the two-point method, place one dot at the center of the lesion (*point A*) and a second dot at the point where the lesion most closely abuts a pial or an ependymal surface (*point B*). **(d)** Then extend that line to the surface of the skull (*arrow*). This line indicates the approach necessary to remove the lesion.

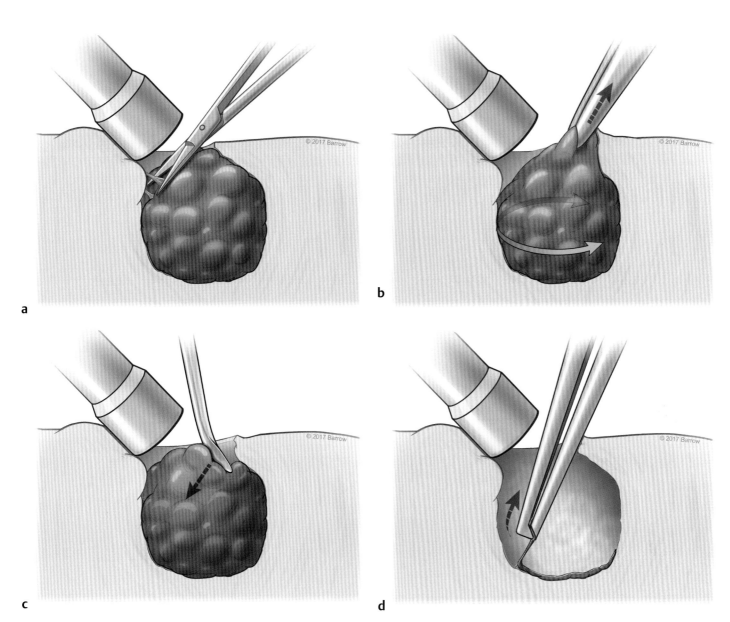

Figure 3.9. Techniques of sharp dissection, mobilization, and peeling. When operating in the brainstem or the confines of eloquent nuclei, the surgeon should meticulously adhere to the basic tenets of microneurosurgery. **(a)** When possible, sharp dissection should be used to free the lesion from the adjacent eloquent structures. Sharp dissection minimizes compression, retraction, and manipulation of eloquent structures. **(b,c)** Sharp dissection should be alternated with techniques of blunt mobilization. In cases of intrinsic brainstem pathologies, such as cavernous malformations, the atraumatic mobilization of remnants and the circumferential development of planes with the adjacent brain enable the lesion to be removed safely. **(d)** More so than in any other location, remnants of the lesion adherent to the brainstem may be peeled away using specialized instruments without disturbing adjacent tracts.

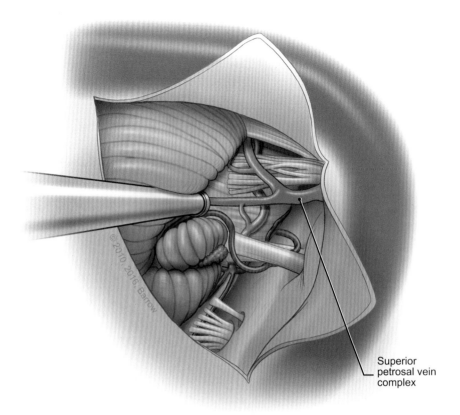

Superior
petrosal vein
complex

a

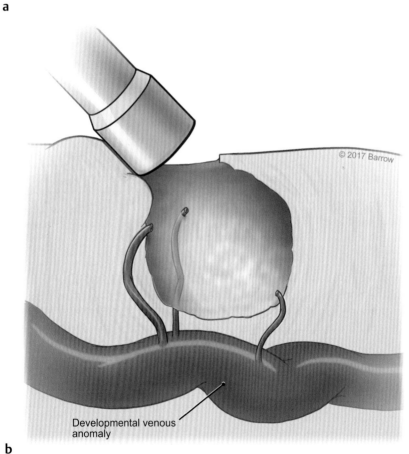

Developmental venous
anomaly

b

Figure 3.10. Preservation of the venous anatomy. **(a)** The preservation of venous outflow is key to preventing venous congestion and infarction within the confines of the posterior fossa. Superficial veins on the brainstem should be mobilized and preserved when possible. Every attempt should be made to preserve veins, such as the superior petrosal vein complex, while approaching the cerebellopontine angle. Naturally, a vein is better coagulated in a controlled fashion rather than being avulsed during surgery, but generous mobilization of veins is possible without the need to sacrifice them in most cases. **(b)** The successful removal of cavernous malformations depends on the preservation of any associated developmental venous anomalies. Care must be taken to preserve the integrity of these venous structures while removing the cavernous malformation in its entirety.

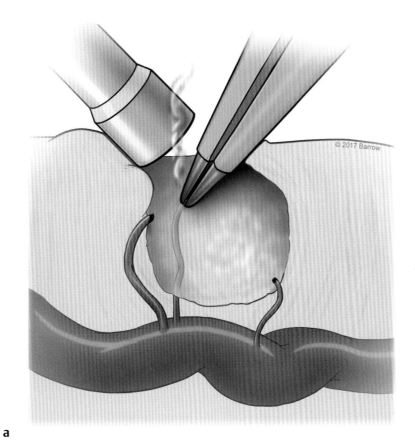

a

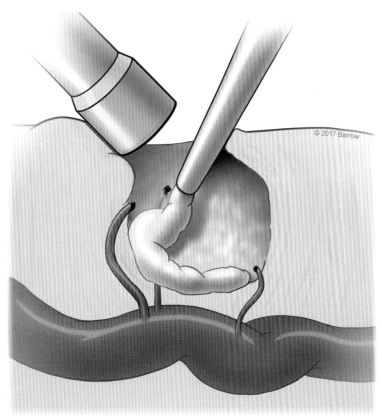

b

Figure 3.11. Hemostasis. **(a)** When hemostasis is undertaken in the brainstem, it is critical to avoid uncontrolled coagulation of adjacent eloquent tissues, as this can cause injury to the nuclei within the limited surgical working space. Careful and deliberate coagulation of bleeding points should be conducted under direct visualization with the cautery on a low setting. Oozing can be controlled with simple compression and patiently repeated irrigation with saline. **(b)** Rarely, a small amount of hemostatic agent may be placed in the resection cavity and washed out to obtain hemostasis.

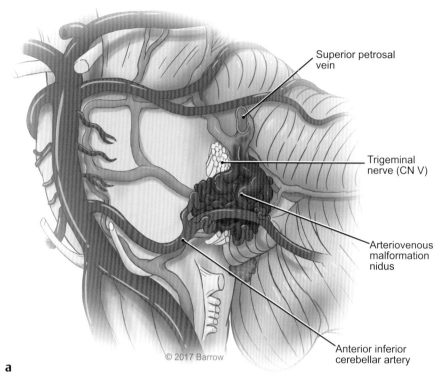

Superior petrosal vein

Trigeminal nerve (CN V)

Arteriovenous malformation nidus

Anterior inferior cerebellar artery

© 2017 Barrow

a

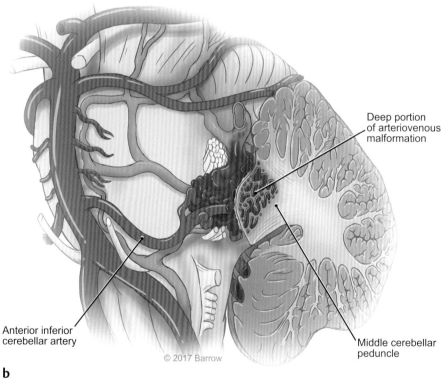

Deep portion of arteriovenous malformation

Anterior inferior cerebellar artery

Middle cerebellar peduncle

© 2017 Barrow

b

Figure 3.12. Steps for resection of arteriovenous malformations in non-eloquent regions of the brainstem. A lateral pontine arteriovenous malformation is used to illustrate this technique. **(a)** Anterolateral view of lateral pontine arteriovenous malformation in the middle cerebellar peduncle lateral to the trigeminal nerve, with arterial feeders from the anterior inferior cerebellar artery and major venous drainage to the superior petrosal vein complex. **(b)** Parasagittal section through the lateral pontine arteriovenous malformation shows deep vascular structures in the fiber tracts of the middle cerebellar peduncle, where it is relatively safe to resect arteriovenous malformations.

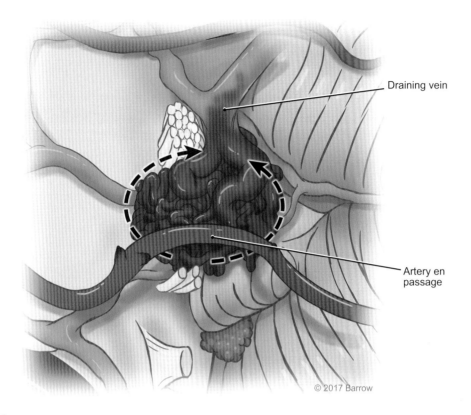

Draining vein

Artery en passage

c

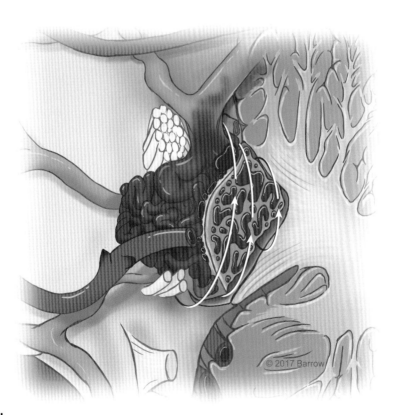

d

Figure 3.12. **(c)** The feeding arteries are cauterized and divided circumferentially. Arteries en passage and the draining vein are left intact, but feeders contributing to the arteriovenous malformation are cauterized.

(d) Circumferential conical dissection is performed to fully devascularize the arteriovenous malformation and disconnect it from the parenchyma.

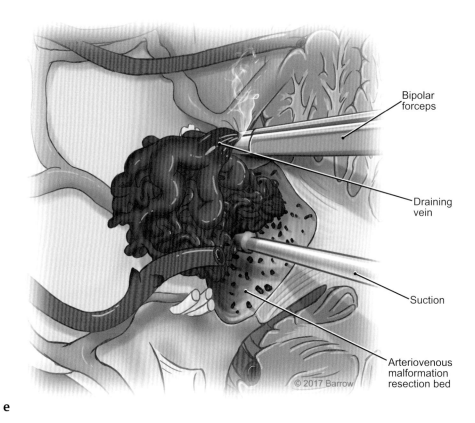

e

Figure 3.12. (e) The final draining vein (no longer turgid) is cauterized and divided, and the arteriovenous malformation is removed. The resection bed is inspected to ensure complete hemostasis.

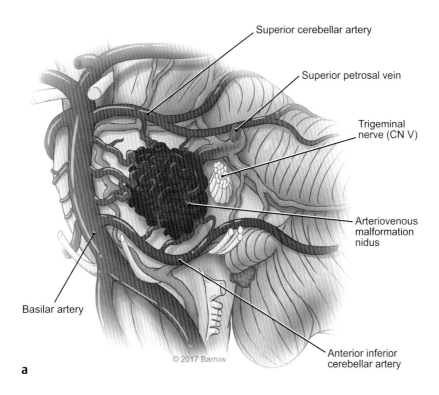

a

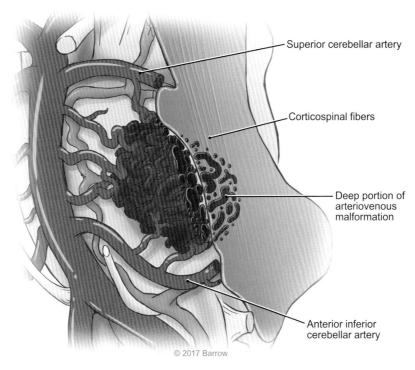

b

Figure 3.13. Steps for resection of arteriovenous malformations in eloquent regions of the brainstem. An anterior pontine arteriovenous malformation is used to illustrate this technique. **(a)** Anterolateral view of anterior pontine arteriovenous malformation medial to the trigeminal nerve, with arterial feeders from the basilar artery, superior cerebellar artery, and anterior inferior cerebellar artery, and a major draining vein to the superior petrosal vein complex. **(b)** Parasagittal section through the anterior pontine arteriovenous malformation shows the association of the arteriovenous malformation vessels with the corticospinal fibers in the pons, where they cannot be safely removed.

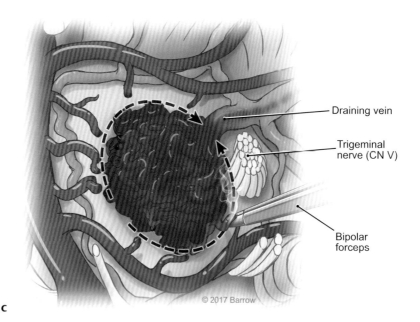

Draining vein

Trigeminal
nerve (CN V)

Bipolar
forceps

© 2017 Barrow

c

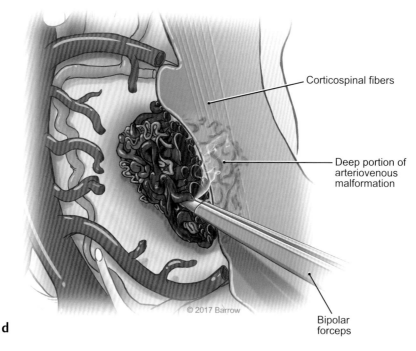

Corticospinal fibers

Deep portion of
arteriovenous
malformation

© 2017 Barrow

Bipolar
forceps

d

Figure 3.13. (c) The feeding arteries are cauterized and divided circumferentially. Arteries en passage and the draining vein are left intact, but feeders contributing to the arteriovenous malformation are cauterized. Illustrations show one of two options for obliterating the arteriovenous malformation without damaging eloquent brainstem tissue. **(d)** Option 1: Parasagittal section through the arteriovenous malformation shows all the surface vessels of the arteriovenous malformation cauterized, with the draining vein left until last. Vessels deep in the pons collapse.

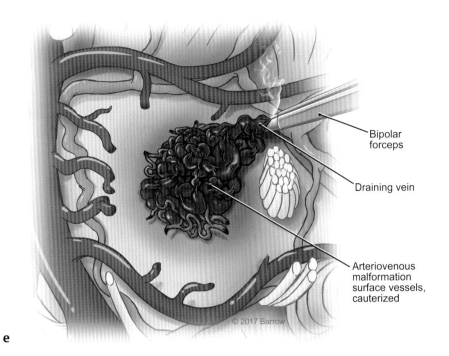

e

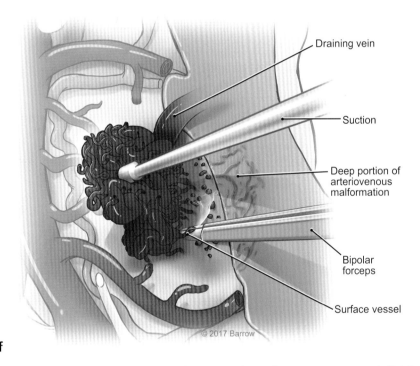

f

Figure 3.13. (e) Anterolateral view shows cauterization and division of draining vein (no longer turgid). **(f)** Option 2: Parasagittal section through arteriovenous malformation shows peeling of the surface arteriovenous malformation vessels, with cauterization and division of the vessels entering the pons. Deep arteriovenous malformation channels collapse. The parenchyma is not entered. The draining vein is left until last.

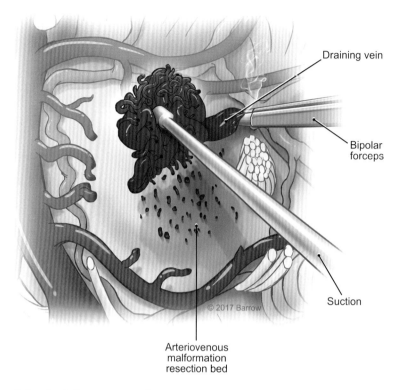

g

Figure 3.13. (g) Anterior view of the final draining vein being cauterized and divided before removal of the surface arteriovenous malformation.

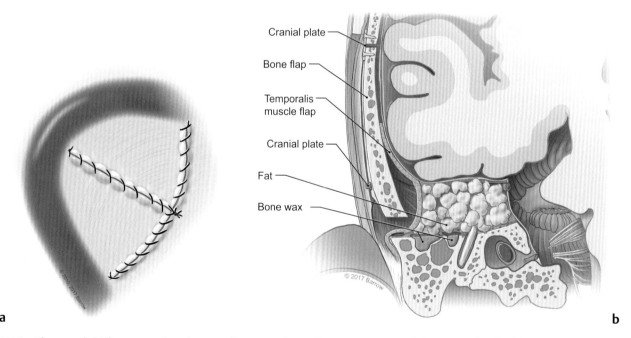

a   b

Figure 3.14. Closure. **(a)** The operative closure of a wound in the posterior fossa is particularly important. A meticulous watertight closure minimizes the likelihood of a cerebrospinal fluid leak, infection, and intracranial hypotension. Although we do not routinely use a lumbar drain for cerebrospinal fluid removal, in cases where it is used, the lumbar drain can aid the healing of the posterior fossa incision and decrease the likelihood of a delayed cerebrospinal fluid leak. **(b)** Care must be taken during closing to obliterate air cells that allow communication with the extracranial compartment. This is best accomplished by aggressive waxing of air cells and the use of a multilayered closure (using muscle, fat, and fascia), especially in cases of large skull base approaches.

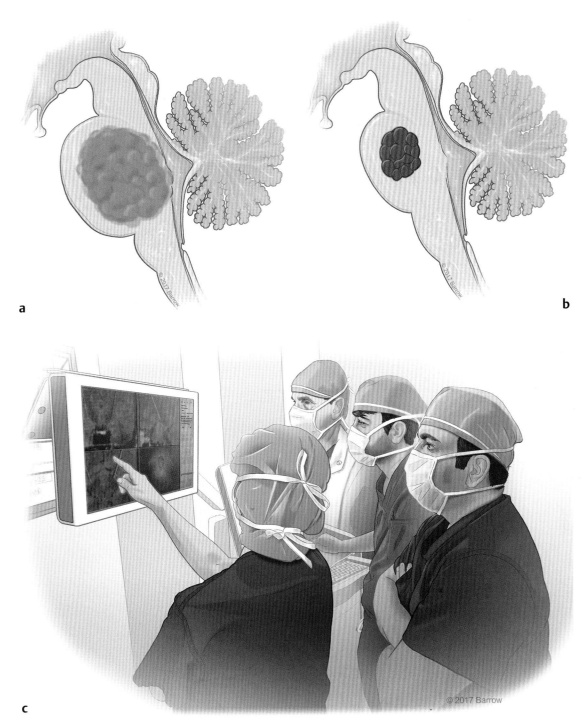

Figure 3.15. Patient selection and timing of surgery. Patient selection is of utmost importance for optimizing surgical results, decreasing morbidity, and giving the patient the best chance for good long-term quality of life. Certain lesions in the brainstem and thalamus have aggressive and poor natural histories, and despite attempts at surgical extirpation, result in poor long-term survival and outcomes. In such cases, a biopsy may be a more appropriate course of action than aggressive surgery that is unlikely to help the patient. **(a)** The importance of patient selection is illustrated by the case of a diffuse intrinsic pontine glioma. **(b)** If the natural history of the lesion permits aggressive resection, an attempt should be made to remove it surgically if its removal can be done safely. An example of one such pathology is a surgically accessible pontine cavernous malformation in a patient who presents with multiple hemorrhages. **(c)** The timing of surgery is another important consideration. It depends greatly on the individual presentation of the patient. Although repeated hemorrhages and precipitous decline require emergent intervention, most patients can be observed after a hemorrhage and allowed to recover from the acute event. They may then be considered for observation or surgical intervention, depending on lesion location, accessibility, and possible neurologic deficits.

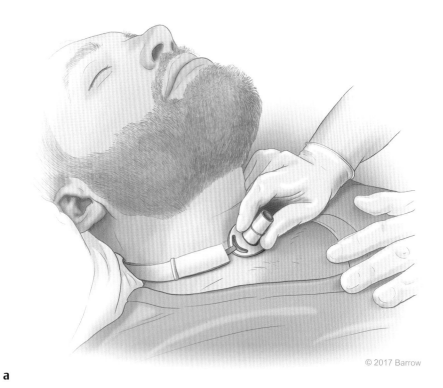

a

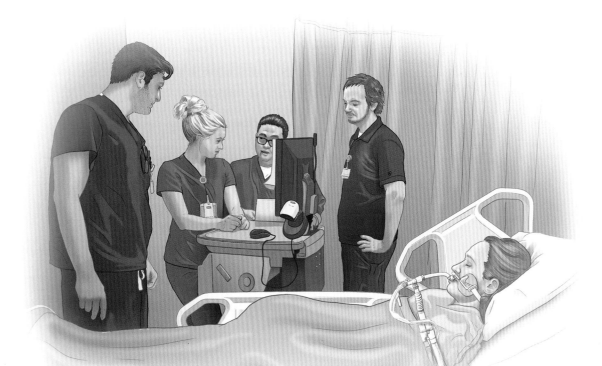

b

Figure 3.16. Other considerations. **(a)** Patients undergoing brainstem operations often experience transient or permanent cranial nerve deficits. These deficits are often exacerbations of the deficits with which the patient originally presented. The patient should be warned of this risk, and the surgeon and medical team should be prepared to deal with the sequelae of these events. At times, early placement of a temporary tracheostomy may be necessary when dealing with medullary lesions. **(b)** An experienced team familiar with the care of patients with neurovascular pathologies improves the overall care of patients. The team should consist of members of the medical critical care team, the nursing staff, and the rehabilitation staff.

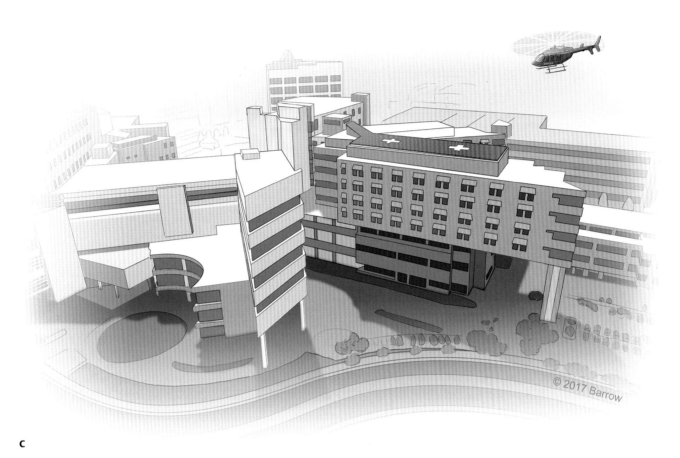

c

Figure 3.16. (c) The importance of practice and experience in achieving good outcomes with lesions in the brainstem cannot be overemphasized. Patients should be referred to treatment centers with experience in the surgical resection of brainstem and thalamic pathology.

4 Approaches to Thalamic, Pineal, and Brainstem Lesions

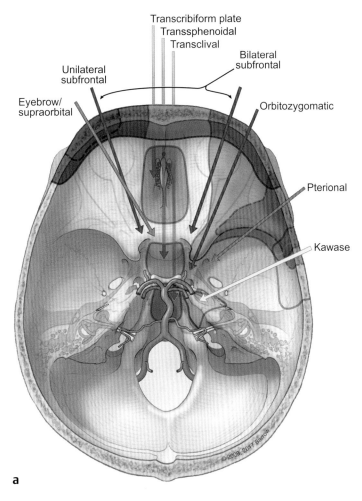

Figure 4.1. Anterior skull base approaches. **(a)** The various anterior and anterolateral skull base approaches that can be used to access lesions in the brainstem. These approaches constitute a continuum, and they include unilateral and bilateral subfrontal, eyebrow/supraorbital or orbitopterional, pterional, orbitozygomatic, and Kawase approaches. With improvements in endoscopy, anterior transclival approaches can be used for ventral pontine and pontomedullary lesions.

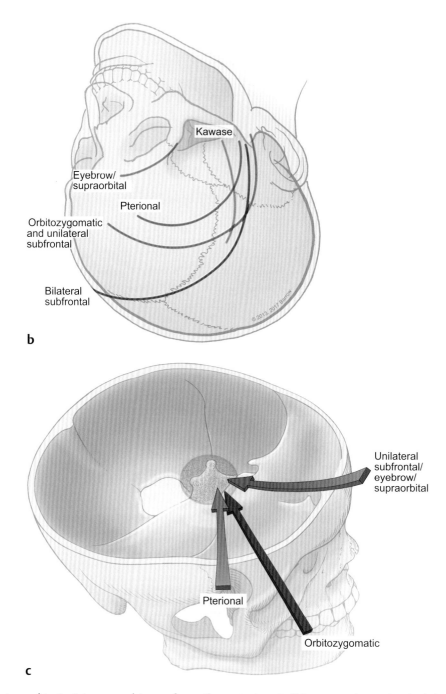

b

c

Figure 4.1. **(b)** The various skin incisions used to perform the anterior skull base craniotomies in **(a)**. **(c)** The various working trajectories afforded by anterior skull base approaches to the top of the brainstem. The extent of the lesion plays an important role in the choice of actual approach used and the degree of bony removal necessary to achieve the exposure. All of the various approaches to the brainstem are summarized at the end of the section **(Table 4.1)**.

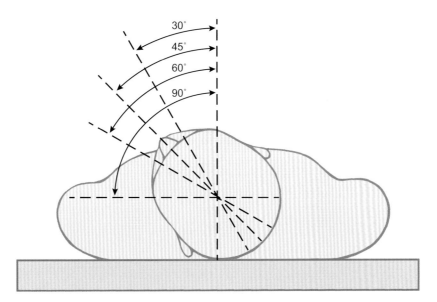

Figure 4.2. Patient positioning used for various anterior skull base approaches. The exact degree of head rotation depends on the approach selected, the specific target of interest, and the extent of the pathology. The patient is positioned to enable gravity to retract the frontal and temporal lobes from the floor of the anterior and middle fossae. When possible, head rotation enables the surgeon to obtain the necessary view down the longest axis of the lesion. The head should be placed above the level of the heart, and kinking of the neck resulting in venous congestion should be avoided.

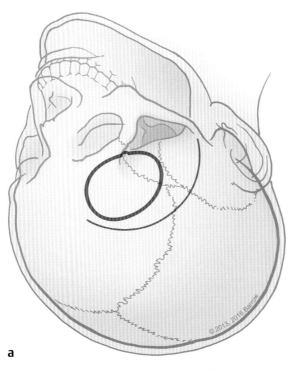

a

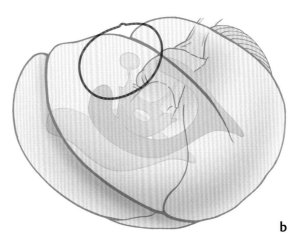

b

Figure 4.3. Unilateral subfrontal or frontolateral approach. **(a)** The patient's head is rotated 30 degrees off the vertical axis, with the neck slightly extended. The skin incision should be placed behind the hairline from the midline to the zygomatic process. This craniotomy is performed along the floor of the frontal fossa, extending to the pterion. Drilling the anterior fossa floor flush provides a flat and unhindered exposure to the basal cisterns. **(b)** The relationship between the craniotomy and the underlying neural structures.

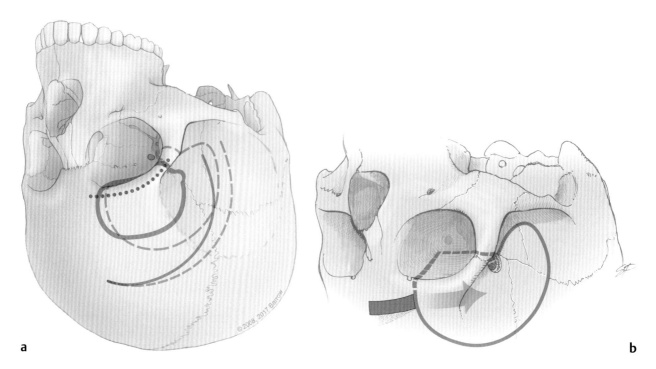

Figure 4.4. Orbitopterional approach. **(a)** An alternative to the unilateral subfrontal approach is the orbitopterional approach. The patient is positioned with the head rotated 30 degrees off the vertical axis with the neck slightly extended. Extension of the neck enables gravity to displace the frontal lobe off the floor of the anterior fossa, minimizing the need for fixed retraction. The skin incision is similar to that used for the unilateral subfrontal approach and can be placed behind the hairline. Alternatively, the incision can be made above or within the eyebrow (*dotted line*) of patients with generous eyebrows or a receding hairline, and it can be extended laterally to the corner of the eye for a more lateral

approach. The orbitopterional craniotomy (*solid circular outline*) is performed along the floor of the frontal fossa, and the frontal fossa floor is drilled flush to enhance the exposure. The amount of pterional bony removal (*circular dashed line*) depends on the lateral extent of pathology and the amount of lateral visualization and the working trajectory necessary to approach the lesion. **(b)** The orbitopterional craniotomy is outlined (*orange line*). The pterional portion of the craniotomy can be extended as necessary to accommodate the lesion and site of involvement. The direction of the last cut across the frontal fossa floor is demonstrated (*arrow*).

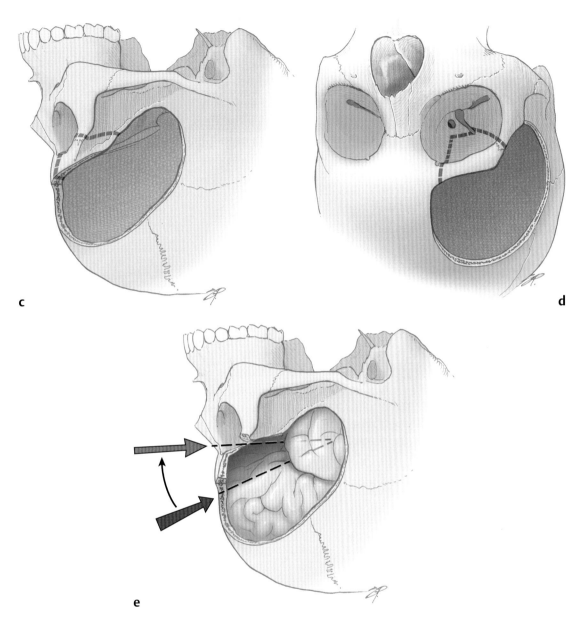

Figure 4.4. (c) The orbitopterional craniotomy extends into the orbit and provides access to the ventral mesencephalon and the sellar/parasellar region. **(d)** The extent of the removal of the orbital wall can be better appreciated from an anterior view. Removal of this bony prominence minimizes the need for frontal lobe retraction while providing the surgeon an improved view for high-riding lesions at the level of the basilar apex and the mesencephalon. **(e)** When orbital bar removal is combined with tailored removal of the pterion, the orbitopterional approach (*orange arrow*) can be used for aneurysms in the proximal circle of Willis and lesions in the midbrain. The removal of the orbital bar provides a greater degree of working angle than a simple pterional approach (*purple arrow*), notably in the superior direction. When properly closed, this exposure provides a cosmetically outstanding outcome for the patient.

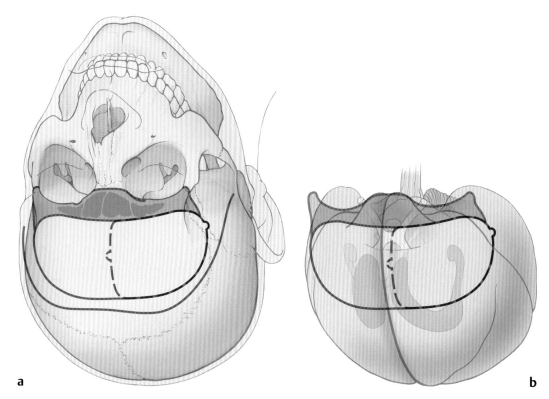

Figure 4.5. Bilateral subfrontal approach. **(a)** The head is often placed in the midline with some extension of the neck to enable gravity retraction of the frontal lobes. When enhanced superior exposure is necessary, the orbital bandeau (*shaded area*) may be removed to increase the surgical working space. **(b)** The relationship of the craniotomy relative to the underlying neural structures.

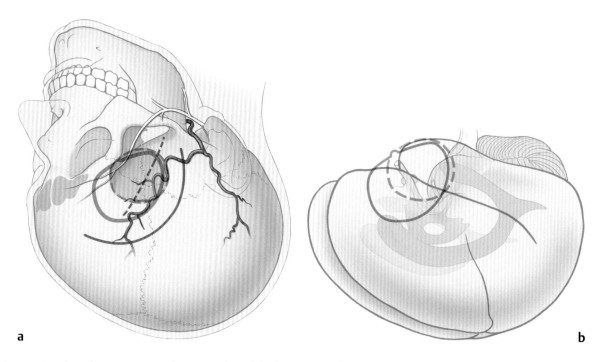

Figure 4.6. Pterional and mini-pterional approaches. **(a)** The pterional craniotomy is the mainstay skull base approach for lesions in the anterior cranial fossa and for ventral mesencephalic lesions. The skin incision and craniotomies for the standard (*solid line*) and mini-pterional (*dashed line*) approaches are illustrated. **(b)** The relationship between the craniotomy and the underlying neural structures.

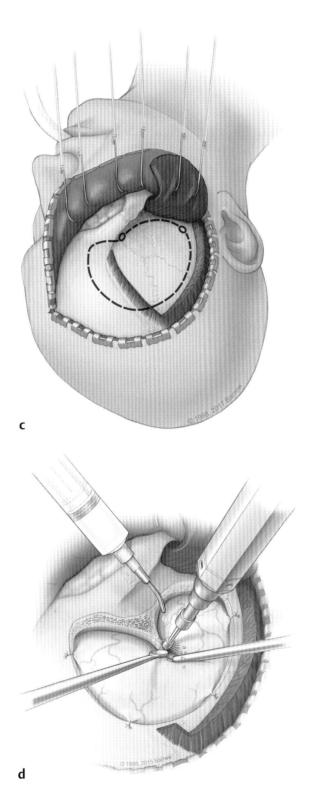

c

d

Figure 4.6. **(c)** The scalp is elevated to expose the zygomatic root posteroinferiorly and the keyhole anteriorly. The fat pad superficial to the temporalis fascia should not be entered because the frontalis branch of the facial nerve (CN VII) lies in the interfascial plane and can be injured by manipulation. The temporalis muscle is incised and reflected anteroinferiorly, leaving a cuff of fascia and muscle along the superior temporal line for eventual suturing at closure. **(d)** Extradural drilling of the sphenoid wing can enhance working room.

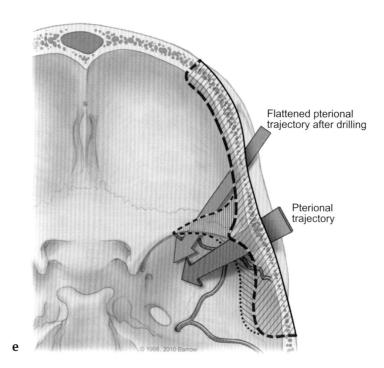

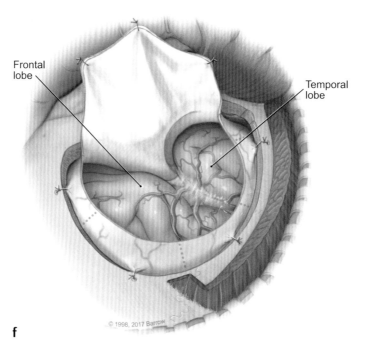

Figure 4.6. (e) When the pterional bone flap is removed, the working trajectory to the middle fossa is steep (*thick arrow*). Removal of the lesser wing of the sphenoid bone medially to the superior orbital fissure and the anterior clinoid process provides a flat surface over the orbit connecting the anterior and middle cranial fossae (*thin arrow*). **(f)** The dura is opened in a semicircular fashion, extending from the floor of the middle cranial fossa at the posterior-inferior aspect of the exposure to the floor of the anterior cranial fossa at the anterior-inferior aspect of the exposure. This opening provides an unobstructed view of the carotid cistern.

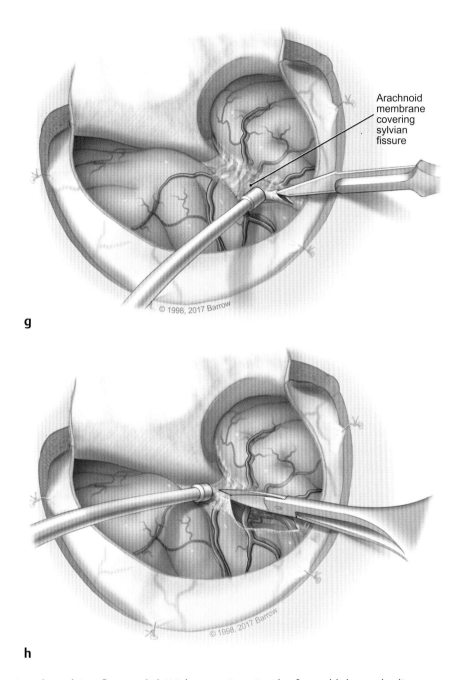

Arachnoid
membrane
covering
sylvian
fissure

© 1998, 2017 Barrow

g

© 1998, 2017 Barrow

h

Figure 4.6. (g–k) Opening the sylvian fissure. **(g)** With a suction tip, the frontal lobe and adjacent temporal lobe are retracted to place the arachnoid membrane over the fissure under tension. The arachnoid membrane is then incised using a knife. **(h)** Sharp dissection is used to cut the arachnoid membrane to gradually open the sylvian fissure. Large sylvian veins must be preserved; if venous pruning is necessary, veins should be preferentially mobilized with the temporal lobe.

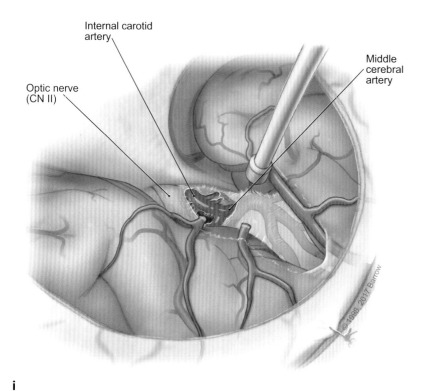

Internal carotid artery

Optic nerve (CN II)

Middle cerebral artery

i

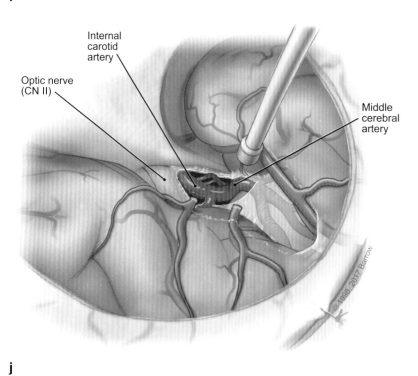

Internal carotid artery

Optic nerve (CN II)

Middle cerebral artery

j

Figure 4.6. (i) Removal of cerebrospinal fluid allows for brain relaxation. However, removal of excess cerebrospinal fluid early in the splitting of the sylvian fissure may complicate opening of the fissure by allowing the frontal and temporal opercula to adhere to each other. The judicious use of saline irrigation can aid with the dissection of the sylvian fissure. **(j)** The arachnoid membrane overlying the internal carotid artery is opened and arachnoid bands connecting the internal carotid artery and anterior cerebral artery to the optic nerve (CN II) are sharply cut to enable mobilization of the frontal and temporal lobes to arrive at the deep cisterns used to access the brainstem. For exposure of the basilar apex and ventral brainstem, the carotid and optic cisterns must be maximally opened to enable cerebrospinal fluid release.

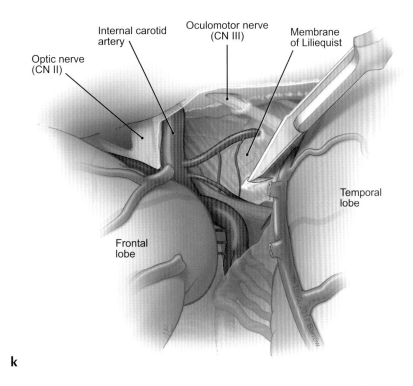

k

Figure 4.6. (k) The membrane of Liliequist is opened to release the cerebrospinal fluid from the interpeduncular cistern. In total, three working corridors could be utilized to visualize the contents of the interpeduncular cistern. These corridors include the carotico-oculomotor, opticocarotid, and supracarotid working corridors.

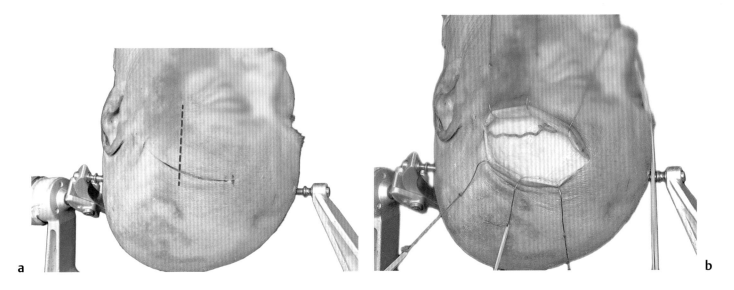

a   b

Figure 4.7. Cadaveric dissection demonstrating the mini-pterional craniotomy. **(a)** A curvilinear incision is centered on the extension line of the sphenoid groove (*blue dashed line*) 1 cm behind the hairline. **(b)** The subcutaneous tissue, frontal branch of the superficial temporal artery, and superficial fat pad are exposed after the galeal flap is reflected toward the temporal fossa.

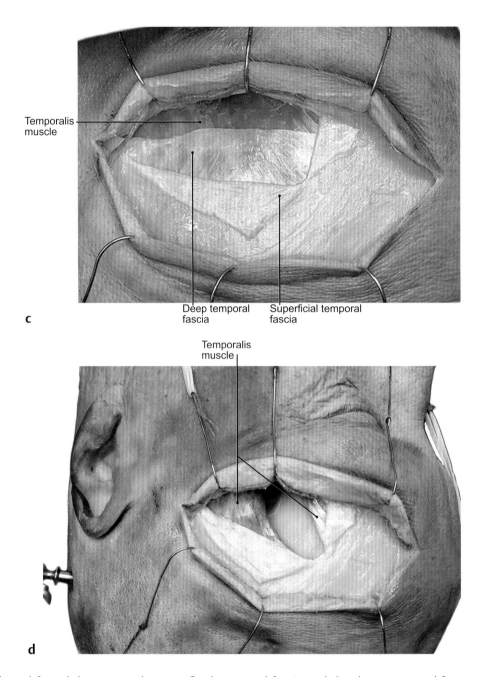

Temporalis muscle

Deep temporal fascia

Superficial temporal fascia

c

Temporalis muscle

d

Figure 4.7. (c) In the subfascial dissection, the superficial temporal fascia and the deep temporal fascia are cut to expose the temporalis muscle fiber bundles. **(d)** The temporalis muscle is split in the same direction as its fiber bundles to expose the pterion and the sphenoid groove.

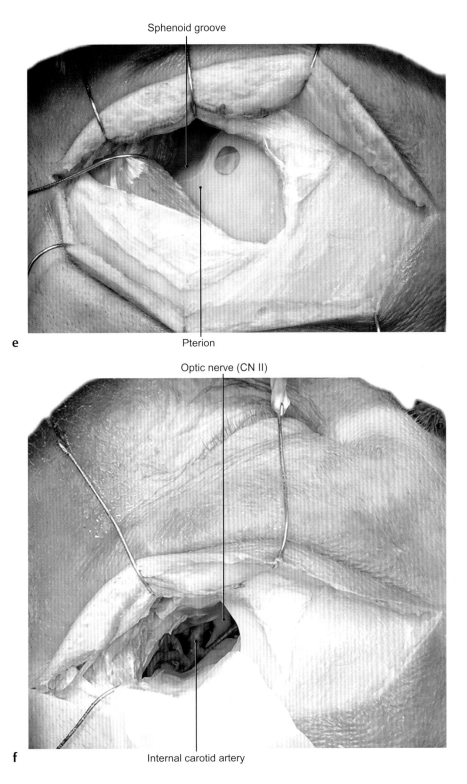

Sphenoid groove

e

Pterion

Optic nerve (CN II)

f

Internal carotid artery

Figure 4.7. (e) A bur hole is placed just anterior to the pterion in the frontal bone. **(f)** After the craniotomy, the dura is opened and the sylvian fissure is dissected, exposing the opticocarotid complex.

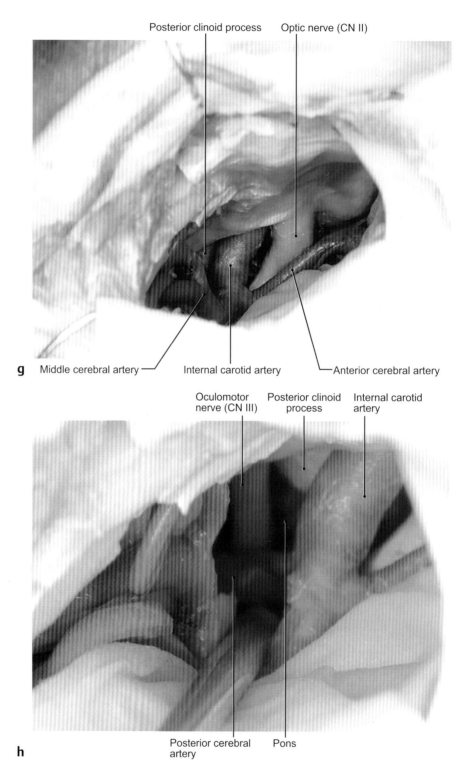

Posterior clinoid process   Optic nerve (CN II)

g   Middle cerebral artery   Internal carotid artery   Anterior cerebral artery

Oculomotor   Posterior clinoid   Internal carotid
nerve (CN III)   process   artery

h   Posterior cerebral   Pons
        artery

Figure 4.7. (g) Enlarged view of the opticocarotid complex, showing the exposure of the internal carotid artery, the anterior cerebral artery (A1 segment and anterior communicating artery), the middle cerebral artery (M1 and M2 segments), and the optic nerve (CN II). **(h)** Exposure of the oculomotor nerve (CN III) and the ventral midbrain and pons.

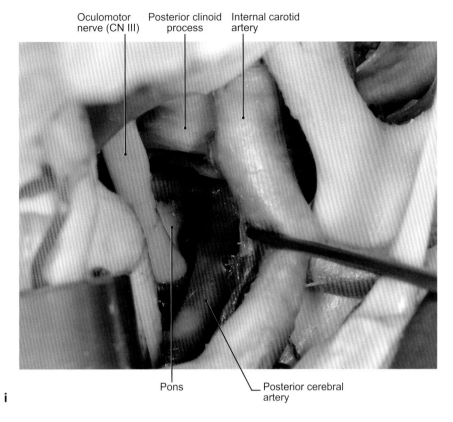

i

Figure 4.7. (i) View of the pons and the posterior cerebral artery from the carotico-oculomotor working corridor.

Figure 4.8. Orbitozygomatic craniotomy. **(a)** The scalp incision and the craniotomy cuts for the orbitozygomatic craniotomy. The patient positioning and skin incisions are identical to those used for the pterional craniotomy. **(b)** The orbitozygomatic craniotomy can be performed as a one- or two-piece craniotomy. The orbitozygomatic complex consists of the orbital rim, orbital roof, lateral orbital wall, and zygomatic process. In the two-piece orbitozygomatic craniotomy, a pterional craniotomy is first turned, and the orbitotomy and zygomatic arch removal are then performed with an oscillating saw. The shaded areas can be drilled to enhance the exposure. **(c)** The relationship of the craniotomy to the top of the brainstem. **(d–j)** The steps of temporalis muscle elevation and specific cuts for an orbitozygomatic approach. **(d)** The first major difference between the pterional craniotomy and the orbitozygomatic craniotomy is in the method of soft tissue mobilization.

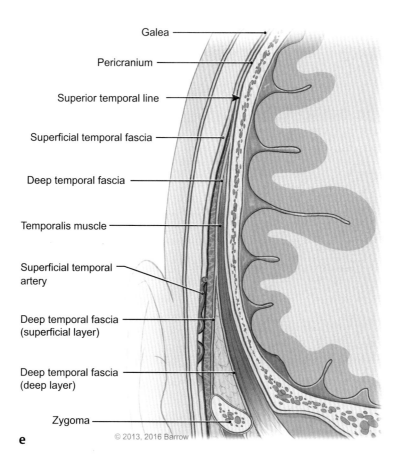

Galea

Pericranium

Superior temporal line

Superficial temporal fascia

Deep temporal fascia

Temporalis muscle

Superficial temporal artery

Deep temporal fascia (superficial layer)

Deep temporal fascia (deep layer)

Zygoma

© 2013, 2016 Barrow

e

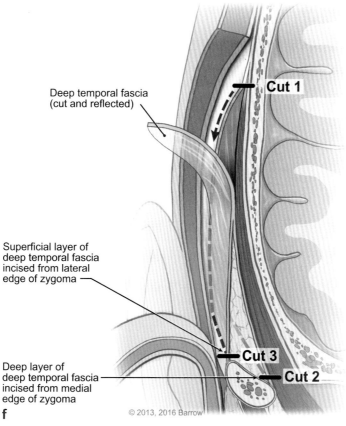

Deep temporal fascia (cut and reflected)

Cut 1

Superficial layer of deep temporal fascia incised from lateral edge of zygoma

Deep layer of deep temporal fascia incised from medial edge of zygoma

Cut 3

Cut 2

© 2013, 2016 Barrow

f

Figure 4.8. (e) The zygoma and orbital rim are covered by two layers of temporal fascia, which must be **(f)** incised and **(g)** mobilized to enable the osteotomies to be performed. In total, six osteotomies must be performed to enable removal of the orbitozygomatic unit.

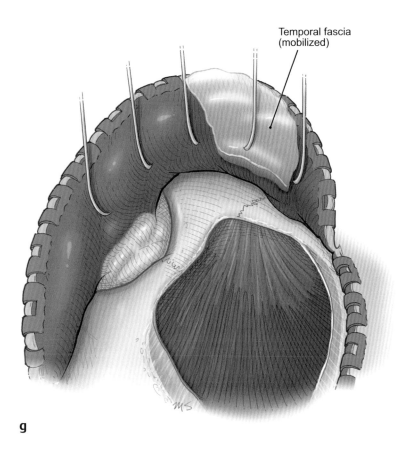

Temporal fascia
(mobilized)

g

Figure 4.8. (*Continued*)

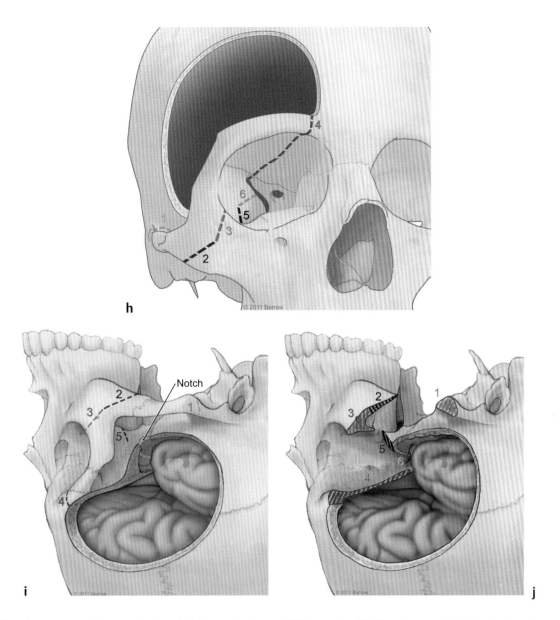

Figure 4.8. The six osteotomies are depicted **(h)** anteriorly and **(i)** laterally. **(j)** The six completed osteotomies.

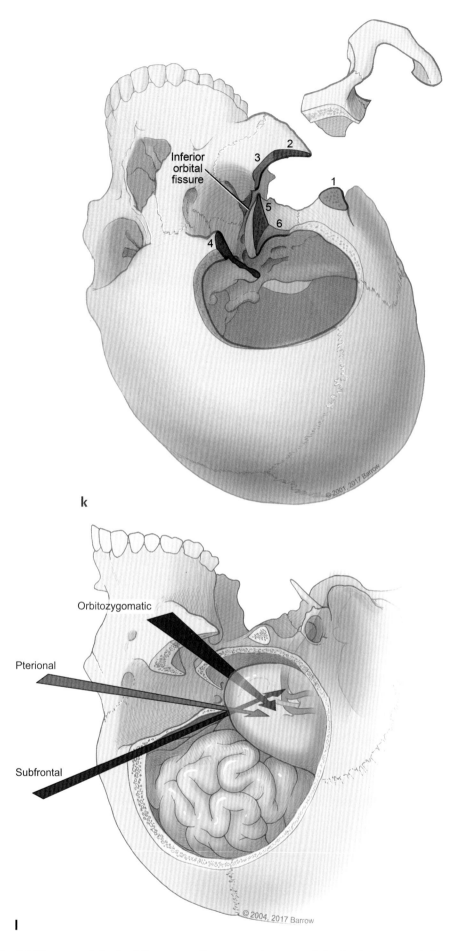

k

l

Figure 4.8. (k) The completed orbitozygomatic approach provides a view of the upper clivus, perimesencephalic cisterns, and the top of the basilar artery. With a subtemporal variant of the approach, the temporal lobe can be displaced posterolaterally by widely splitting the sylvian fissure to obtain an excellent subtemporal ventrolateral view of the brainstem and the top of the basilar artery. **(l)** The three arrows demonstrate the angles to the perimesencephalic cistern obtained via the subfrontal, pterional, and orbitozygomatic approaches. The removal of the orbital rim provides an enhanced upward view.

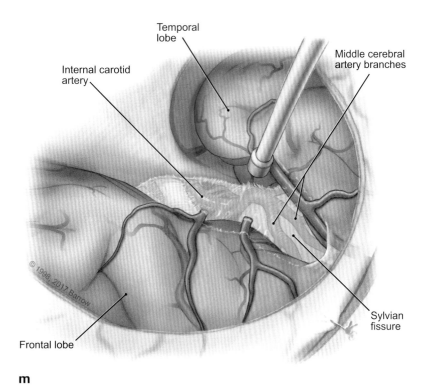

Figure 4.8. (m) The sylvian fissure is opened, and the distal middle cerebral artery branches are followed proximally to arrive at the carotid artery and the carotid and chiasmatic cisterns. **(n)** The carotid and chiasmatic cisterns are opened and the carotico-oculomotor triangle is explored to arrive at the crural and interpeduncular cisterns.

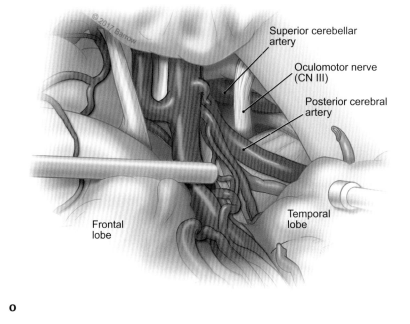

o

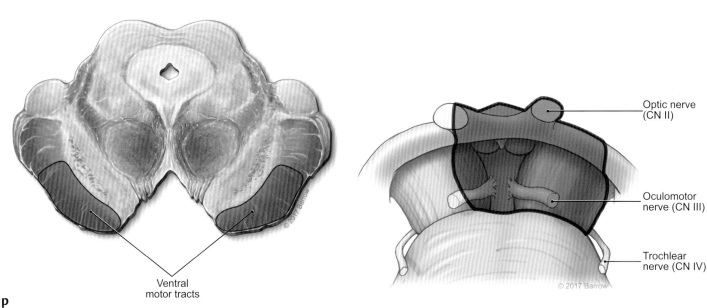

p   q

Figure 4.8. (o) Once the crural and interpeduncular cisterns are opened, the oculomotor nerve is traced back to the cerebral peduncle. **(p)** Axial view of the midbrain. The ventral approaches are often avoided due to the rich motor tracts that travel ventrally in the brainstem; nonetheless, in select cases, anterior approaches may be used to resect lesions in the midbrain. The motor tracts reside in the middle three-fifths of the cerebral peduncle. Care must be taken to avoid these fibers to minimize the morbidity of ventral approaches. Two ventral safe entry zones have been described for accessing lesions in the midbrain. Both of these safe entry zones make use of the location of the motor tracts. **(q)** Anterior view. Schematic depiction of the region of brainstem exposed by the orbitozygomatic and pterional (and variant) approaches (*shaded area*).

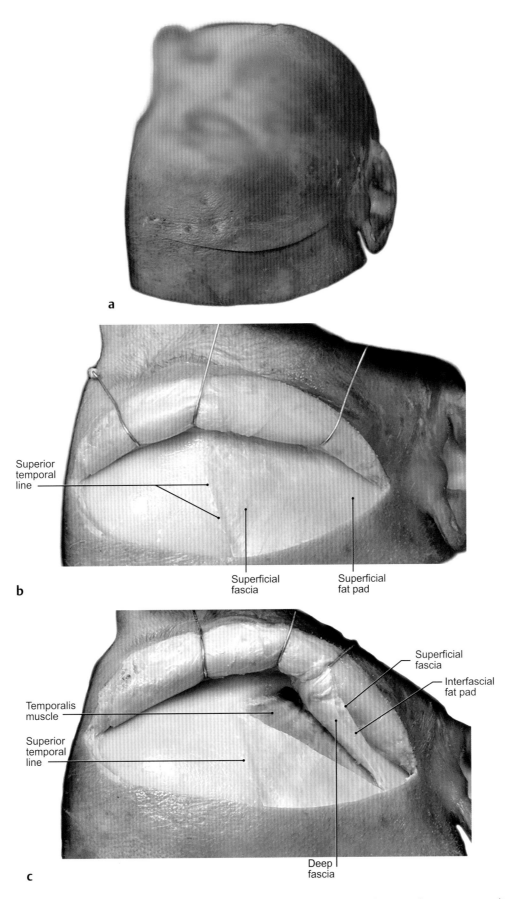

a

Superior
temporal
line

Superficial
fascia

Superficial
fat pad

b

Temporalis
muscle

Superior
temporal
line

Superficial
fascia

Interfascial
fat pad

Deep
fascia

c

Figure 4.9. Cadaveric dissection of the modified orbitozygomatic craniotomy. **(a)** The curvilinear incision line extends from 1 cm anterosuperior to the tragus and ends at the same sagittal level as the midpupillary line. **(b)** The galeal flap is reflected toward the temporal fossa. The superficial fascia and the superficial fat pad are also exposed. **(c)** The superficial and deep fascia are dissected to expose the temporalis muscle.

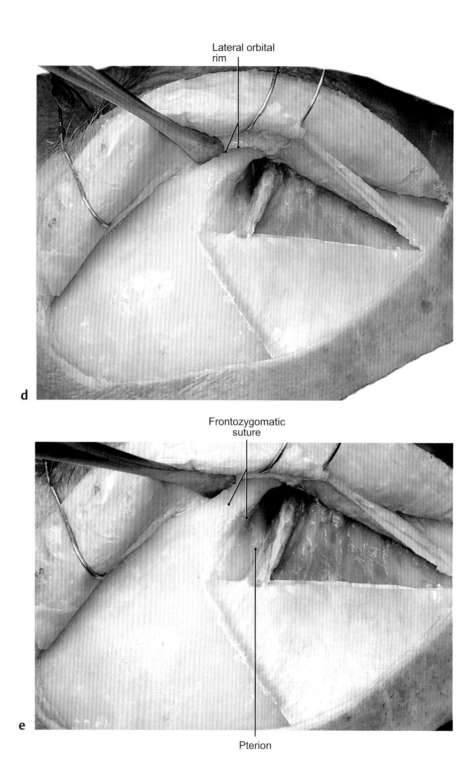

Figure 4.9. (d) The anterosuperior edge of the temporalis muscle and fascia are mobilized subperiosteally from the superior temporal line and retracted toward the temporal fossa to expose the lateral orbital rim and frontozygomatic suture. **(e)** The frontozygomatic suture is the junction of the zygomatic process of the frontal bone and the frontal process of the zygomatic bone.

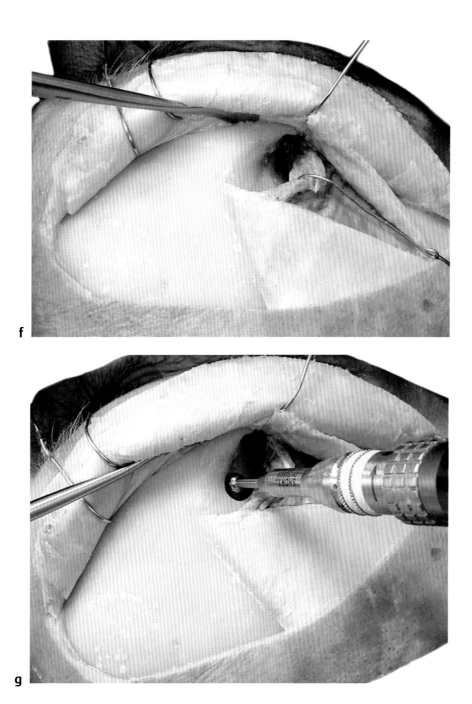

Figure 4.9. (f) A fishhook retractor can be used for retracting the muscle, thereby minimizing muscle elevation in cases where a great deal of lateral exposure is not necessary. **(g)** A bur hole is placed at the MacCarty keyhole, located 5 mm superior and 5 mm posterior to the frontozygomatic suture, by holding the drill at a 45-degree angle to the temporal squamous bone.

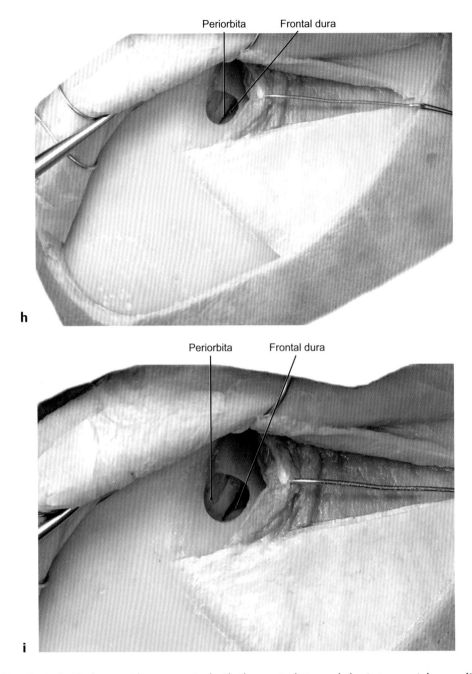

Figure 4.9. (h) The MacCarty keyhole provides access to both the periorbita and the intracranial area. (i) Stripping the periorbita enables the surgeon to use this single bur hole to complete the craniotomy.

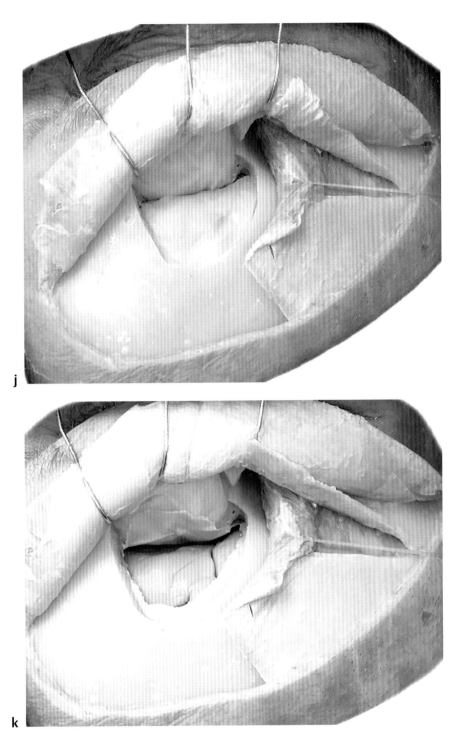

Figure 4.9. (j) Removal of the orbital rim and frontal fossa floor provides a flat subfrontal exposure, whereas selective removal of the pterion enables lateral exposure. **(k)** Opening the dura reveals the intracranial subfrontal and lateral views afforded by the modified orbitozygomatic approach.

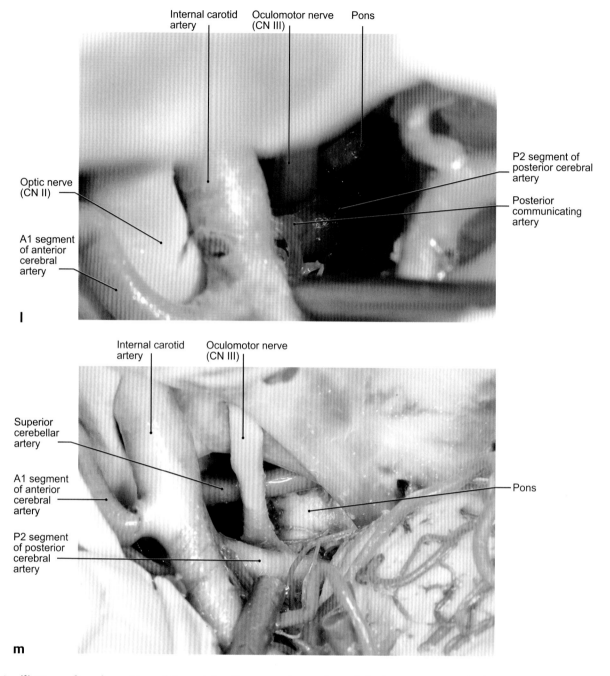

Figure 4.9. (l) View after dissection of the sylvian fissure and opening of the basal cisterns. **(m)** Lower magnification view after exposure of the pons from this approach.

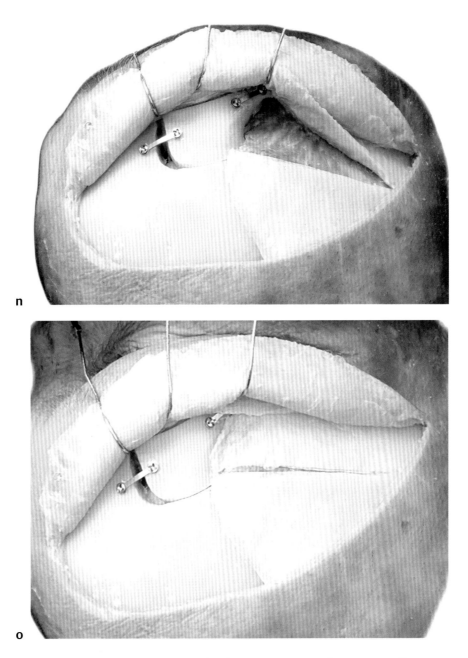

Figure 4.9. (n) Repair of the craniotomy using a low-profile plating system results in an excellent cosmetic outcome in most cases. **(o)** The temporalis muscle and fascia are reapproximated to minimize muscle wasting.

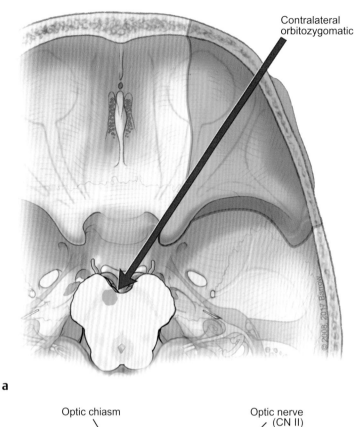

Contralateral
orbitozygomatic

a

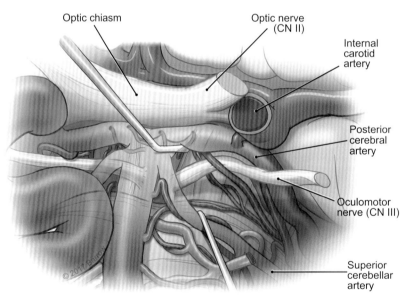

Optic chiasm

Optic nerve
(CN II)

Internal
carotid
artery

Posterior
cerebral
artery

Oculomotor
nerve (CN III)

Superior
cerebellar
artery

b

Figure 4.10. Contralateral orbitozygomatic approach. **(a)** In select cases, depending on the anteroposterior extension of the lesion, its proximity to pial surfaces, and its relation to the oculomotor nerve (CN III) nucleus and motor fibers, a contralateral orbitozygomatic approach can be used. This approach is used here to resect a centromedian lesion in the midbrain that resides medial to the oculomotor nerve and the motor fibers via the interpeduncular safe entry zone.

(b) Opening the membrane of Liliequist enables the surgeon to explore the interpeduncular cistern and provides access to the basilar artery bifurcation, both posterior cerebral arteries and superior cerebellar arteries, the medial posterior choroidal artery, and the thalamoperforating arteries, and direct perforators of the proximal superior cerebellar artery.

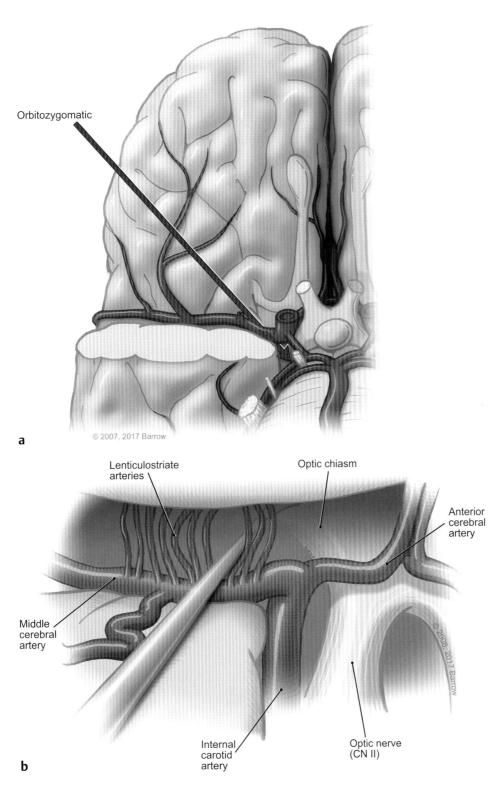

Figure 4.11. Thalamomesencephalic orbitozygomatic approach. **(a)** Inferior view depicting the orbitozygomatic approach to lesions in the thalamomesencephalic junction. **(b)** Anterior view. Wide dissection of the sylvian fissure enables the surgeon to develop a small corridor between the labyrinth of lenticulostriate arteries, between the posterior limits of the gyrus rectus and medial orbital gyrus, and the M1 segment of the middle cerebral artery.

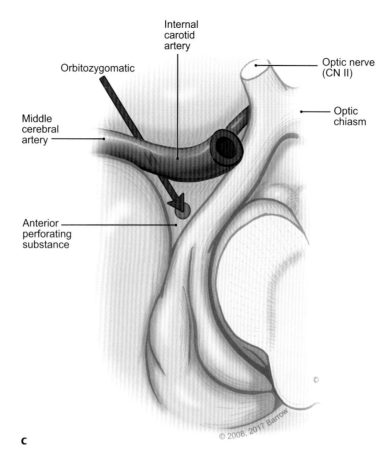

c

Figure 4.11. (c) Inferior view. This approach requires a small opening on the anterior perforating substance, posterior to the olfactory stria and near the optic tract.

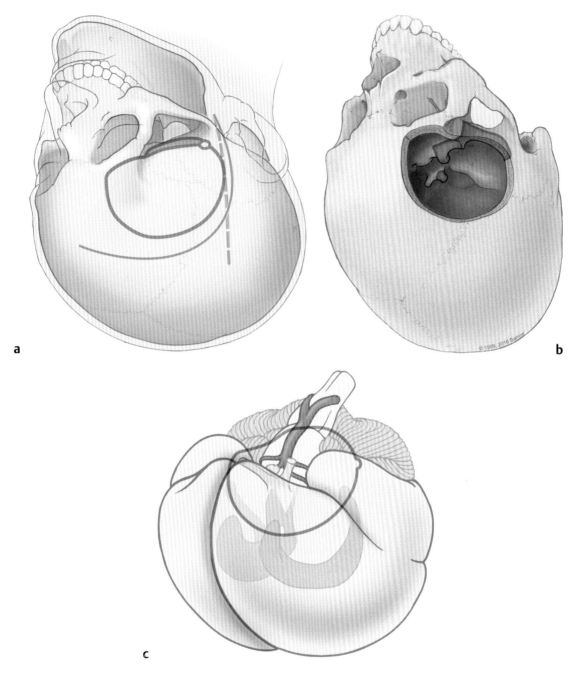

Figure 4.12. Kawase/anterior petrosectomy. **(a)** The skin incision and craniotomy for the Kawase (anterior petrosectomy) approach. Alternatively, a linear skin incision (*dashed line*) may be used. **(b)** The craniotomy performed is similar to that for a temporal craniotomy. At times an orbitozygomatic craniotomy can be combined with drilling of the anterior petrous apex (*shaded area*) to increase the working area to the top of the basilar artery complex. The additional bone drilling to remove the anterior petrous ridge (*shaded area*) provides enhanced exposure of the ventral brainstem to reach lesions anterior to the trigeminal nerve (CN V) and basilar artery complex. The exposure is limited anteriorly by the V3 segment of the trigeminal nerve and laterally by the greater superficial petrosal nerve. **(c)** Anterior view depicting the relationship of the craniotomy to the ventral brainstem.

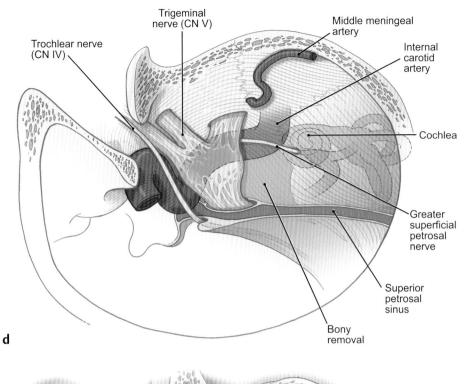

d

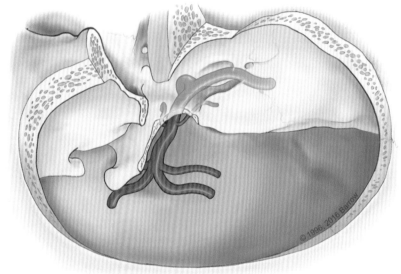

e

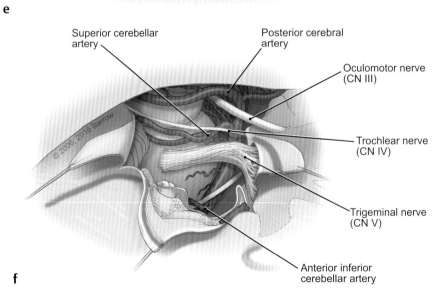

f

Figure 4.12. (d) Anatomic landmarks for drilling of the Kawase approach. The anterior margin for drilling is the trigeminal nerve, the lateral margin is the greater superficial petrosal nerve, the inferior margin is the internal carotid artery, and the medial margin is the inferior petrosal sinus. Posteriorly, the cochlea should be preserved to prevent injury to hearing. The extent of bony removal is depicted (*green area*). **(e)** The anterior petrosectomy provides enhanced exposure to the ventrolateral brainstem. Drilling of the medial apex of the petrous bone increases exposure to the clivus and the upper basilar artery. **(f)** Final anatomic exposure afforded by the anterior petrosectomy.

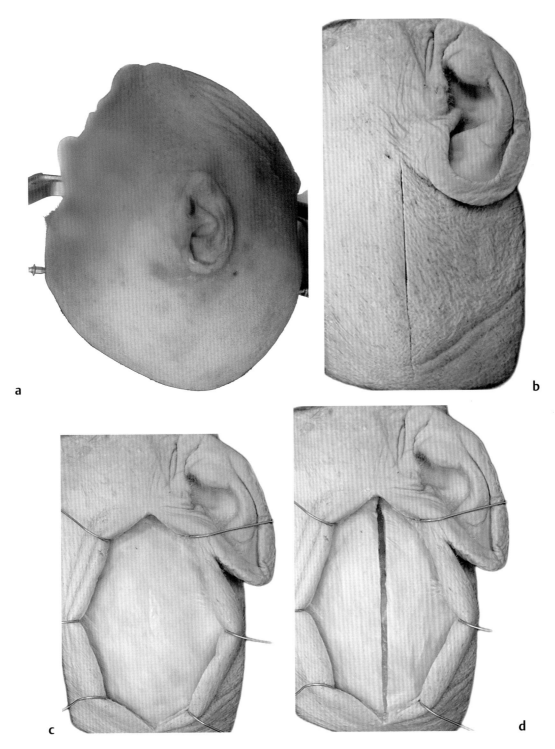

Figure 4.13. Cadaveric dissection of an anterior petrosectomy. **(a)** The patient is placed supine with the head turned to the contralateral side. **(b)** A linear skin incision is made anterior to the ear, extending from the zygoma to the level of the parietal suture. **(c)** The scalp flap is retracted laterally. **(d)** A linear incision is made through the fascia and temporalis muscle.

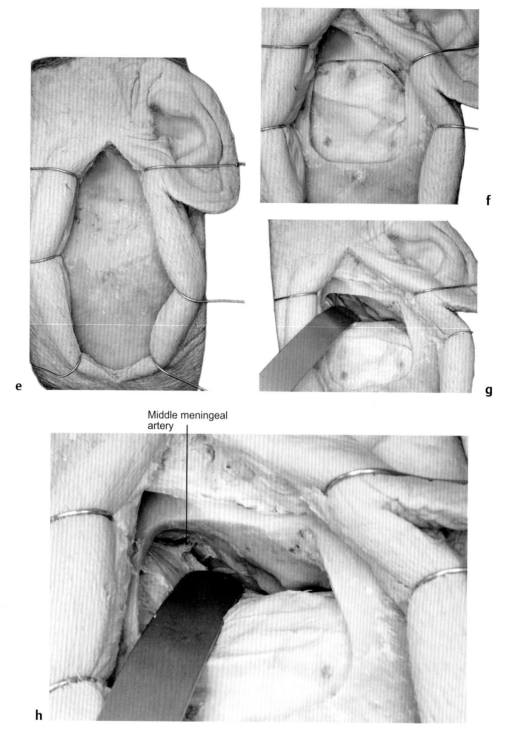

Figure 4.13. (e) The temporalis muscle and fascia are retracted laterally. **(f)** A temporal craniotomy flap reaching the skull base is performed. **(g)** Under the microscope, the dura mater is peeled away from the floor of the middle fossa, taking care to preserve the greater superficial petrosal nerve. **(h)** The middle meningeal artery is located and then cut.

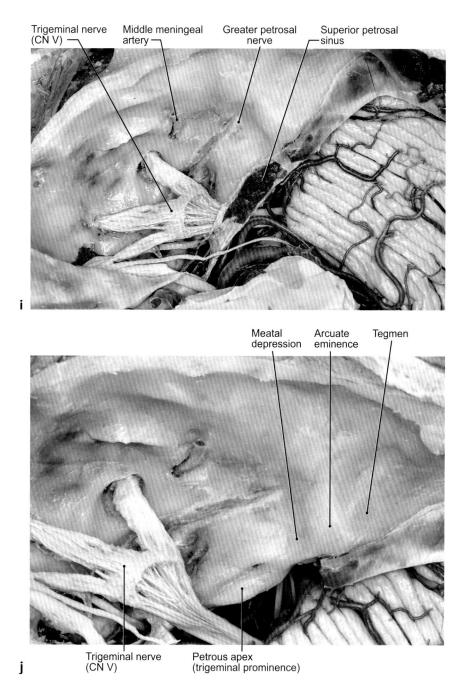

Figure 4.13. (i) The superior petrosal sinus is located on the petrosal ridge. **(j)** The trigeminal depression, trigeminal prominence, meatal depression, arcuate eminence, and tegmen are situated on the petrous ridge, in order from medial to lateral.

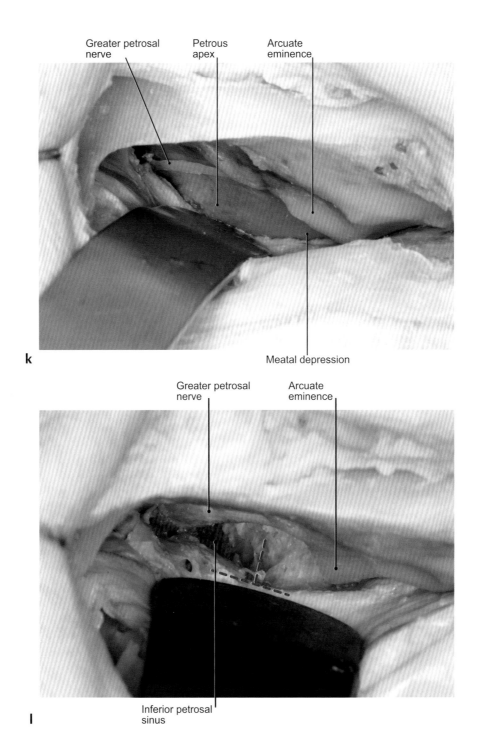

Greater petrosal
nerve

Petrous
apex

Arcuate
eminence

k

Meatal depression

Greater petrosal
nerve

Arcuate
eminence

l

Inferior petrosal
sinus

Figure 4.13. (k) The arcuate eminence is identified. **(l)** The petrous apex is drilled. The lateral margin of the drilling is delineated medial to the greater petrosal nerve and arcuate eminence. The inferior margin of the drilling is the inferior petrosal sinus. Care must be taken to avoid damaging the abducens nerve (CN VI). The dural incision is started 2 cm lateral to the superior petrosal sinus in a T-shaped fashion (*dashed line*).

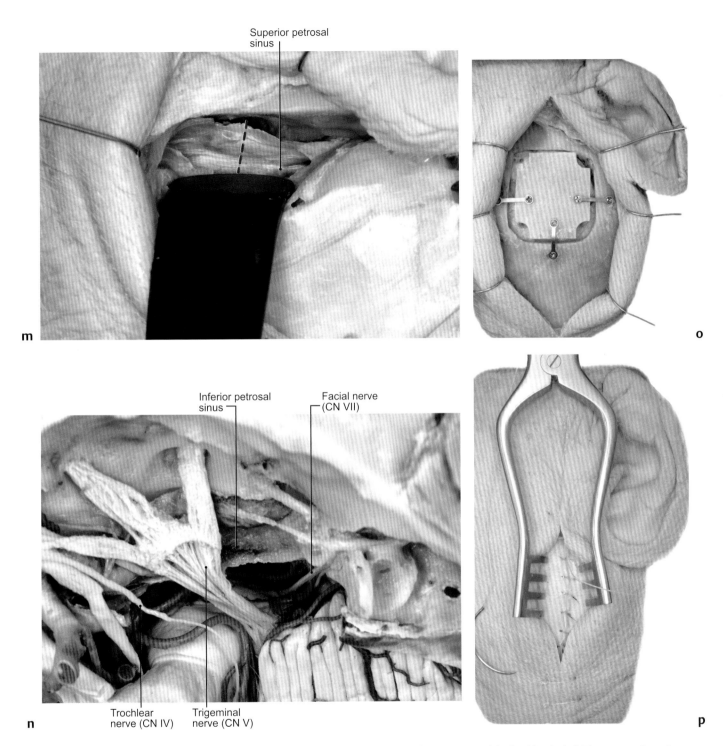

Figure 4.13. (m) The superior petrosal sinus is ligated or coagulated before cutting (*dashed line*). **(n)** The tentorium is cut completely, taking care not to injure the trochlear nerve (CN IV) at the tentorial notch. **(o)** The bone flap is reattached using titanium plates after closing the dura. **(p)** The temporal fascia and scalp are sutured.

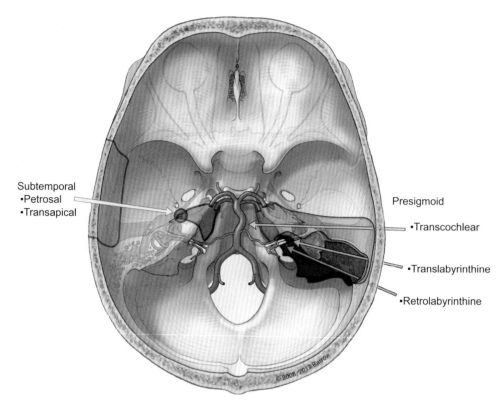

Subtemporal
∙Petrosal
∙Transapical

Presigmoid

∙Transcochlear

∙Translabyrinthine

∙Retrolabyrinthine

Figure 4.14. Approaches to the middle cranial fossa. This axial view illustrates the approaches to the middle cranial fossa and the combined middle and posterior fossa approaches. The subtemporal approach can be used to access lesions in the lateral brainstem. Variations of the subtemporal approach (*yellow arrow*), including the petrosal (*light orange area*) and transapical (*dark orange area*) approaches, provide exposure of the petrous portion of the internal carotid artery and the midclival region of the posterior fossa. Because of the risk of injury to the vein of Labbé and the facility of exposure gained by using the orbitozygomatic approach with or without an anterior petrosectomy, these approaches are rarely used to access lesions in the ventral or ventrolateral brainstem. The presigmoid approaches, which include the retrolabyrinthine (*purple arrow*), translabyrinthine (*blue arrow*), and transcochlear (*green arrow*) approaches, enable graded removal of the posterior petrous ridge, enhancing exposure to the posterior fossa, but with added potential morbidity of facial nerve (CN VII) injury or loss of hearing. Given the robust exposure afforded by the retrosigmoid craniotomy and its variations, we rarely use the presigmoid approaches. The combination of subtemporal and presigmoid approaches constitutes the combined supra- and infratentorial approaches. These large approaches are rarely needed for access to intrinsic brainstem lesions.

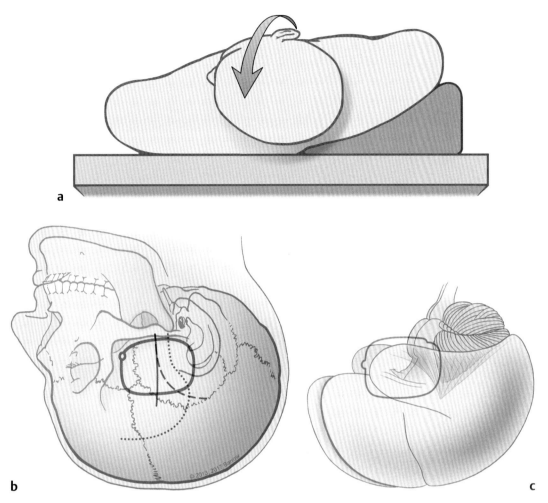

Figure 4.15. Subtemporal approach. **(a)** The patient is positioned supine with the ipsilateral shoulder elevated and the head in the horizontal position. The neck is slightly extended to allow for gravity retraction of the temporal lobe. Adequate release of cerebrospinal fluid upon dural opening obviates the need for permanent retractors and minimizes the likelihood of injury to the vein of Labbé, a major consideration with this approach. **(b)** The scalp incision(s) and craniotomy for the subtemporal approach. It is important to place the craniotomy as anterior as possible and to extend it inferiorly to be flush with the floor of the middle fossa. Failure to be flush with the middle fossa floor limits the superior exposure made possible by this approach. Alternatively, a posteriorly pointing scalp incision (*dashed line*) can be used in cases where a more posterior view into the posterior fossa may be required. **(c)** The relationship between the craniotomy and the temporal lobe and midbrain.

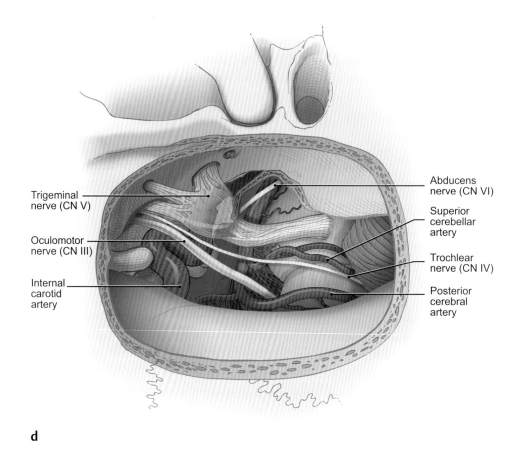

Trigeminal nerve (CN V)

Oculomotor nerve (CN III)

Internal carotid artery

Abducens nerve (CN VI)

Superior cerebellar artery

Trochlear nerve (CN IV)

Posterior cerebral artery

d

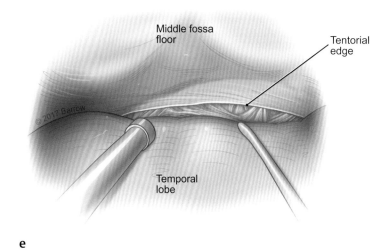

Middle fossa floor

Tentorial edge

Temporal lobe

e

Figure 4.15. (d) The removal of the petrous ridge, the so-called transapical variant, provides enhanced ventrolateral exposure to the brainstem. **(e)** The dura is opened in a U-shaped fashion, and dissection is continued to the tentorial edge. Upon removal of cerebrospinal fluid and elevation of the temporal lobe, the edge of the tentorium comes into view.

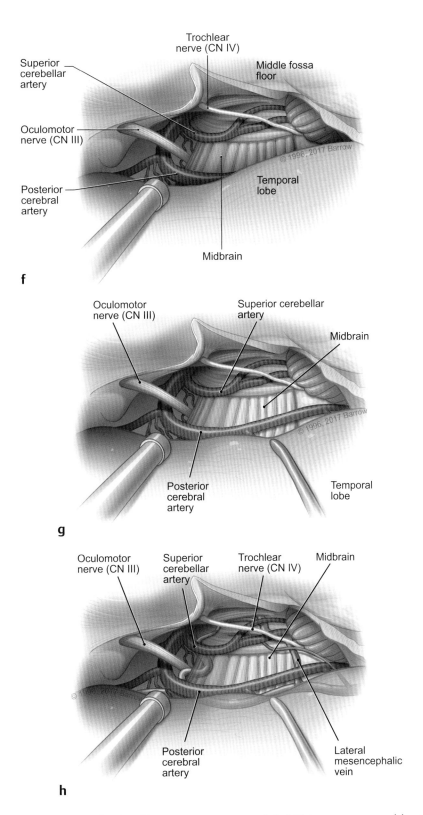

Figure 4.15. **(f)** Next, the tentorium is incised, taking care to avoid injury to the trochlear nerve (CN IV) that runs in the medial edge of the tentorium. The anterior and middle incisural spaces are visualized. The arachnoid membrane over the ambient, crural, and interpeduncular cisterns is opened. **(g)** This exposure enables the surgeon to visualize the lateral surface of the midbrain down to the pontomesencephalic junction. **(h)** The lateral mesencephalic vein generally covers the lateral mesencephalic sulcus.

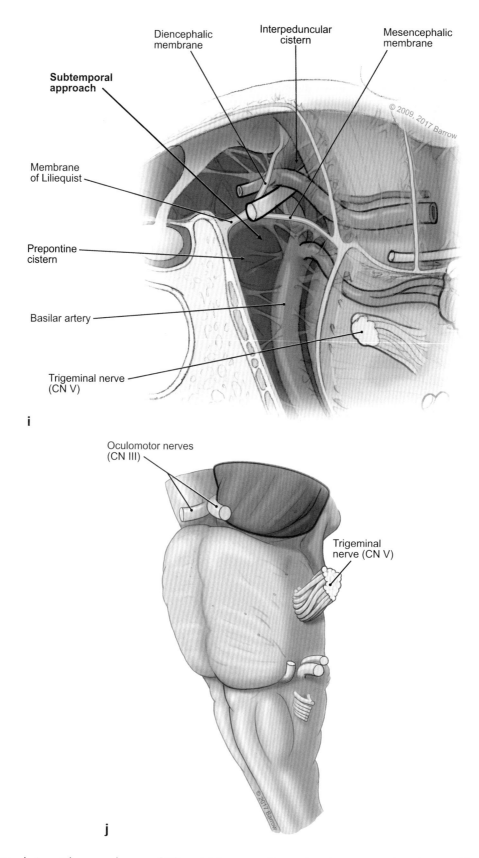

Figure 4.15. (i) Lateral view. The membrane of Liliequist is opened to enter the prepontine cistern. **(j)** Anterolateral view depicting the anatomy exposed by the subtemporal approach (*shaded area*).

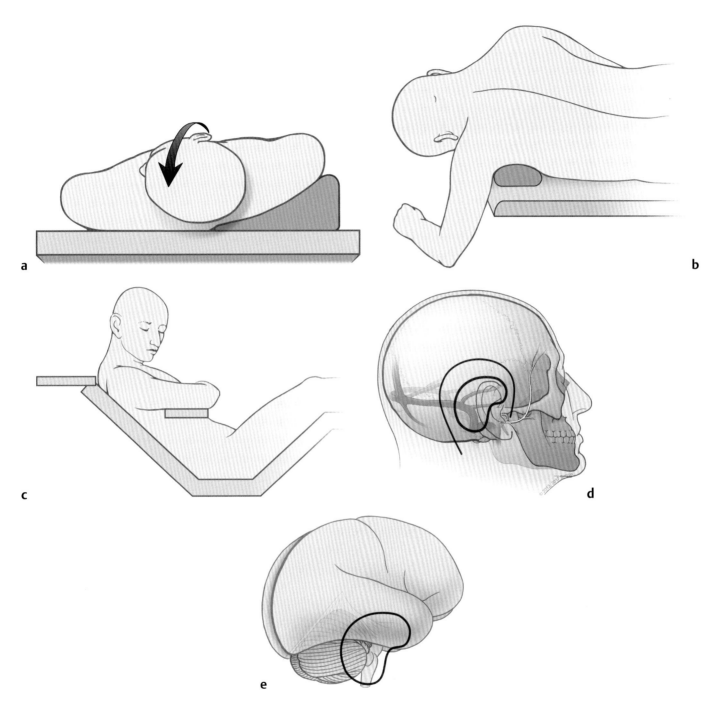

Figure 4.16. Combined supra- and infratentorial approaches. These approaches are appropriate for lesions with extension both above and below the tentorium along the petrous ridge, the clivus, or both. Often a team approach including a neurosurgeon and neuro-otologist is necessary to perform these approaches. The patient can be placed in a variety of positions: **(a)** supine position with the ipsilateral shoulder elevated by a wedge and the head turned contralaterally; **(b)** modified park bench position; or **(c)** modified semi-sitting position. **(d)** The incision for this approach begins in front of the ear below the zygomatic arch, above and behind the frontalis branch of the facial nerve (CN VII). The incision curves over the ear to end behind and below the tip of the auditory meatus. The skin incision can be modified depending on the location and type of lesion exposed. The scalp and underlying muscle are mobilized in two directions. The scalp and temporalis muscle are mobilized anteriorly to expose the zygomatic process and the middle fossa floor. Mobilization is best performed with fishhook retractors attached to rubber bands and fixed by a Leyla bar. The remainder of the soft tissue is retracted posteroinferiorly to expose the rim of the external auditory canal and the auditory meatus. **(e)** The combined supra- and infratentorial approach provides access to the cerebellopontine angle and the supratentorial compartment.

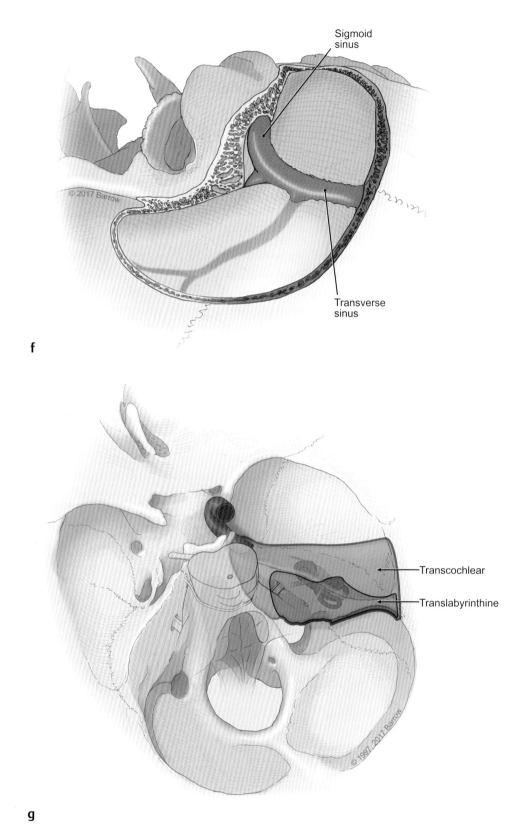

Figure 4.16. (f) The petrous bone is drilled to expose the dura of the posterior fossa and the sigmoid sinus. **(g)** The extent of petrous bone removal is dependent on the approach used and the necessary exposure. Graded removal of the bone provides increased lateral exposure of the brainstem but with added risk to hearing and facial nerve integrity. A petrous resection that spares the labyrinth is depicted. A translabyrinthine petrous resection would include the *blue area*; the transcochlear approach would additionally include the *green area*.

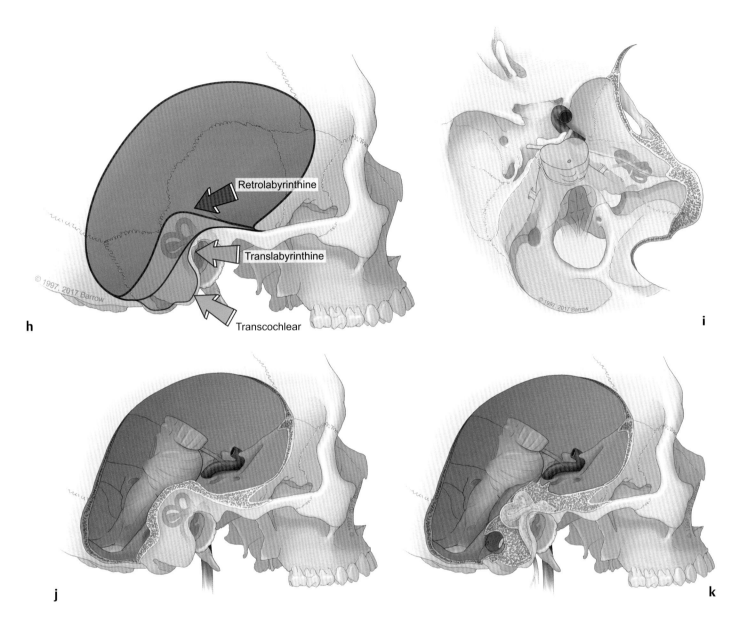

Figure 4.16. (h) A lateral view of the three approaches: the combined supra- and infratentorial retrolabyrinthine (*purple area*), the combined supra- and infratentorial translabyrinthine (*blue area*), and the combined supra- and infratentorial transcochlear approaches (*green area*). **(i)** In the retrolabyrinthine approach, which preserves the labyrinth, hearing is preserved but **(j)** limited exposure of the ventrolateral brainstem is obtained. **(k)** The extended retrolabyrinthine approach, which skeletonizes the posterior and superior semicircular canals and removes the mastoid, provides an enhanced lateral view of the brainstem.

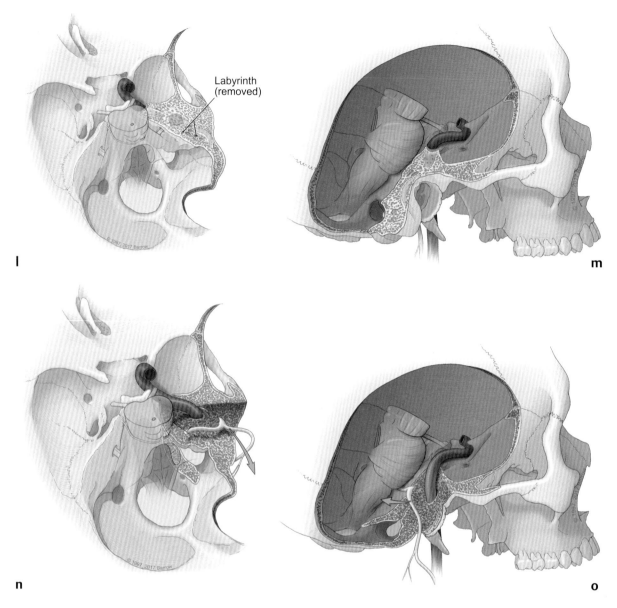

Labyrinth
(removed)

l

m

n

o

Figure 4.16. **(l)** The translabyrinthine approach removes the labyrinth and hearing is sacrificed on the ipsilateral side; **(m)** an enhanced and direct ventrolateral exposure to the top of the brainstem is obtained. **(n)** Alternatively, in the transcochlear approach, the entire cochlea and the remainder of the petrous pyramid are removed, and the facial nerve is mobilized (*arrow*) by disconnecting it from the superior petrosal branch. **(o)** The transcochlear approach is rarely needed but provides substantial exposure of the ventral and ventrolateral brainstem.

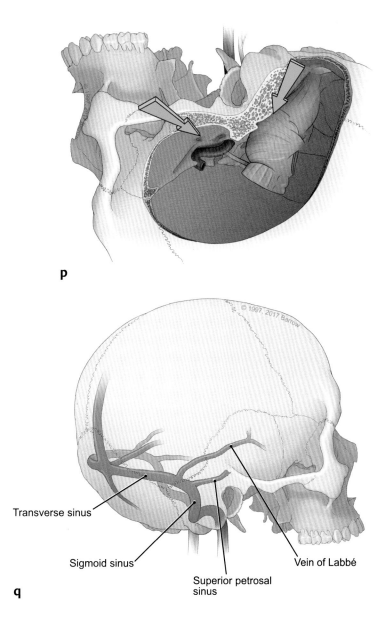

p

q

Transverse sinus

Sigmoid sinus

Superior petrosal
sinus

Vein of Labbé

Figure 4.16. (p) The extent of bone resection in an extended combined supra- and infratentorial approach (*arrows*). The enhanced subtemporal exposure facilitates visualization of the petrous tip and clivus. **(q)** As with the subtemporal approach and its variants, this combined supra- and infratentorial approach places the vein of Labbé at risk for retraction injury or avulsion. Judicious release of cerebrospinal fluid is necessary to enable brain relaxation. Use of dynamic and gravity retraction obviates the need for placement of permanent retractors in most cases.

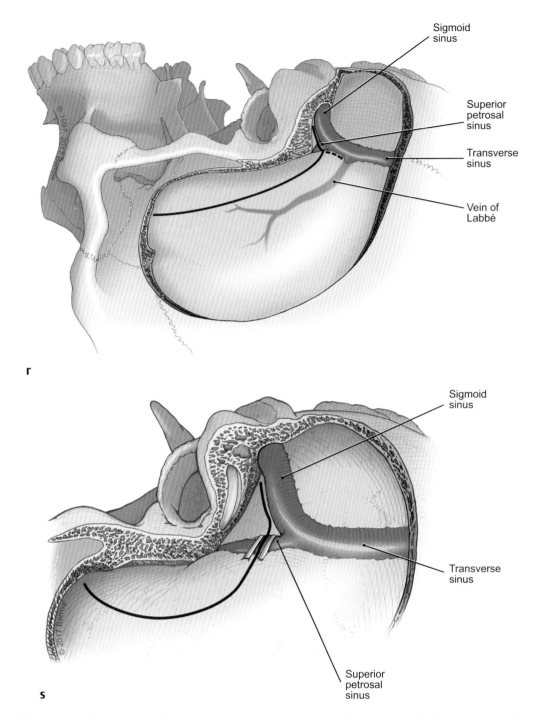

Figure 4.16. **(r)** The vein of Labbé enters the transverse sinus proximal to the junction of the sigmoid and superior petrosal sinuses. **(s)** Recognizing this anatomic relationship is important because it enables the entire width of the tentorium to be incised below this junction, sacrificing the superior petrosal sinus while preserving the important drainage of the vein of Labbé into the transverse sinus.

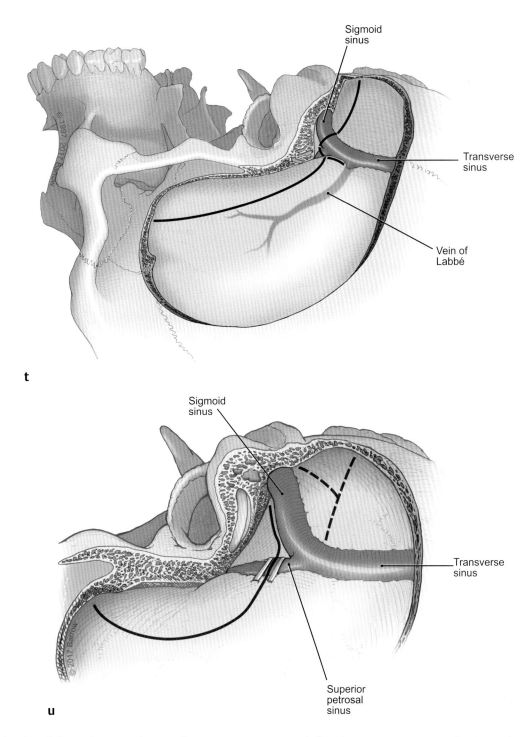

Figure 4.16. (t) When bilateral sigmoid sinus drainage is present, or venous drainage is primarily through the contralateral sigmoid sinus, the ipsilateral sinus can be sacrificed. This maneuver enables almost unlimited retraction of the incised tentorium, along with the lateral sinus, the vein of Labbé, and the base of the temporal lobe. The need for this retraction is reduced with aggressive petrous bone resection. If the facial nerve is drilled out of its canal, facial paresis can persist for 6 to 12 months. If less exposure is adequate, the facial nerve can be protected with a rim of bone and left in its normal anatomic course to avoid facial palsy. **(u)** Alternatively, the dura can be opened in a presigmoid fashion (*solid line*), with preservation of the sigmoid sinus. The jugular bulb forms the caudal limit of this alternative approach. A retrosigmoid opening (*dashed line*) can be used to access the cerebellopontine angle cistern.

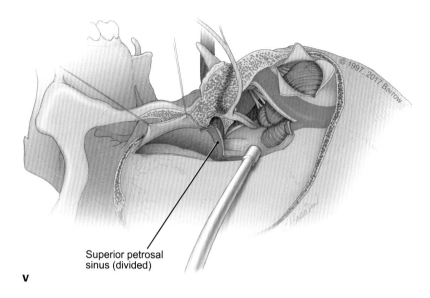

Superior petrosal
sinus (divided)

v

Figure 4.16. (v) The ultimate view provided by a combined supra- and infratentorial exposure that preserves the sigmoid sinus.

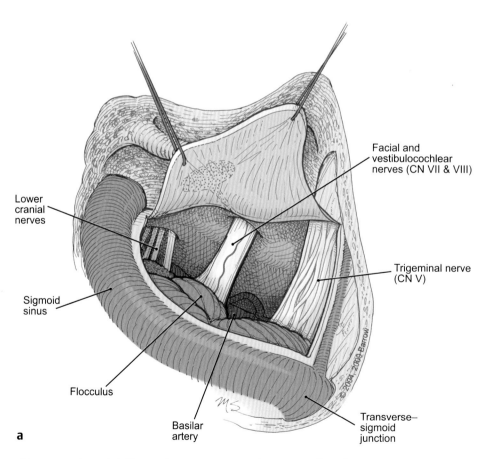

Facial and
vestibulocochlear
nerves (CN VII & VIII)

Lower
cranial
nerves

Trigeminal nerve
(CN V)

Sigmoid
sinus

Flocculus

Transverse–
sigmoid
junction

Basilar
artery

a

Figure 4.17. Presigmoid approaches. **(a)** The various presigmoid craniotomies are illustrated in **Figure 4.16** (combined supra- and infratentorial approaches). After the desired craniotomy is performed, the dura is opened along the transverse and sigmoid sinuses and retracted anteriorly. The petrosal surface of the cerebellum is initially exposed and the cerebrospinal fluid is drained; the flocculus behind the facial–vestibulocochlear nerve (CN VII-VIII) complex and the anterior inferior cerebellar artery become visible.

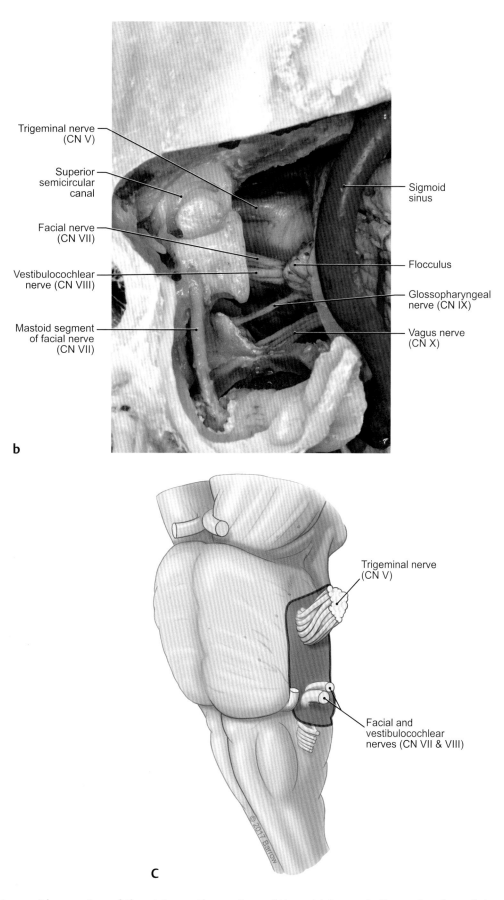

b

Trigeminal nerve
(CN V)

Superior
semicircular
canal

Facial nerve
(CN VII)

Vestibulocochlear
nerve (CN VIII)

Mastoid segment
of facial nerve
(CN VII)

Sigmoid
sinus

Flocculus

Glossopharyngeal
nerve (CN IX)

Vagus nerve
(CN X)

c

Trigeminal nerve
(CN V)

Facial and
vestibulocochlear
nerves (CN VII & VIII)

Figure 4.17. (b) Upon wide opening of the cisterns, the surface of the middle cerebellar peduncle and the root entry zone of the trigeminal nerve (CN V) can be seen. The motor root of the trigeminal nerve exits the pons superomedial to the larger sensory root. **(c)** Anterolateral view. The presigmoid approaches provide direct lateral access to the supratrigeminal, peritrigeminal, and lateral pontine safe entry zones (*shaded area*).

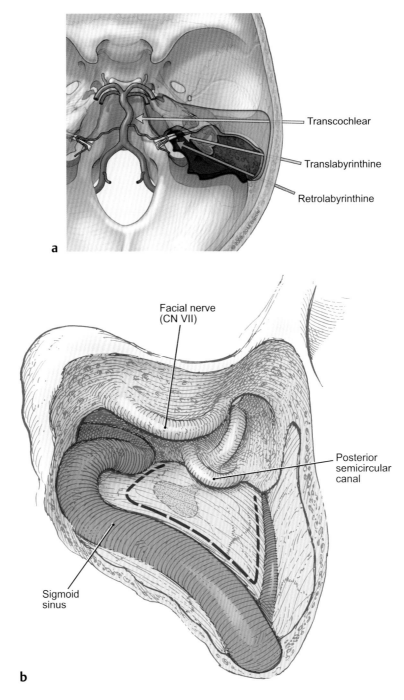

Figure 4.18. Posterior petrosectomy. **(a)** Superior view of posterior petrous approaches. **(b)** Bony removal and dural opening (*dashed lines*) for a retrolabyrinthine approach.

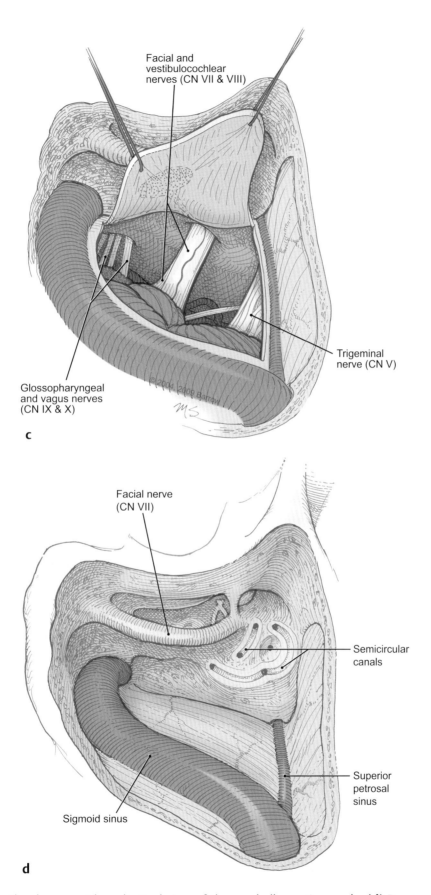

Figure 4.18. **(c)** Opening the dura provides a limited view of the cerebellopontine angle. **(d)** Bony removal for a translabyrinthine approach.

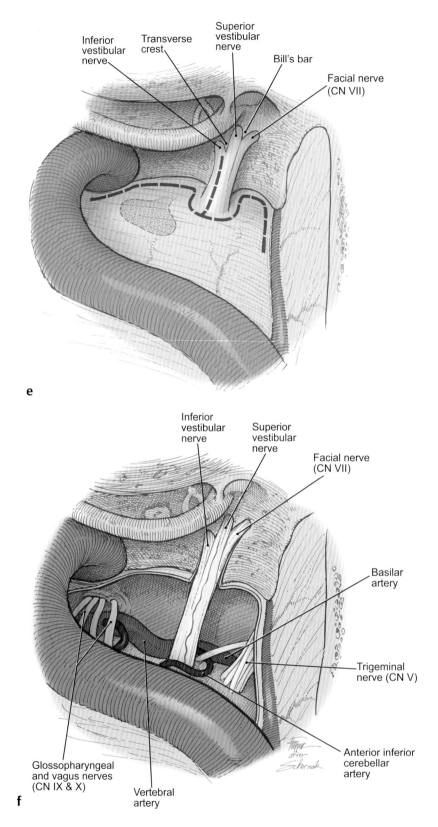

Figure 4.18. (e) Dural opening (*dashed lines*) for a translabyrinthine approach. **(f)** Opening the dura provides an extensive view of the cerebellopontine angle cistern and the facial–vestibulocochlear nerve (CN VII-VIII) complex.

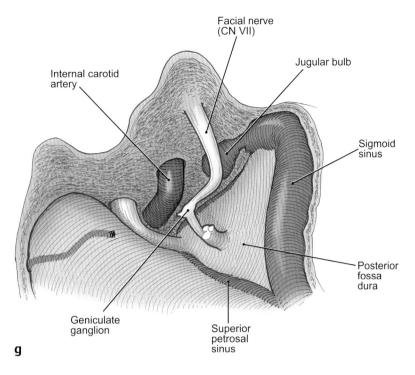

Internal carotid
artery

Facial nerve
(CN VII)

Jugular bulb

Sigmoid
sinus

Posterior
fossa
dura

Geniculate
ganglion

Superior
petrosal
sinus

g

Figure 4.18. (g) Further bony removal via a transcochlear approach enables mobilization of the facial nerve and better visualization of the brainstem.

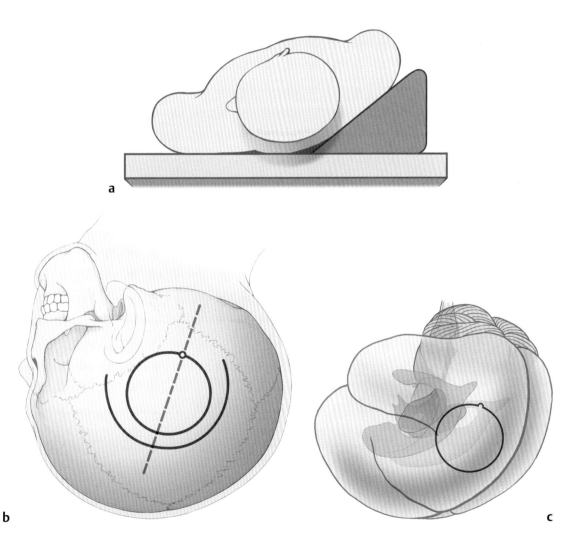

a

b

c

Figure 4.19. Parieto-occipital transventricular approach. **(a)** The patient is positioned supine on the operating table with the ipsilateral shoulder elevated carotid and the head turned horizontally to the contralateral side. Alternatively, a modified park bench position can be used **(Figure 4.16b)**. **(b)** Two alternative scalp incisions and the craniotomy for a parieto-occipital transventricular approach. The linear skin incision is preferred when possible, as it is the shortest incision that provides the needed exposure for the craniotomy. **(c)** Relationship of the craniotomy to the lateral ventricle and the thalamus.

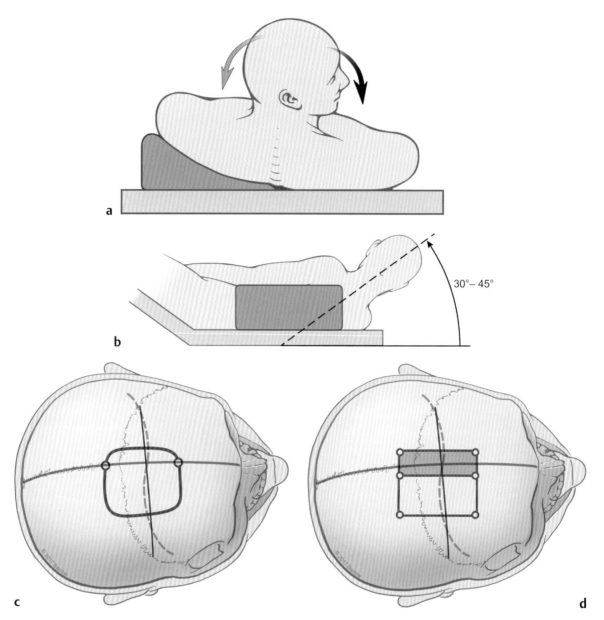

30°– 45°

Figure 4.20. Anterior interhemispheric transcallosal approach. **(a)** The interhemispheric approach can be performed with the patient's head in either the vertical or horizontal position. Placing the patient's head in a horizontal position enables the surgeon to dynamically retract the frontal lobe using the falx. The patient is placed supine with the ipsilateral shoulder raised and the head turned horizontally. For lesions at the rostrum and genu of the corpus callosum, the neck should be flexed (*black arrow*) to optimize the angle of the approach to the ventral corpus callosum. For lesions in the body and splenium of the corpus callosum, the head should be extended (*blue arrow*) to optimize the view of the posterior corpus callosum. **(b)** The head can be raised 30 to 45 degrees from the table. This position enables the surgeon to use both hands in the same horizontal plane along the interhemispheric fissure and allows the ipsilateral hemisphere to be retracted by gravity,

obviating the need for a retractor. Raising the head above the heart also improves venous drainage and cerebral relaxation. **(c)** Two alternative skin incisions (*straight and dashed purple lines*) and the craniotomy for the interhemispheric approach with the patient in the horizontal position are depicted. In most cases the linear incision provides adequate exposure with the least soft tissue disruption. The head should be elevated above the heart to enhance venous drainage. Bur holes may be placed directly over the sinus. This technique enables the surgeon to dissect the sinus off the skull and to ensure that the exposure is extradural prior to completing the craniotomy. Note that the craniotomy is two-thirds in front and one-third behind the coronal suture. **(d)** Alternatively, the bur holes may be placed on the sides of the sinus, and the sinus can be dissected off the skull (*shaded area*) prior to completing the cuts of the craniotomy.

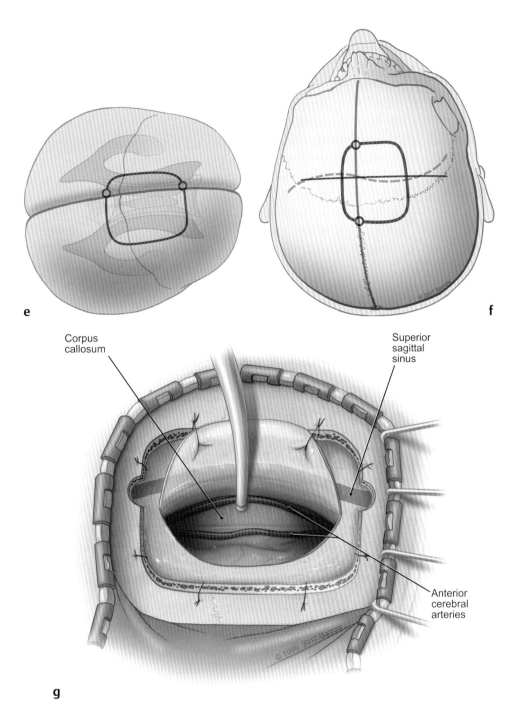

Figure 4.20. (e) The interhemispheric approach provides access to the pericallosal and callosomarginal arteries. Opening of the corpus callosum provides exposure of the lateral and third ventricles. This approach is particularly useful for access to thalamic lesions. **(f)** The skin incision and craniotomy for vertical head positioning are identical to those for horizontal positioning. Placing the patient's head in the vertical position does not enable the surgeon to use the falx for gravity retraction, but it does provide the surgeon with a more familiar view of the anatomy. **(g)** The anatomic view obtained after splitting of the interhemispheric fissure. Note that the dura is retracted with sutures to the edge of the craniotomy. The exposure facilitates complete visualization of the sinus, and the sinus can be gently retracted with tack-up sutures to provide a flush view against the falx. Dissection of the interhemispheric fissure facilitates visualization of the bilateral anterior cerebral arteries and the corpus callosum.

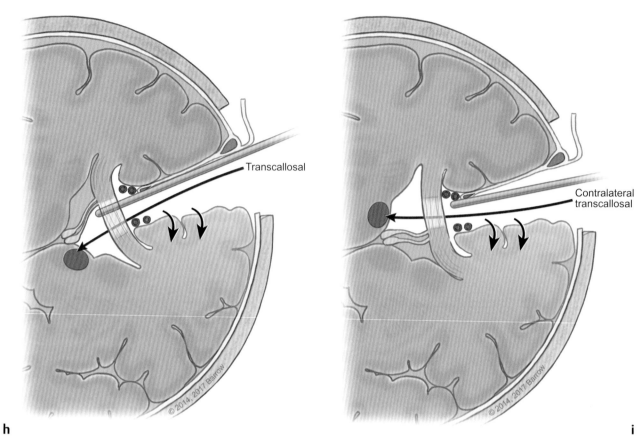

h

i

Figure 4.20. (h) The transcallosal approach to the ipsilateral lateral ventricle and thalamus. The contralateral hemisphere is dynamically retracted by the falx. The shafts of the suction and bipolar forceps enable dynamic retraction when necessary. The ipsilateral lobe is retracted by gravity (*black arrows*). Care is taken to keep the superior sagittal sinus moist and minimally retracted to prevent sinus occlusion or thrombosis. Covering the sinus with a piece of saline-soaked Gelfoam without thrombin serves the purpose well. **(i)** The contralateral transcallosal approach to the lateral ventricle and thalamus (*blue arrow*). The falx can be resected to enhance exposure of this approach. This approach is particularly useful for lesions in the dominant hemisphere. Placing the dominant hemisphere up allows the falx to gently retract the lobe and minimizes trauma. The contralateral lobe is retracted by gravity (*black arrows*). For more laterally situated lesions, a trans-cingulate gyrus approach can be used to obtain the more lateral trajectory necessary.

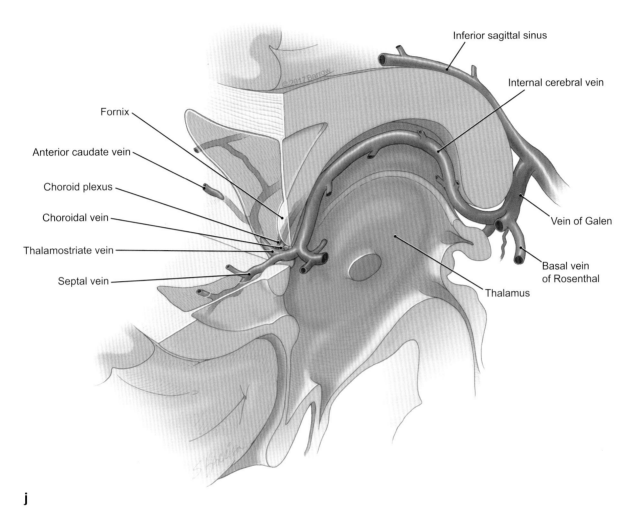

j

Figure 4.20. **(j)** The intraventricular anatomy and the relation of the ventricular veins to the thalamus. The choroid plexus is the first anatomic landmark identified upon entry into the lateral ventricle. The choroid plexus overlies the choroidal fissure. The choroid plexus rests between the body of the fornix and the thalamus, which forms the floor of the lateral ventricle.

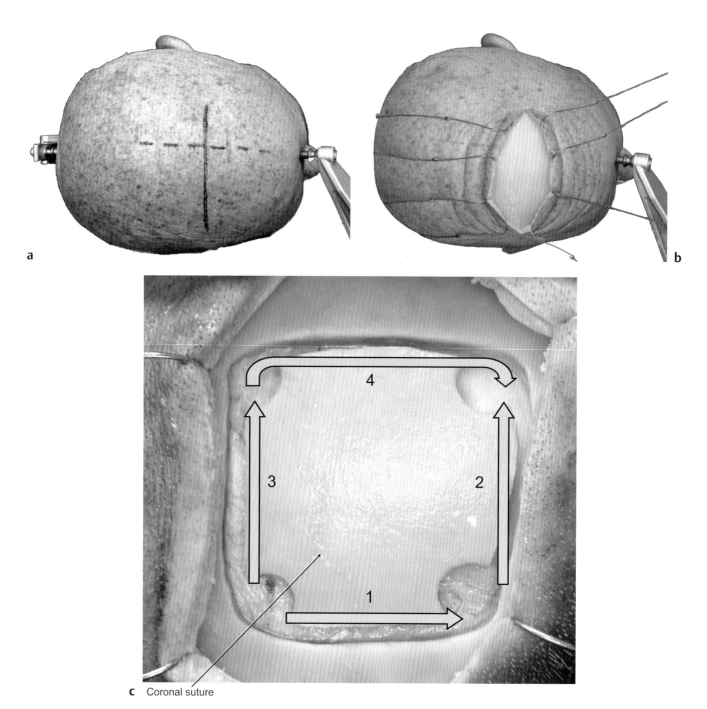

c   Coronal suture

Figure 4.21. Anterior interhemispheric approach. **(a)** The patient is placed in the supine position with the sagittal plane (*dashed line*) of the head turned parallel to the floor and the lesion side in the up position. The head is elevated 30 to 45 degrees. A linear skin incision (*solid line*) is made pre-coronally, one-third contralateral to the craniotomy side and two-thirds to the ipsilateral side. **(b)** The scalp flap is retracted and the coronal suture is observed. **(c)** The craniotomy is placed two-thirds in front of and one-third behind the coronal suture. This area usually has few draining veins to the superior sagittal sinus and it facilitates access to the interhemispheric fissure. There are many ways to perform the craniotomy over the superior sagittal sinus. Bur holes may be placed directly over the sinus, and the bone flap is reflected after stripping the sinus free. Alternatively, bur holes may be placed adjacent to the sinus in the manner shown here. The *yellow arrows,* as numbered, indicate the order in which the cuts are made when performing the craniotomy.

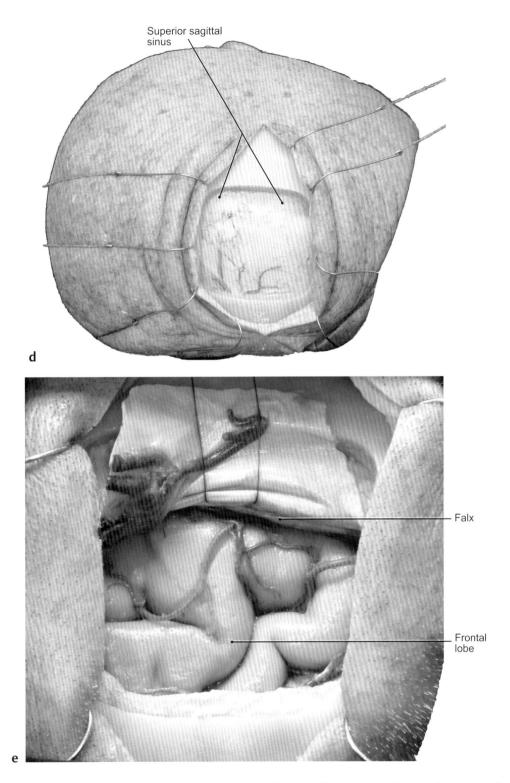

Superior sagittal
sinus

d

Falx

Frontal
lobe

e

Figure 4.21. (d) Removal of the bone exposes the superior sagittal sinus, allowing it to be gently retracted with sutures upon opening the dura. **(e)** The dura is opened in a U shape, with the flap protecting the sinus. The dural flap is reflected and retracted with retention sutures over the sinus. Note that gentle retraction of the sinus provides the surgeon with a flat view against the falx.

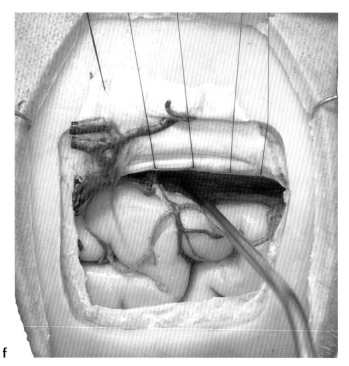

f

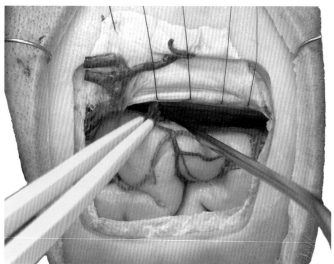

g

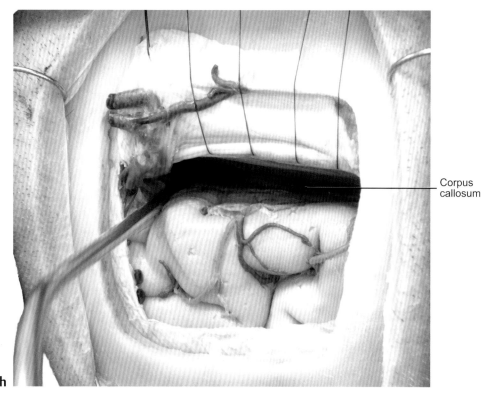

Corpus callosum

h

Figure 4.21. (f) The interhemispheric fissure is easily opened and accessed, without the need for fixed retraction. The falx serves as a natural retractor to prevent sagging of the contralateral frontal lobe. **(g)** Care should be taken to preserve bridging veins or venous lakes draining into the sinus. Although the classic teaching dictates that veins in the anterior one-third of the superior sagittal sinus may be sacrificed, every effort should be made to preserve these veins with careful microdissection. One may be able to work in between and around them, rather than sacrificing them, which may require multiple slits in the dural flap. **(h)** The white corpus callosum appears deep in the interhemispheric fissure. The paired anterior cerebral arteries can be seen lying upon the corpus callosum.

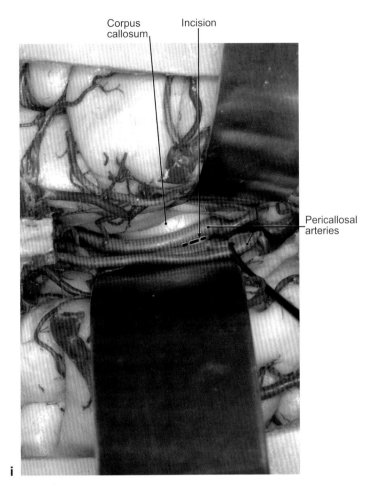

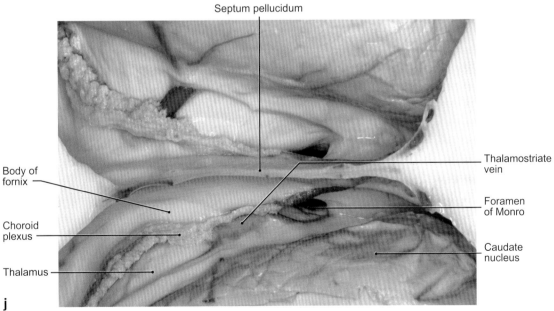

Figure 4.21. (i) For a transcallosal approach, the anterior cerebral arteries should be dissected and mobilized laterally. A small callosotomy can be placed in the corpus callosum to enter the ventricle (*dashed line*). The opening in the corpus callosum can be performed in the horizontal or vertical plane. It is important to keep this opening as small as possible to minimize the risk of disconnection syndrome. **(j)** Intraventricular anatomy from a transcallosal approach. Note the relation of the fornix, thalamus, and choroid plexus.

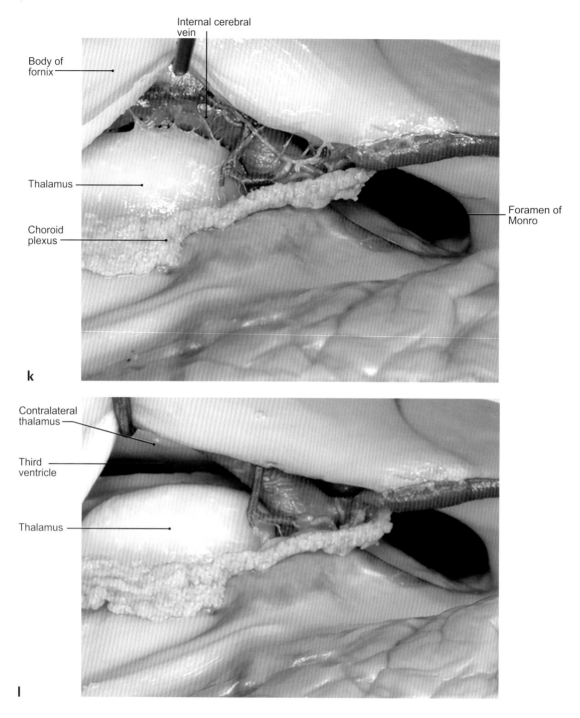

Figure 4.21. (k) View of the lateral ventricle and its relation to the thalamus, fornix, and choroid plexus. The choroidal fissure can be opened between the fornix and the choroid plexus or between the thalamus and the choroid plexus. **(l)** View of a transchoroidal approach with opening of the choroid fissure on the forniceal side. Opening the fissure on the thalamic side minimizes possible injury to the fornix. The choroid plexus is used as a cushion to minimize forniceal retraction while opening the choroid fissure on the thalamic side.

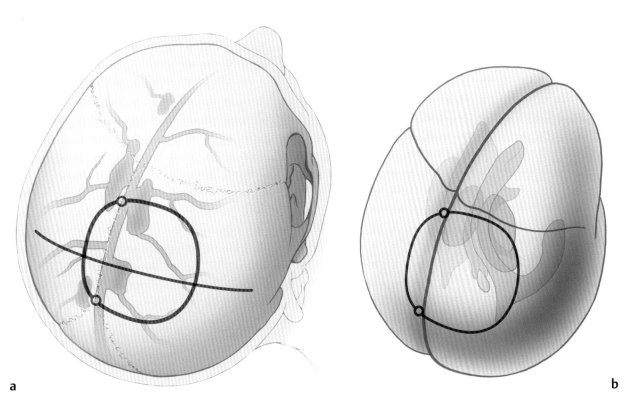

a

b

Figure 4.22. Posterior interhemispheric transcallosal approach. **(a)** The posterior interhemispheric transcallosal approach can be used to access lesions in the splenium of the corpus callosum. This approach is rarely used, given the unforgiving rich venous anatomy in the middle half of the superior sagittal sinus. The skin incision and craniotomy are depicted. Similar to the anterior interhemispheric approach, the posterior interhemispheric approach can be performed with the patient's head in the horizontal or vertical position. **(b)** The relationship between the craniotomy and the ventricular system and thalami.

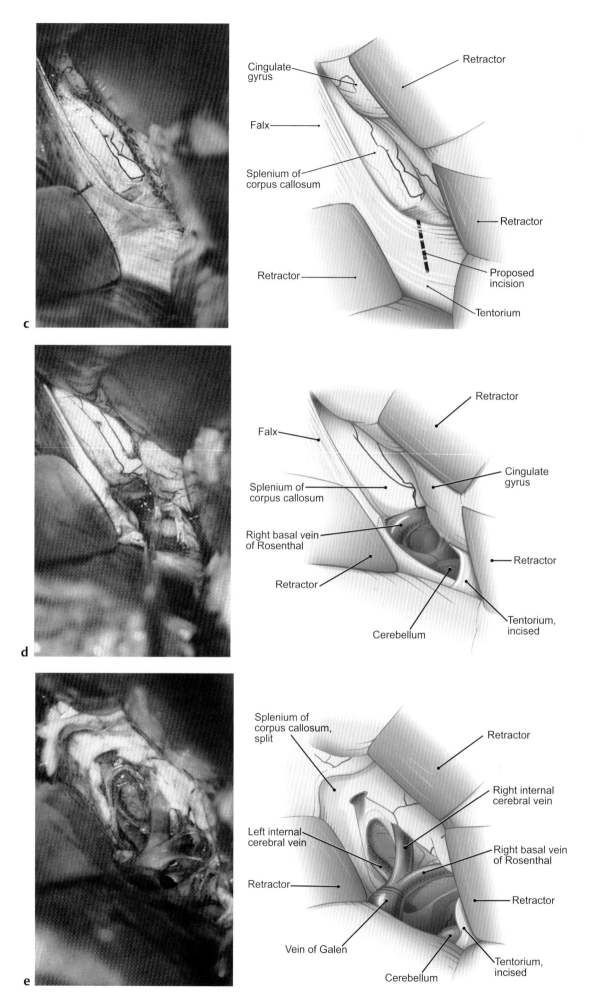

Figure 4.22. (c) The approach along the falx exposes the splenium of the corpus callosum. Opening of the falcotentorial junction (*dashed line*) facilitates visualization of the deep venous complex. **(d)** The falx and tentorial junction are opened, exposing the pineal region and the deep venous circulation. **(e)** An incision into the splenium of the corpus callosum anteriorly facilitates visualization of the pineal region between the paired internal cerebral veins as they join with the basal vein of Rosenthal and the internal occipital veins to form the vein of Galen.

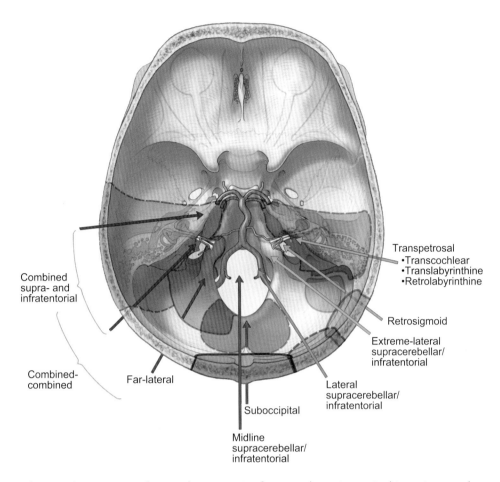

Figure 4.23. Approaches to the posterior fossa. The posterior fossa and craniocervical junction can be accessed via the approaches depicted: suboccipital, retrosigmoid, far-lateral, transpetrosal, and combined supra- and infratentorial.

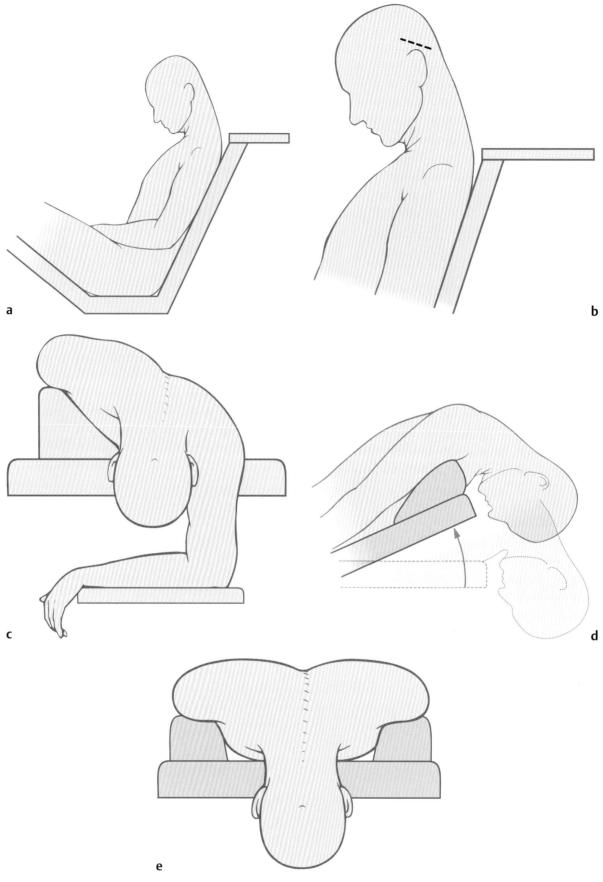

Figure 4.24. Patient positioning for access to posterior fossa lesions. Approaches to the posterior fossa can be performed from several positions. The ultimate position depends on surgeon preference and comfort, the patient's body habitus, and the location and extent of the lesion. **(a)** The patient's neck is commonly flexed in the sitting position. The sitting position and its modifications provide excellent access to the posterior fossa. This position enables gravity retraction of the cerebellum. With this approach, blood pooling in the surgical field is rare, as gravity drains it away, and the risk of venous air embolism is minimized. When a sitting position is considered, a preoperative echocardiogram with a bubble study to evaluate the heart for a patent foramen ovale is necessary. An anesthesia team comfortable with the use of this position and capable of dealing with complications associated with its use is essential. **(b)** The degree of neck flexion required depends on the relationship of the lesion to the straight sinus (*dashed line*). The straight sinus should be optimally placed parallel to the floor. **(c–e)** Patient positioning: **(c)** semi-prone; **(d,e)** prone. The amount of neck flexion and rotation depends on the specific location in the posterior fossa and on the extent of the lesion.

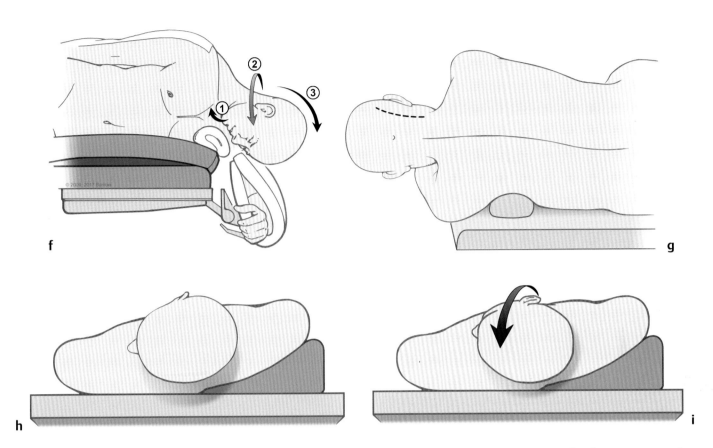

Figure 4.24. (f) The modified park bench position is often used for patients with a large barrel chest or large shoulders. This position provides good exposure of the cerebellopontine angle or midline structures. Pulling the ipsilateral shoulder inferiorly and flexing the chin (*arrow 1*), rotating the neck to the opposite side (*arrow 2*), and maximally extending the neck (*arrow 3*) enable opening of the surgical field to optimally use this approach. **(g)** The lateral position is an alternative position for lesions in the cerebellar hemisphere and the cerebellopontine angle. The *dashed line* demonstrates the site of the skin incision for a lateral cerebellar approach. **(h,i)** Alternatively, the patient may be placed supine, with the head turned completely to the contralateral side to position it in a horizontal orientation to the floor. **(h)** The chin may be flexed toward the contralateral side to open the angle with the ipsilateral shoulder, enhancing the exposure of the cerebellopontine angle. **(i)** Extension of the neck toward the floor (*arrow*) is a subtle but very helpful maneuver that provides the surgeon with better exposure up to the level of the tentorium and trigeminal nerve (CN V) complex. This maneuver is not necessary if the lesion is not located high against the tentorial surface.

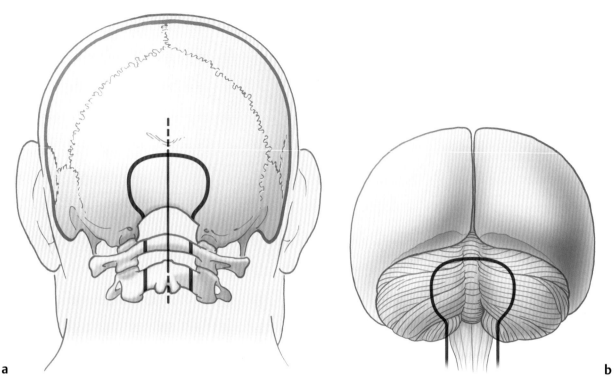

Figure 4.25. Suboccipital approach. **(a)** The skin incision for the midline suboccipital craniotomy. Depending on the location of the lesion, the incision may be made starting several centimeters above the inion and extending down to the level of C2. Removal of the posterior arches of C1 and C2 is usually not necessary. The higher the location of the lesion on the dorsal brainstem surface, the lower the craniotomy and skin incision should extend to obtain the inferosuperior view and necessary trajectory. **(b)** The relationship of the craniotomy to the underlying neural structures.

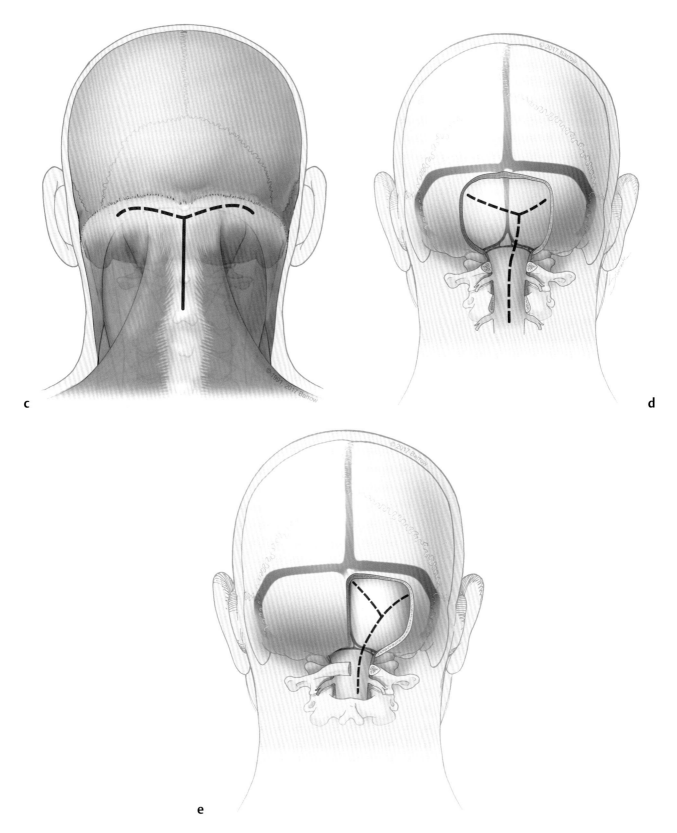

c

d

e

Figure 4.25. **(c)** The nuchal ligament (*dashed line*) and midline (*solid line*) are identified and cut in a T fashion, enabling reattachment of the ligament at the completion of the procedure. **(d)** The midline craniotomy, with removal of the arches of the atlas and axis. The dural opening is marked (*dashed lines*). **(e)** Alternatively, a unilateral craniotomy can be performed.

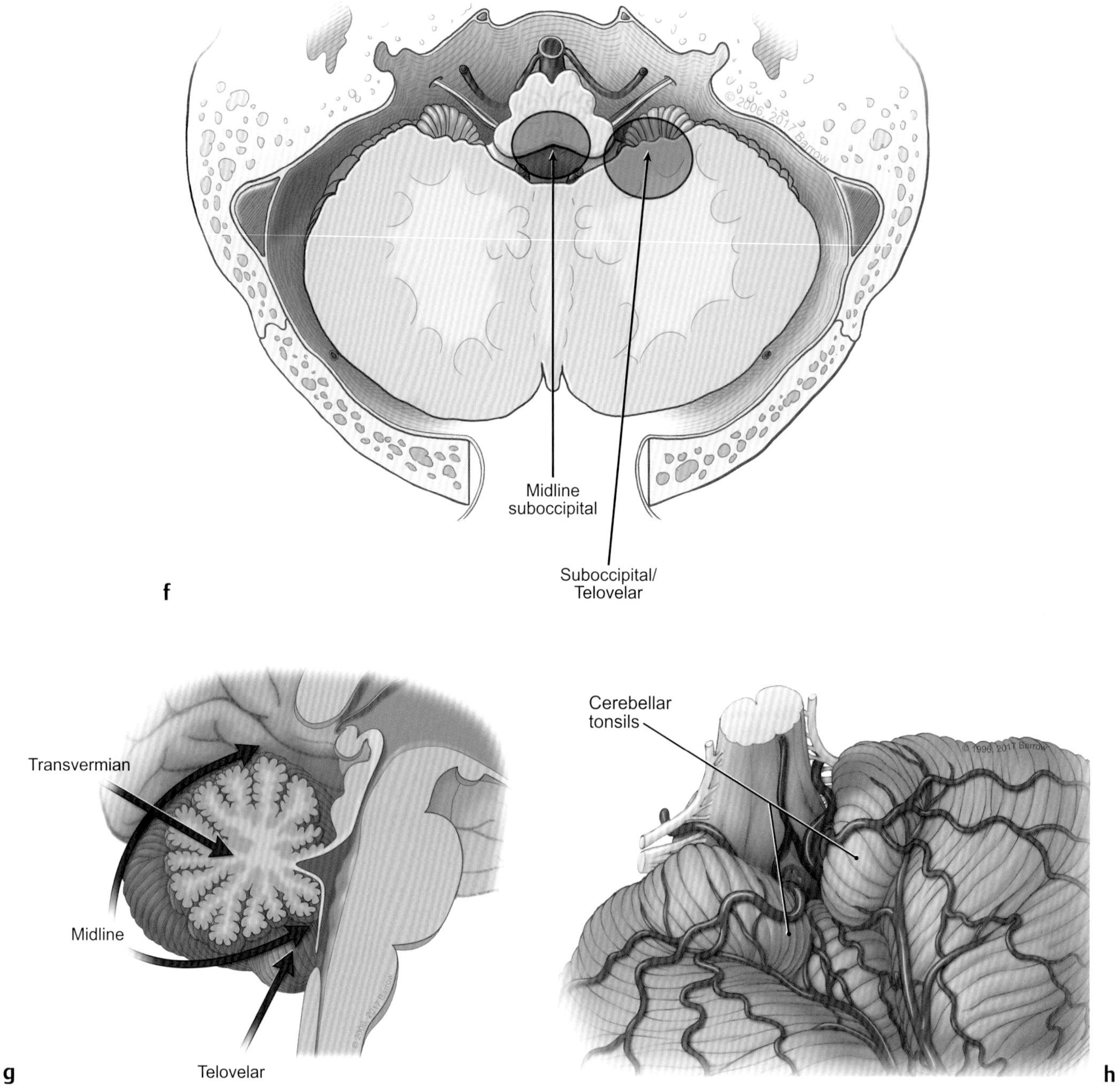

f

Midline
suboccipital

Suboccipital/
Telovelar

g

Transvermian

Midline

Telovelar

h

Cerebellar
tonsils

Figure 4.25. **(f)** Axial view. A midline suboccipital craniotomy provides several routes of entry to remove lesions in the cerebellum or dorsal brainstem. **(g)** Lateral view. Variants include the transvermian and telovelar approaches. **(h)** Posterolateral view. Opening the dura exposes the cerebellar tonsils, which hide the cerebellomedullary fissure.

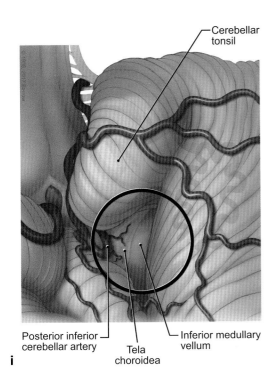

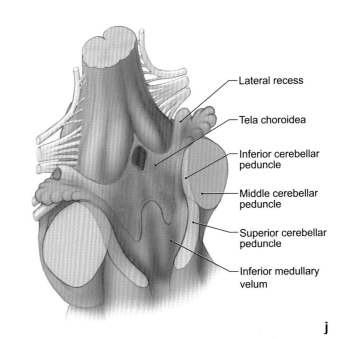

i

j

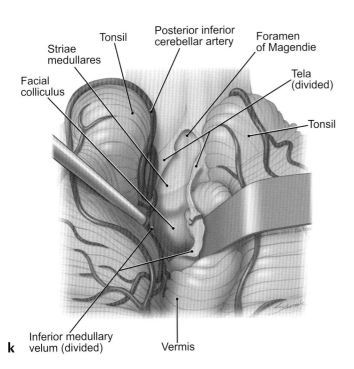

k

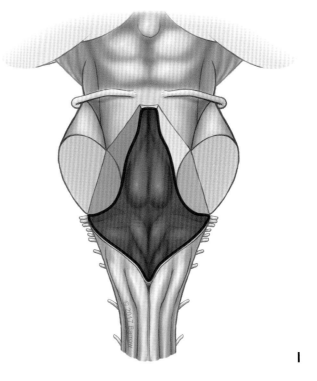

l

Figure 4.25. (i) Posterolateral view. Retraction of the tonsils and mobilization of the telovelotonsillar segment of the posterior inferior cerebellar arteries laterally opens the tela choroidea. **(j)** Posterolateral view. The tela choroidea and the inferior medullary vellum together constitute the inferior half of the roof of the fourth ventricle. **(k)** Dividing the tela bilaterally brings the rhomboid fossa and the lateral recesses into the surgical field. Opening the inferior velum exposes the superior half of the ventricular roof and the superolateral recesses. **(l)** The exposed dorsal surface of the brainstem via the suboccipital approach (*shaded area*).

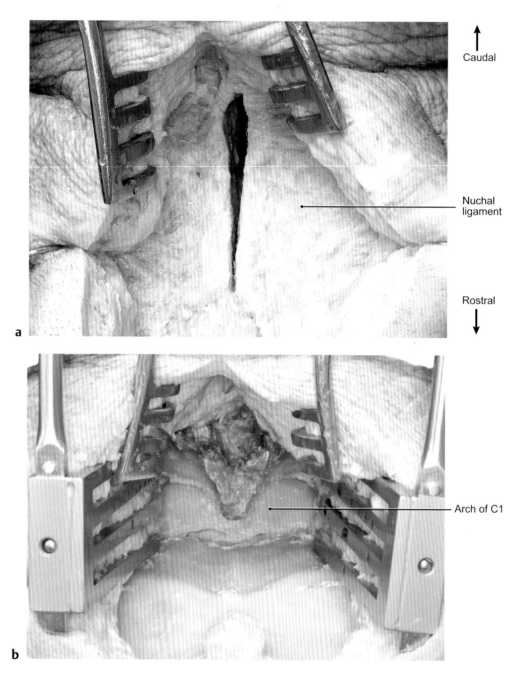

Caudal

Nuchal
ligament

Rostral

a

Arch of C1

b

Figure 4.26. Cadaveric dissection of the midline suboccipital approach, posterior view, with the rostral position at the bottom of the images. **(a)** The suboccipital muscles are stripped off the superior nuchal ligament and retracted laterally. **(b)** The paraspinal muscles are released off the C1 posterior arch using electrocautery, followed by subperiosteal dissection laterally.

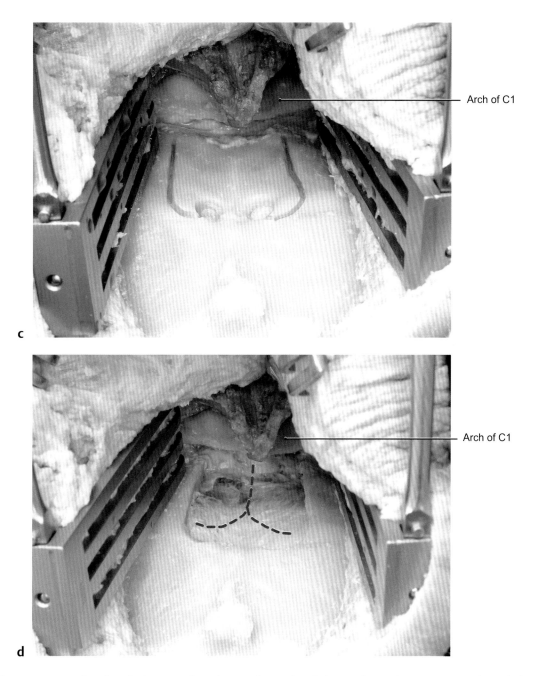

Arch of C1

Arch of C1

Figure 4.26. (c) Two paramedian bur holes are placed on either side of the midline. The posterior edge of the foramen magnum is used as the inferior border of the craniotomy or craniectomy. **(d)** The dural incision is made in an inverse-Y fashion (*dashed line*), starting at the level of the foramen magnum and ascending to the upper corners of the bone flap.

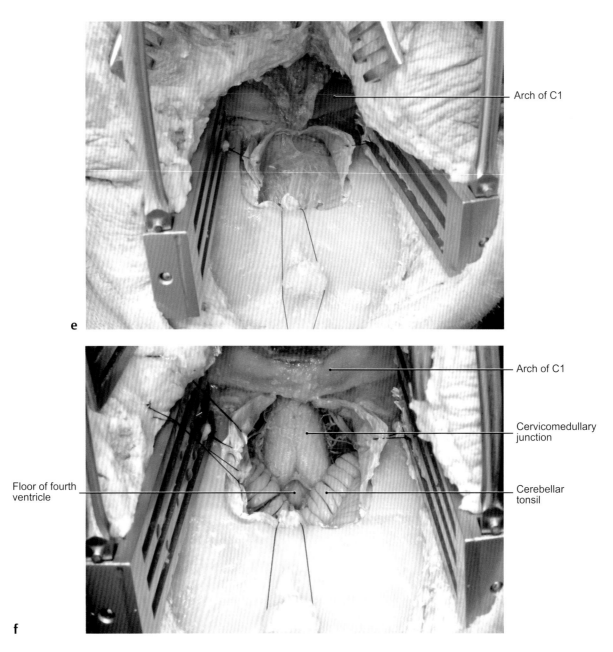

Arch of C1

e

Arch of C1

Cervicomedullary
junction

Floor of fourth
ventricle

Cerebellar
tonsil

f

Figure 4.26. **(e)** After the free edge of the dural flap is tacked up, the cisterna magna (cerebellomedullary cistern) is exposed. **(f)** Opening the cisterna magna and releasing the cerebrospinal fluid relaxes the cerebellum.

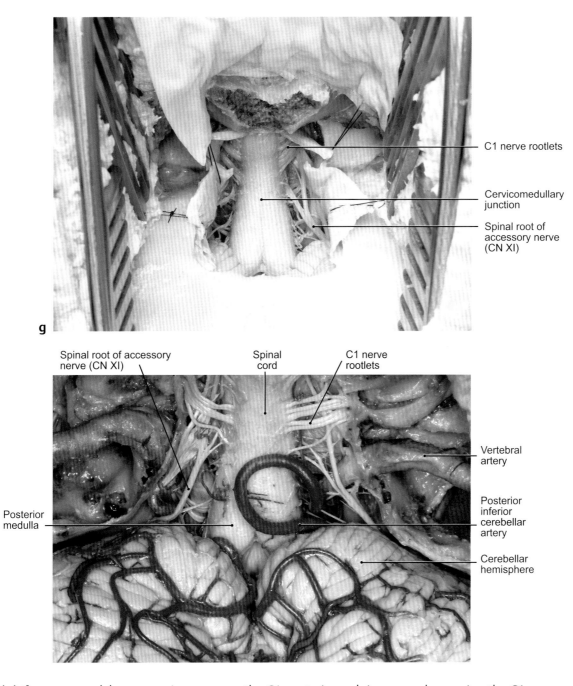

g

C1 nerve rootlets

Cervicomedullary junction

Spinal root of accessory nerve (CN XI)

Spinal root of accessory nerve (CN XI)

Spinal cord

C1 nerve rootlets

Vertebral artery

Posterior inferior cerebellar artery

Cerebellar hemisphere

Posterior medulla

h

Figure 4.26. **(g)** If a more caudal exposure is necessary, the C1 posterior arch is removed, exposing the C1 nerve rootlet, accessory nerve (CN XI) spinal root, cerebellar tonsils, vertebral artery, and posterior medulla and spinal cord. **(h)** Dissection showing the complete exposure of the C1 nerve rootlets, accessory nerve spinal root, cerebellar tonsils, vertebral artery, posterior inferior cerebellar artery, and posterior medulla and spinal cord.

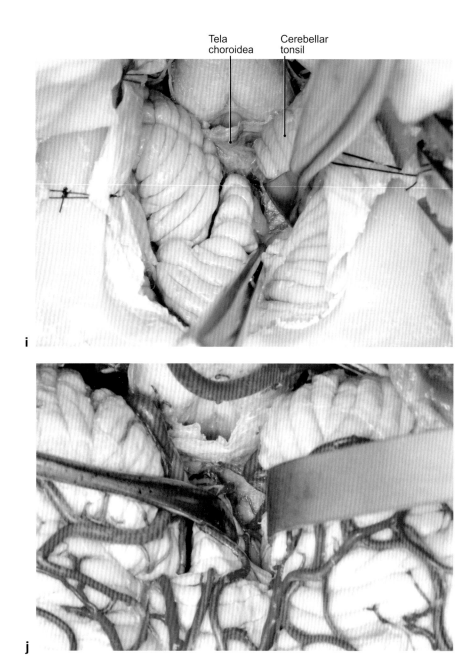

Tela
choroidea

Cerebellar
tonsil

i

j

Figure 4.26. (i) The cerebellar tonsil is retracted superolaterally, exposing the telovelar junction. **(j)** Close-up view of the telovelar junction.

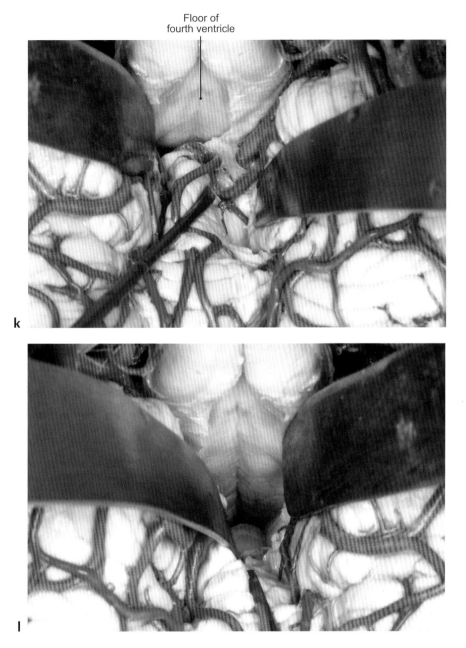

Floor of
fourth ventricle

k

l

Figure 4.26. **(k)** Surgical view after performing a telovelar approach to the dorsal brainstem (floor of the fourth ventricle).
(l) The telovelar approach provides a good exposure to the floor of the fourth ventricle and foramen of Luschka laterally.

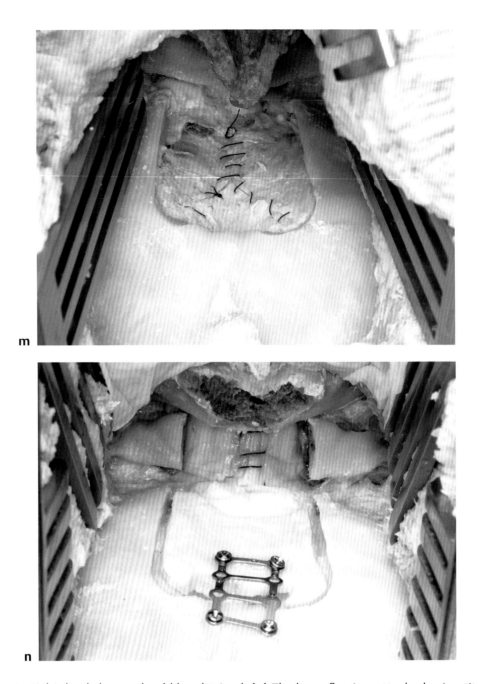

Figure 4.26. (m) A watertight dural closure should be obtained. **(n)** The bone flap is reattached using titanium plates.

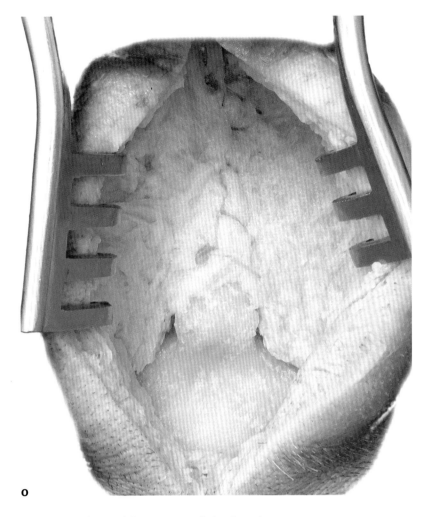

o

Figure 4.26. **(o)** The suboccipital muscles and fascia are tightly closed.

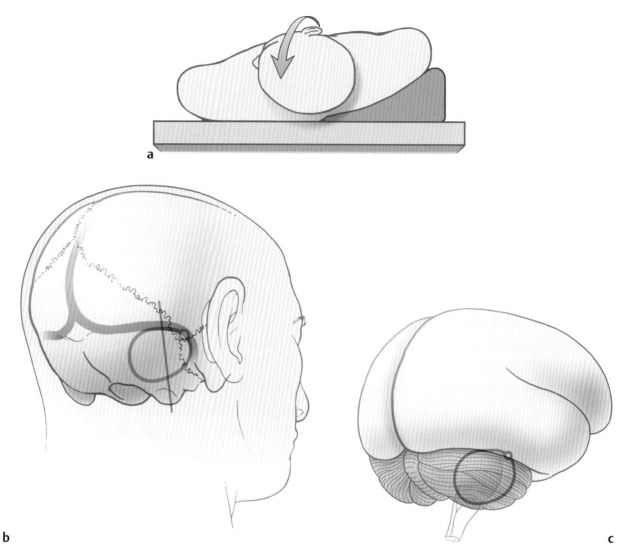

Figure 4.27. Retrosigmoid approach. **(a)** End-on view of the patient positioning for the retrosigmoid approach. The patient should be placed supine, and the ipsilateral shoulder should be elevated and pulled inferiorly. In patients with large shoulders or a barrel chest, a modified park bench position **(Figure 4.24f)** should be used. The head should be turned to the contralateral side and the chin should be tucked. For approaches to lesions at the level of the tentorium, subtle extension of the neck toward the floor (*blue arrow*) greatly assists with visualization. **(b–g)** Posterolateral view. **(b)** The skin incision and craniotomy used for the retrosigmoid approach. Note the placement of the craniotomy at the junction of the transverse and sigmoid sinuses. The caudal extension of this craniotomy depends on the caudal extension of the pathology to be addressed. **(c)** Depiction of the position of the craniotomy in relation to the cerebellum and brainstem.

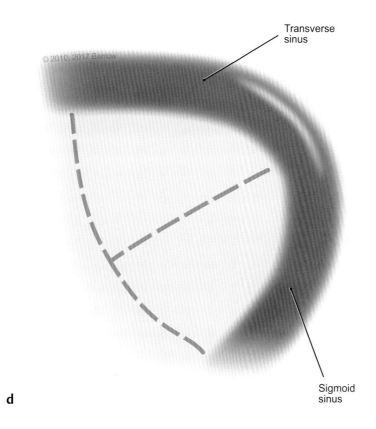

d

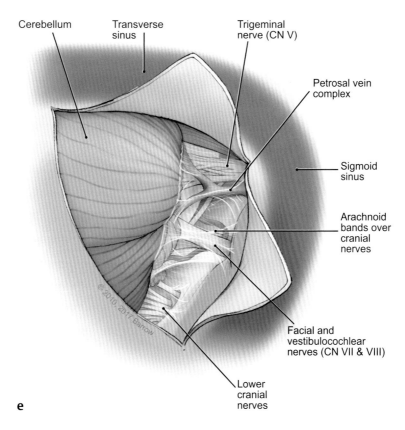

e

Figure 4.27. (d) The dura is opened using an inverted T-shaped incision (*dashed line*), leaving a dural base along the transverse and sigmoid sinuses. These dural leaflets enable the sinuses to be gently retracted, providing a flat view of the cerebellopontine angle. **(e)** Dissection begins along the petrosal surface of the cerebellum, reaching the cerebellopontine cistern. The cranial nerves are covered by dense arachnoid bands. Care should be taken to preserve the petrosal vein complex.

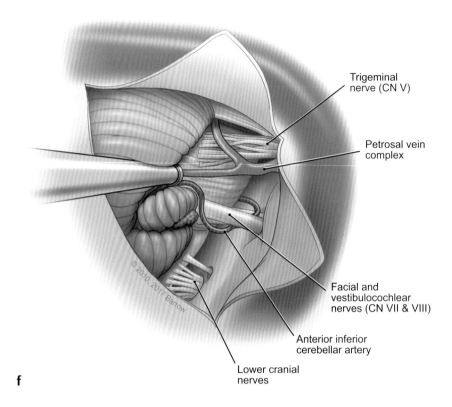

Trigeminal
nerve (CN V)

Petrosal vein
complex

Facial and
vestibulocochlear
nerves (CN VII & VIII)

Anterior inferior
cerebellar artery

Lower cranial
nerves

f

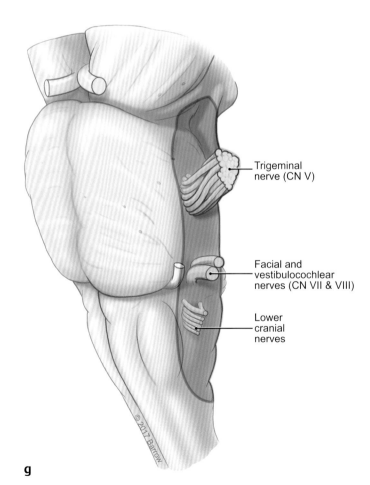

Trigeminal
nerve (CN V)

Facial and
vestibulocochlear
nerves (CN VII & VIII)

Lower
cranial
nerves

g

Figure 4.27. **(f)** Arachnoid bands tethering the petrosal vein complex, as well as those in contact with the trigeminal (CN V), facial (CN VII), and vestibulocochlear (CN VIII) nerves, are cut to enable their mobilization. Next, the middle cerebellar peduncle and the lateral pons are exposed. **(g)** The lateral brainstem surface. The extent of the exposure (*shaded area*) during lateral posterior fossa approaches is shown.

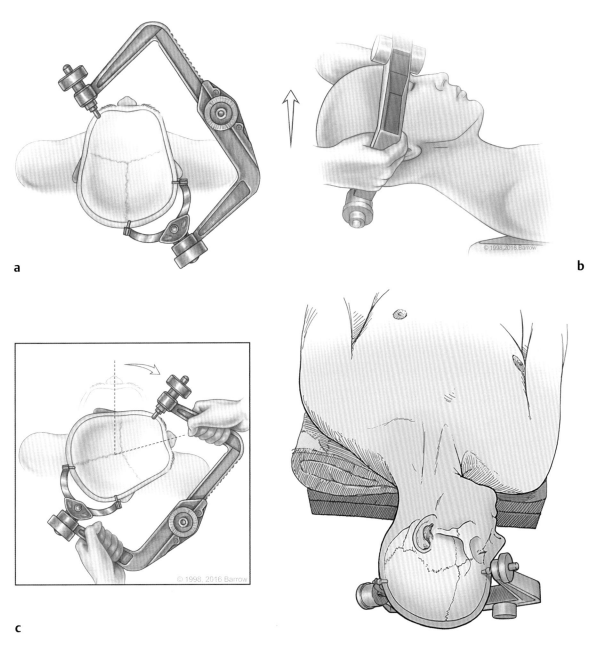

a

b

c

Figure 4.28. Retrosigmoid approach. **(a)** Placement of head pins. Avoid placing the pins of the head holder into the temporalis muscle, which would diminish the stability of the system and potentially allow the head to slip. **(b)** The head should be elevated about 15 degrees above the level of the thorax to improve venous drainage. **(c)** The patient is placed in a supine position with the ipsilateral shoulder elevated (*right*) or in a modified park bench position **(Figure 4.16b)** for patients with large breasts or a barrel chest. The head should be rotated 75 to 100 degrees to the contralateral side (*left*). A rotation angle of 75 degrees is enough for brainstem dissection. An angle of more than 90 degrees is necessary to expose the internal auditory canal and Meckel's cave.

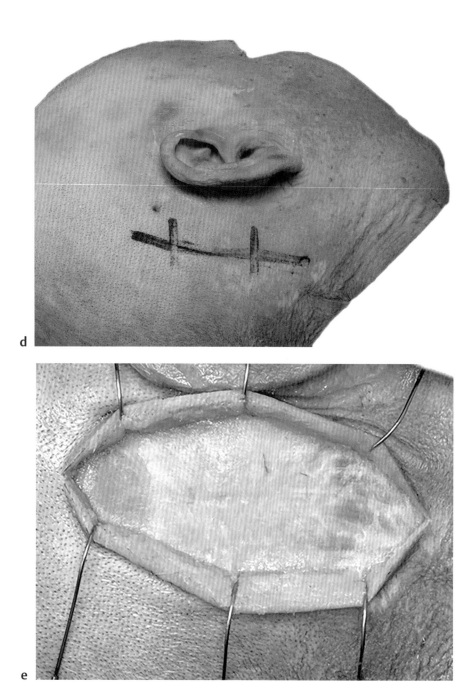

d

e

Figure 4.28. **(d–v)** Cadaveric dissection demonstrating the retrosigmoid approach; posterolateral view with rostral position at left in all images. **(d)** For a retrosigmoid craniotomy, a linear skin incision is placed 5 mm medial to the mastoid notch, extending from 6 cm above the notch to 4 cm below it (*horizontal line*). This approach provides access to the trigeminal nerve (CN V) complex. Alternatively, an incision 5 mm medial to the mastoid notch, extending from 5 cm above the mastoid notch to 5 cm below it, can be used for access to the facial–vestibulocochlear nerve (CN VII-VIII) complex. Finally, an incision 5 mm medial, extending from 4 cm above the notch to 6 cm below it, can be used to approach lesions at the level of the lower cranial nerves. **(e)** After the appropriate skin incision has been made, the fascia overlying the sternocleidomastoid muscle is exposed.

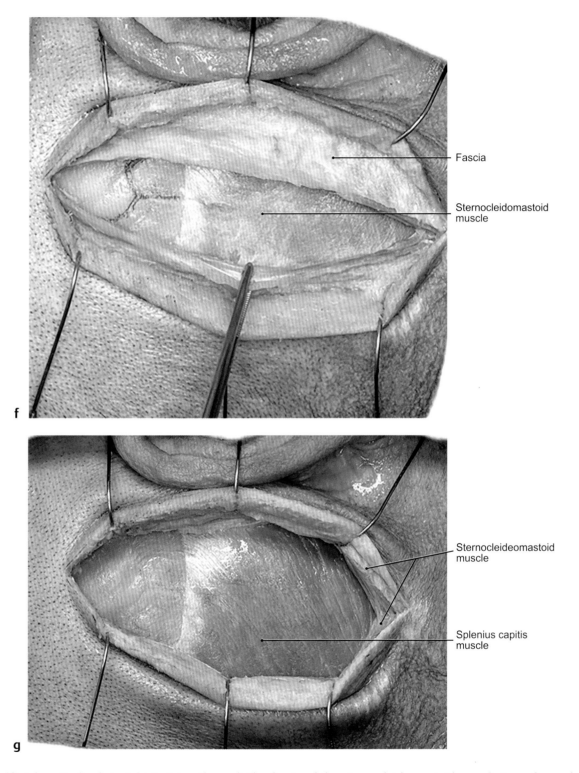

Figure 4.28. (f) A longitudinal straight incision through the fascia of the sternocleidomastoid muscle is performed. **(g)** The sternocleidomastoid muscle is retracted bilaterally, exposing the occipital bone and splenius capitis muscle.

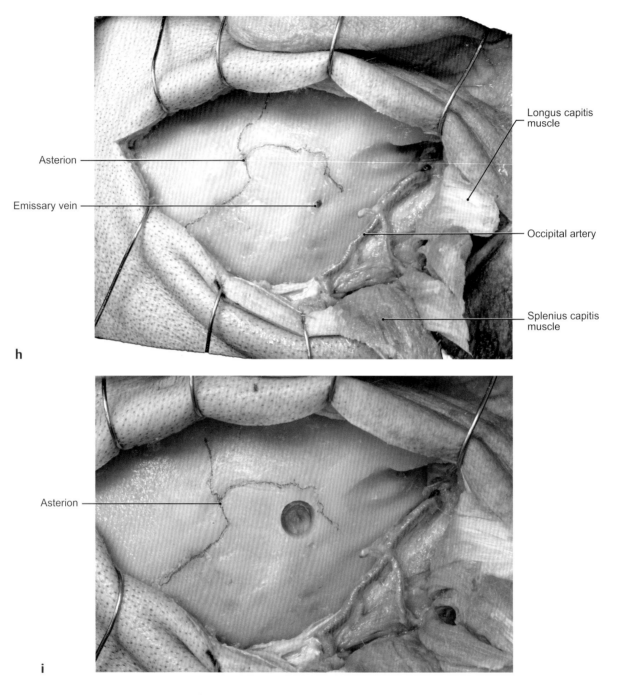

Asterion

Emissary vein

Longus capitis muscle

Occipital artery

Splenius capitis muscle

h

Asterion

i

Figure 4.28. (h) The attachments of the splenius capitis and longus capitis muscles are freed from the occipitomastoid bone. Special attention should be paid to the occipital artery in the inferomedial portion of the exposure, which courses posteriorly. In some cases, the vertebral artery may be exposed after this dissection and care should be taken to avoid injuring it. The periosteum is lifted off using a periosteal elevator. At this point, an emissary vein is usually exposed, resulting in bleeding. This bleeding can be readily controlled with bone wax. **(i)** A single bur hole is made 1 cm below and medial to the asterion using a cranial perforator.

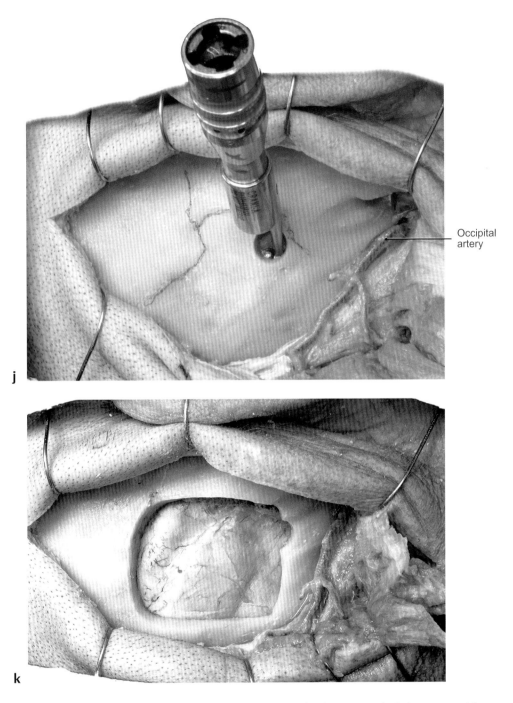

Occipital
artery

j

k

Figure 4.28. (j) The dura is separated from the bone using the tip of a B1 drill bit or a No. 3 Penfield dissector before the craniotomy is performed using a high-speed drill. The use of the craniotome over the sigmoid sinus should be avoided. **(k)** A small craniotomy measuring up to 3 × 3 cm is created. The removal of the mastoid bone and inner edge of the craniotomy results in a remarkable increase in the surgical exposure and visualization. Exposure of the lateral 2 to 3 mm of the sigmoid sinus facilitates visualization by retraction of the sinus with tack-up sutures (not shown).

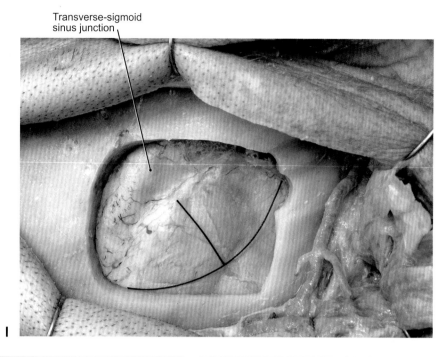

Transverse-sigmoid
sinus junction

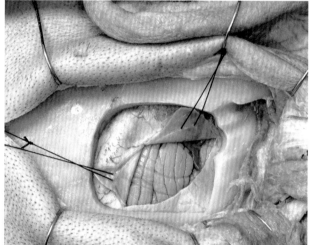

m

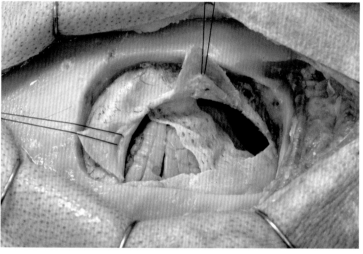

n

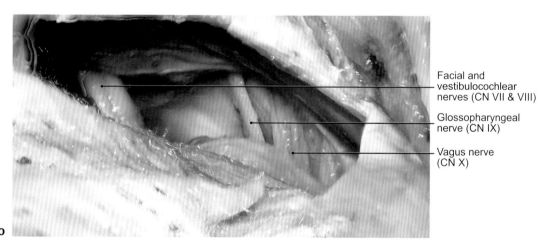

o

Facial and
vestibulocochlear
nerves (CN VII & VIII)

Glossopharyngeal
nerve (CN IX)

Vagus nerve
(CN X)

Figure 4.28. **(l)** A curvilinear dural incision (*black line*), with its base along the transverse–sigmoid sinus junction, is performed. **(m)** Reflecting and tacking the dural triangles over the sinuses with 4-0 Nurolon sutures (Ethicon, Somerville, NJ) enables a flat exposure of the cerebellopontine angle cistern. This maneuver also uses the dural sleeves to protect the sinus. **(n)** Release of cerebrospinal fluid from the cerebellopontine angle enables the cerebellum to relax, provides enhanced exposure of the cerebellopontine angle, and obviates the need for a fixed retractor. **(o)** A low retrosigmoid exposure facilitates visualization of the facial, vestibulocochlear, glossopharyngeal (CN IX), and vagus (CN X) nerves.

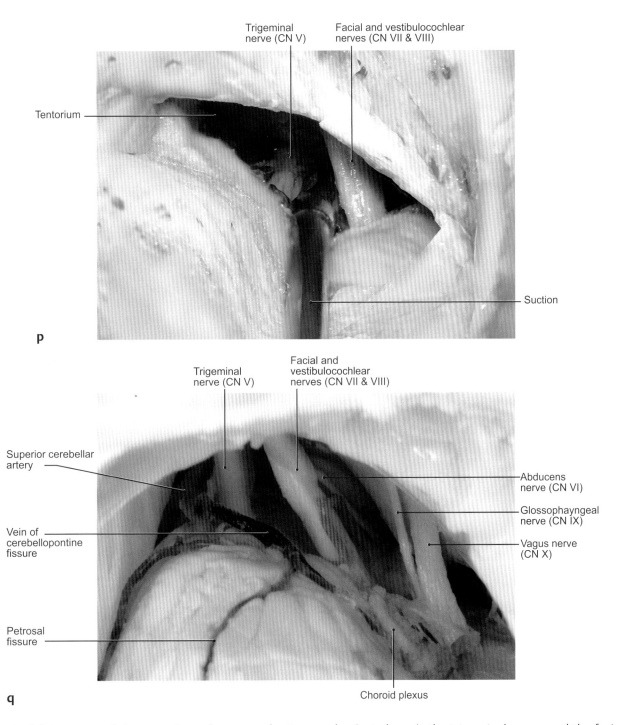

Figure 4.28. (p) Exposure of the tentorium, the petrosal vein complex (not shown), the trigeminal nerve, and the facial–vestibulocochlear nerve complex. **(q)** A generous retrosigmoid exposure facilitates visualization of the tentorium down to the lower cranial nerves.

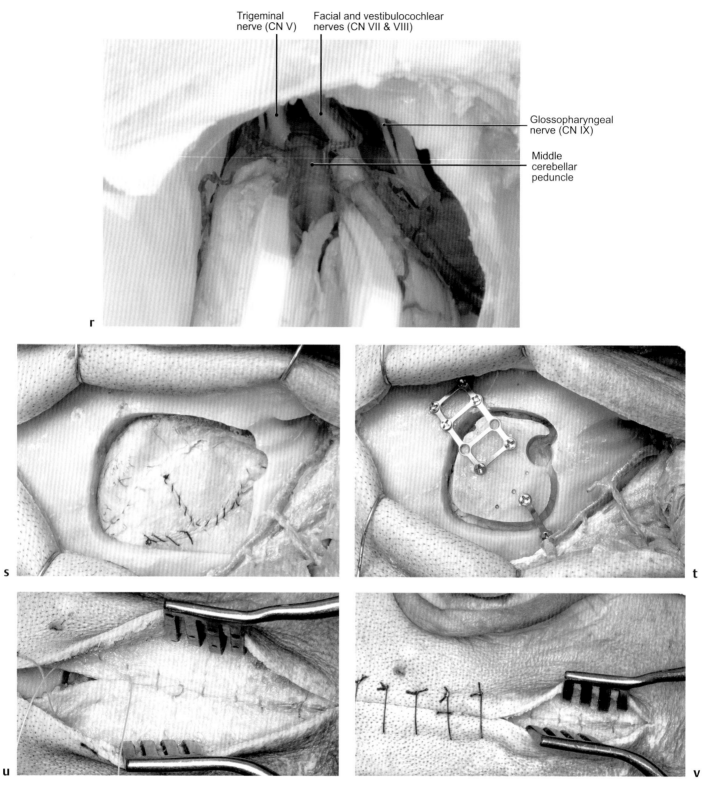

Trigeminal
nerve (CN V)

Facial and vestibulocochlear
nerves (CN VII & VIII)

Glossopharyngeal
nerve (CN IX)

Middle
cerebellar
peduncle

Figure 4.28. (r) Opening the petrosal fissure of the cerebellum provides a flatter and more direct access to the middle cerebellar peduncle. **(s)** A watertight dural closure is necessary in the posterior fossa. If the dura cannot be closed directly, a patch made of autologous or synthetic material should be used. **(t)** The bone flap is replaced using titanium plates. Before closure, it is important to apply bone wax to the mastoid air cells in order to minimize the likelihood of a cerebrospinal fluid leak. **(u)** A stepwise layer-by-layer closure of the muscles and fascia minimizes the risk of a cerebrospinal fluid leak and results in an improved cosmetic outcome. **(v)** Closure of the fascia, subcutaneous tissue, and skin.

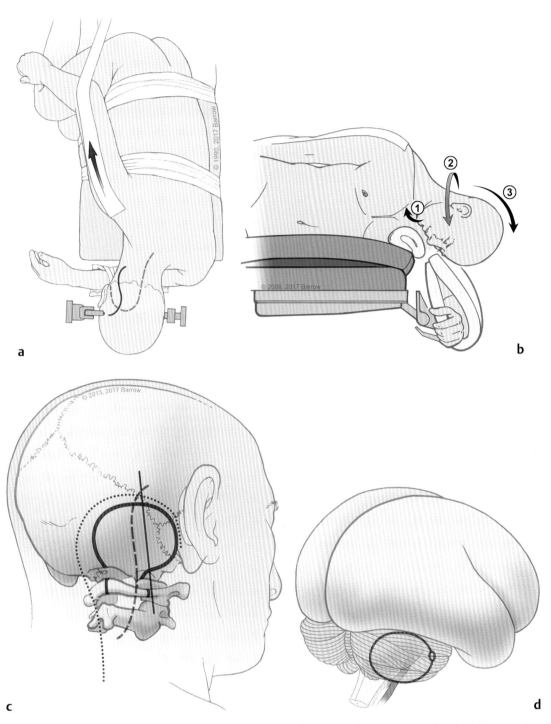

Figure 4.29. Far-lateral approach. **(a)** Patient positioning for the far-lateral approach. The utility of the modified park bench position can be augmented by taping the patient's ipsilateral shoulder (*arrow*) and thigh to the operating table, thus enabling an extended range of positions. **(b)** The head is rotated away from the side with the lesion, positioning the inferior clivus perpendicular to the floor and maximally opening the posterior cervical and suboccipital triangles. Three head and neck positioning maneuvers are required for the park bench position to facilitate exposure: flexion of the neck (*arrow 1*), rotation of the head (*arrow 2*), and downward placement of the head (*arrow 3*). **(c)** The skin incision for the far-lateral approach can be performed using a "lazy-S" incision (*dashed line*), a linear incision (*solid line*), or a hockey-stick incision (*dotted line*). The last of these is the longest incision but has the clearest landmarks and preserves muscular innervation and the occipital artery. **(d)** The craniotomy and its relationship to the cerebellum and brainstem.

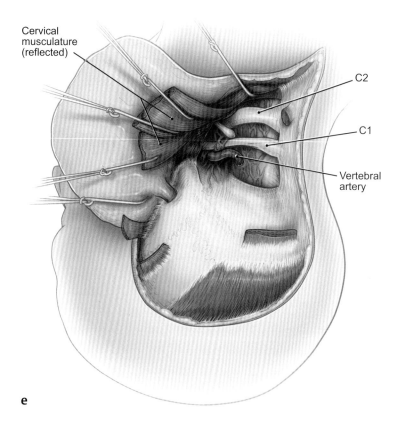

Cervical
musculature
(reflected)

C2

C1

Vertebral
artery

e

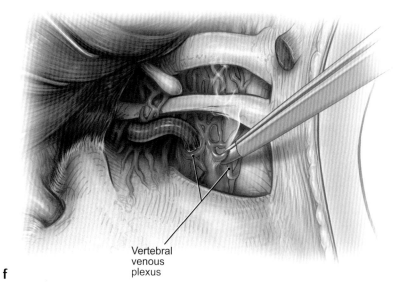

Vertebral
venous
plexus

f

Figure 4.29. (e) An inverted hockey-stick incision is used, starting at the mastoid prominence and proceeding under the superior nuchal line to the midline. The muscle is freed along the nuchal line, leaving a 1-cm edge of nuchal fascia and muscle for closure. During closure, the neck can be extended to help reapproximate the cervical musculature to the nuchal fascia. The incision is extended caudally down to the C6 spinous process when the lesion dictates this caudal extension. The paraspinous muscles are split to expose the C1 and C2 spinous processes. The muscle flap is dissected from the suboccipital bone and the C1 and C2 laminae. The muscle flap is reflected inferiorly and laterally with fishhook retractors to expose the lateral mass of C1 and the vertebral artery from C1 to its dural entry. **(f)** Care is taken in using electrocautery to coagulate the vertebral venous plexus associated with the vertebral artery to avoid injury to the vertebral artery.

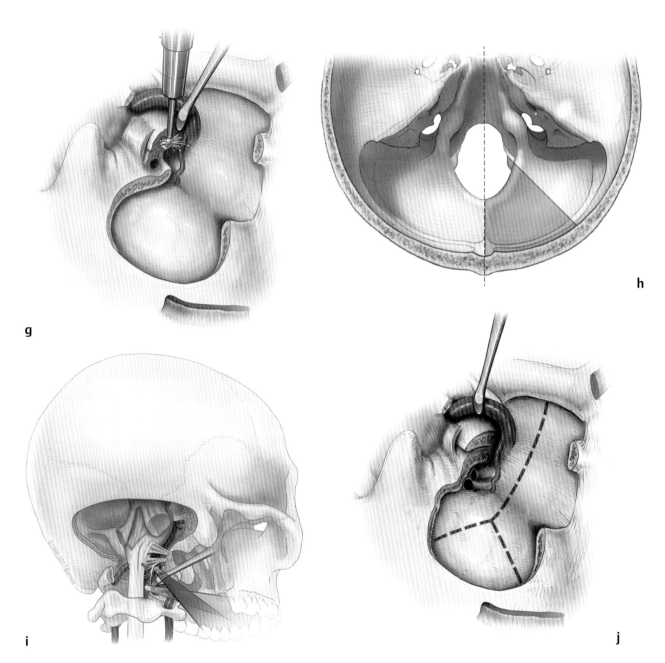

Figure 4.29. **(g)** A high-speed drill is used to remove the posterior occipital condyle. Care is also taken to avoid removing more than 50% of the condyle because excessive removal leads to instability and the need for occipitocervical fusion. The upper and medial part of the condyle may be removed without violating the atlanto-occipital joint, achieving the needed exposure while still preserving stability. Because the hypoglossal canal is situated in the anterior medial third of the occipital condyle, it should remain unharmed by the posterior condylar resection. A C1 laminectomy is performed, and the contralateral lamina is cut across the midline. The excised lamina is preserved for replacement upon completion of the procedure. Ultimately, the craniotomy overlies the lower border of the transverse sinus and courses along the sigmoid sinus. The suboccipital craniotomy is performed starting at the foramen magnum using a drill with a footplate in young patients. In older patients where the dura is adherent to the bone, a bur hole must be placed first to start the craniotomy using a footplate. **(h)** The extent of suboccipital bone removed (*green area*). **(i)** Removal of the C1 arch enables further mobilization of the vertebral artery and facilitates exposure of the lower clivus, anterior foramen magnum, anterior brainstem, and upper cervical spinal cord. **(j)** The dural opening used for the far-lateral approach (*dashed line*).

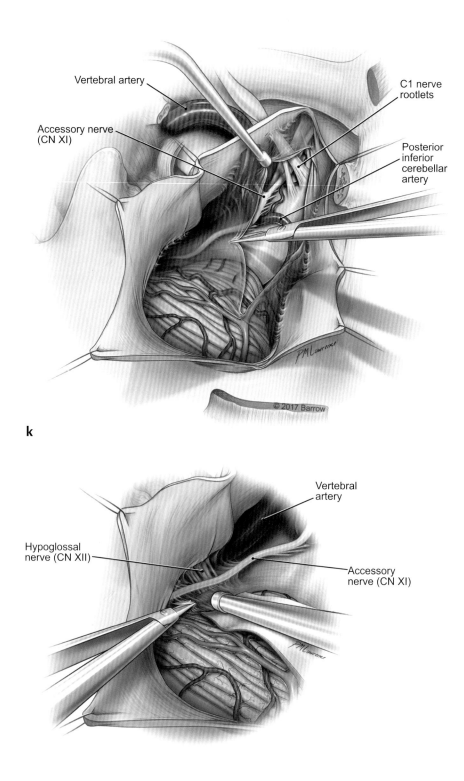

Figure 4.29. (k) The arachnoid membrane over the cisterna magna and the lateral cerebellomedullary cistern is opened. The V4 segment of the vertebral artery courses laterally to the accessory nerve (CN XI) and in front of the hypoglossal rootlets, where the posterior inferior cerebellar artery arises. **(l)** The pontine surface can be approached by dividing the arachnoid membrane covering the cerebellopontine angle cistern. Continuing the dissection ventrally leads to the premedullary cistern, providing access to the anterolateral sulcus and the olivary zone.

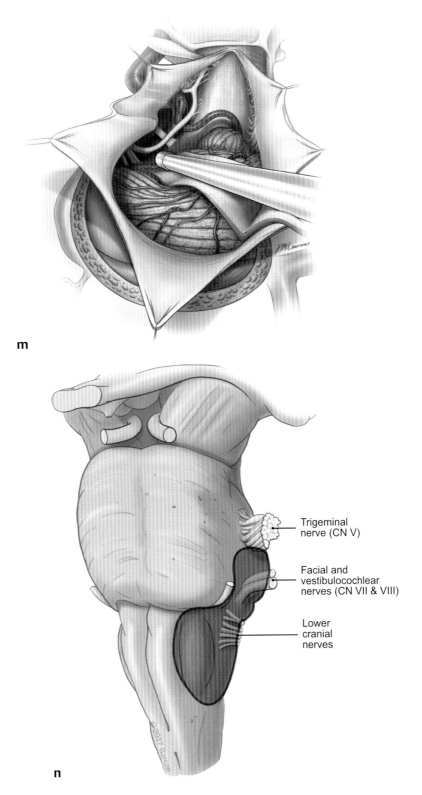

m

n

Figure 4.29. (m) Posterolateral view afforded after opening the dura and releasing cerebrospinal fluid. **(n)** Exposure (*shaded area*) of the brainstem obtained using the far-lateral approach.

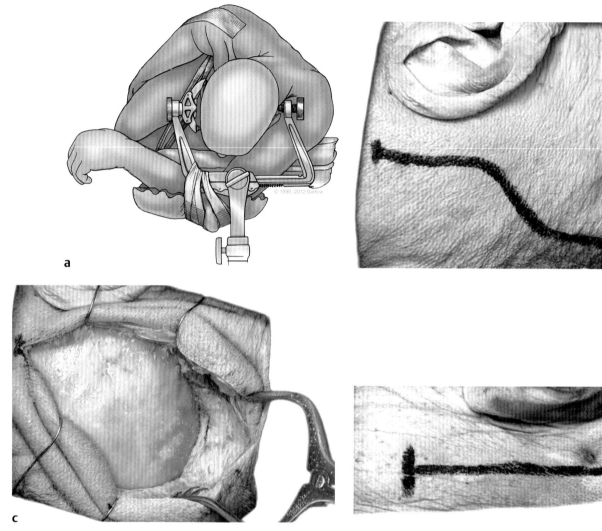

Figure 4.30. Cadaveric dissection using a far-lateral approach. **(a)** With the patient in the park bench position, the thorax is elevated 15 degrees, and the head is placed in a neutral position. Alternatively, the head may be turned 30 degrees to the contralateral side of the lesion. **(b)** The "lazy-S" incision (*black line*) starts over the mastoid, curves toward the midline, and concludes at the C2 level. This incision is typically used for patients with a thick neck.

(c) The suboccipital muscles are cut and retracted laterally to expose the occipital bone. **(d)** The linear incision (*black line*) is an alternative to the lazy-S incision. Depending on the pathology, the linear incision may be started at the level of the external acoustic meatus, pass just behind the posterior border of the sternocleidomastoid muscle, and descend to the C6 level.

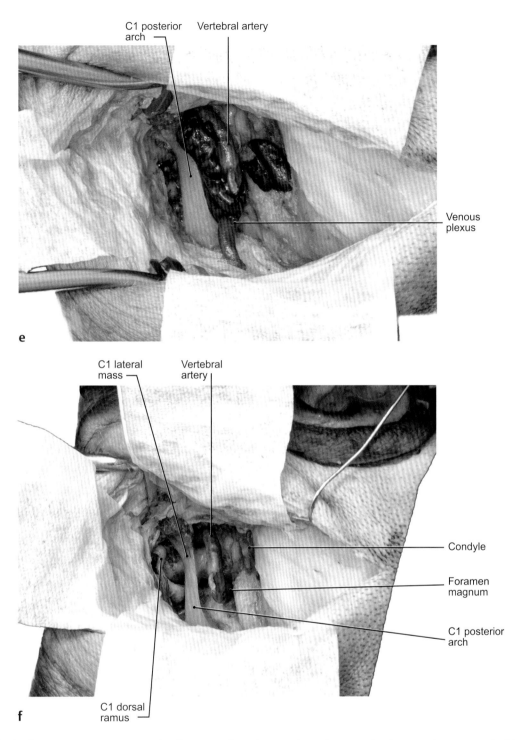

Figure 4.30. (e) The linear incision crosses the fascia and neck muscles. The vertebral artery is surrounded by adipose tissue and a prominent venous plexus. **(f)** After exposure of the vertebral artery, the subperiosteal dissection is performed laterally.

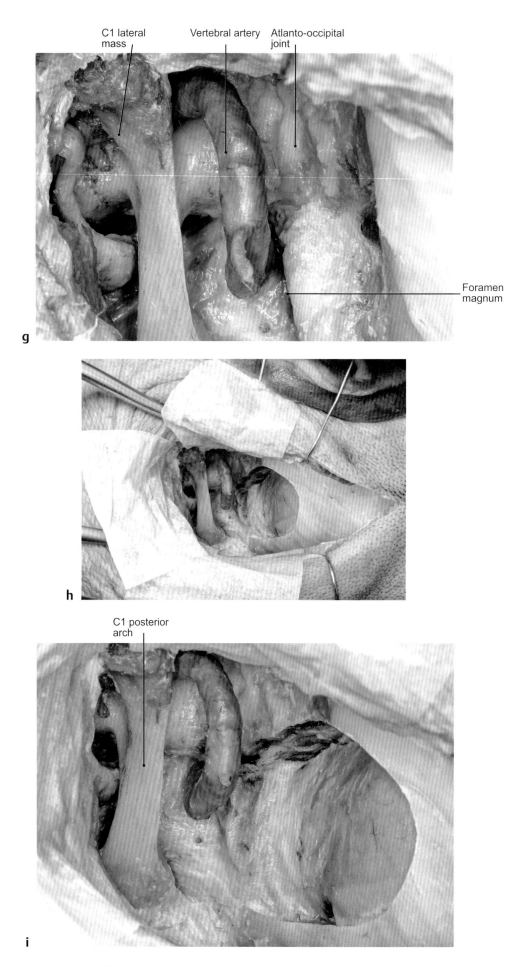

Figure 4.30. (g) Enlarged view of dissection shown in **(f)**. **(h)** The suboccipital craniotomy is performed by starting at the lateral edge of the foramen magnum. **(i)** Enlarged view of dissection shown in **(h)**.

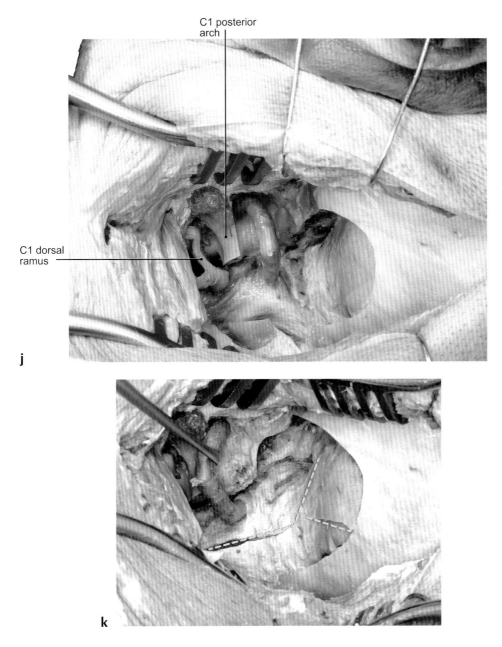

C1 posterior
arch

C1 dorsal
ramus

j

k

Figure 4.30. (j) The C1 posterior arch may be removed to provide more exposure. **(k)** The Y-shaped dural incision (*dashed lines*) is placed between the C1 level and the superolateral edge of the craniotomy.

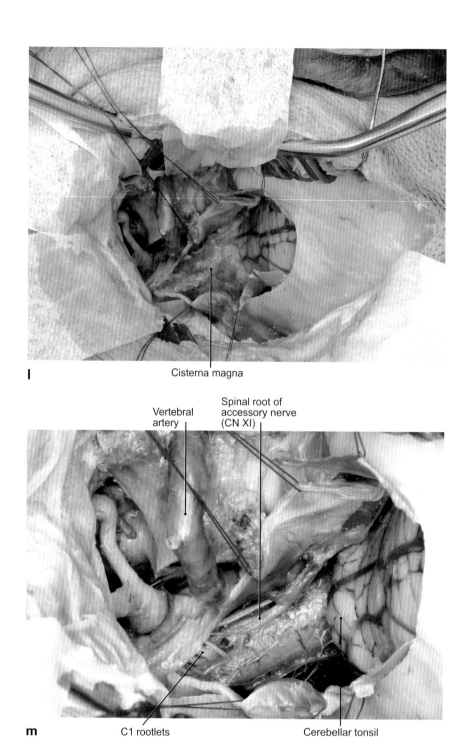

l   Cisterna magna

Vertebral
artery

Spinal root of
accessory nerve
(CN XI)

m   C1 rootlets   Cerebellar tonsil

Figure 4.30. (l) The dura is tacked up and reflected laterally, and cerebrospinal fluid is released from the cisterna magna. **(m)** Exposure of the extradural and intradural vertebral artery, cerebellar tonsil, C1 rootlets, and the spinal root of the accessory nerve (CN XI).

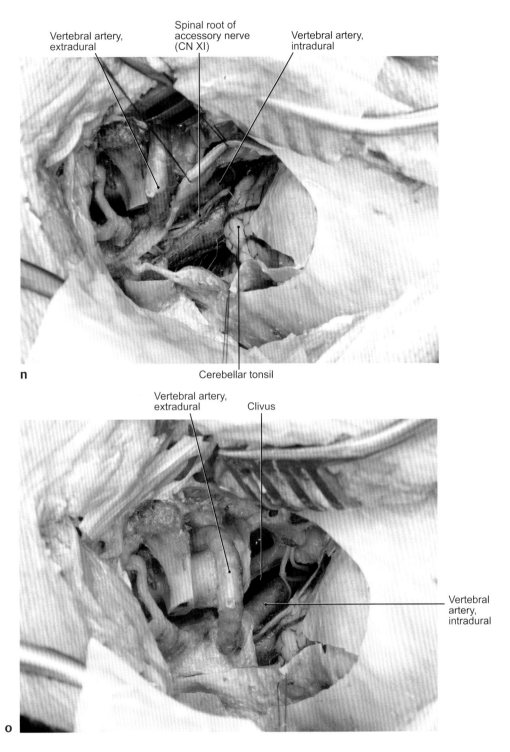

Figure 4.30. **(n)** The far-lateral transcondylar approach is a combination of the far-lateral approach and the removal of one-third of the occipital condyle. This approach provides more anteromedial exposure. **(o)** The far-lateral transcondylar approach provides exposure to premedullary and anterolateral medullary lesions, the lower one-third of the clivus, and the anterior part of the foramen magnum.

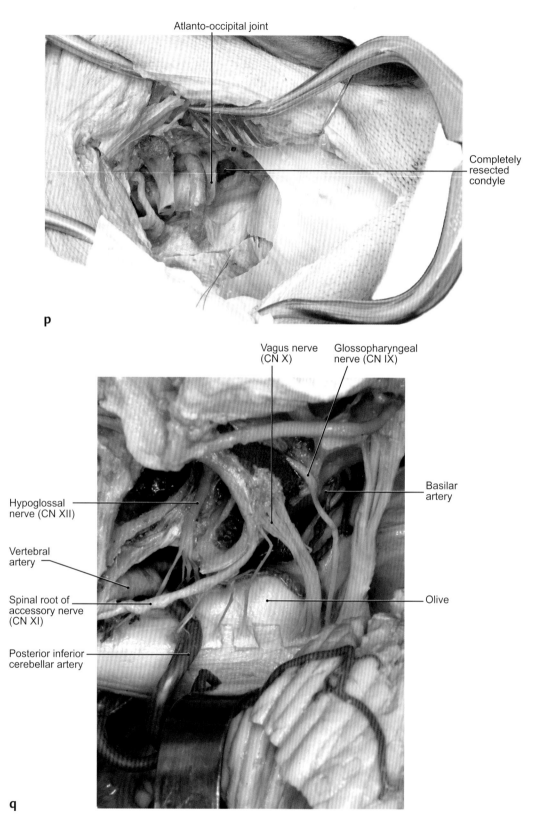

p

q

Figure 4.30. (p) The extreme far-lateral approach is a combination of the far-lateral approach and total removal of the occipital condyle. This approach is rarely needed and results in spinal instability requiring occipitocervical fusion. **(q)** Exposure after total removal of the occipital condyle.

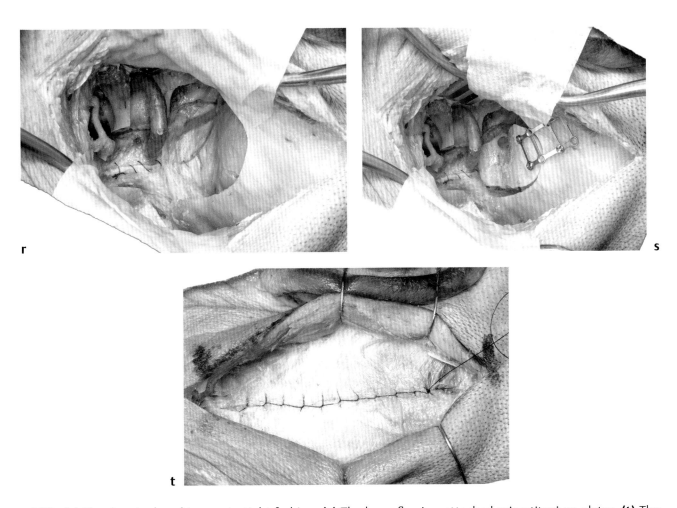

Figure 4.30. (r) The dura is closed in a watertight fashion. **(s)** The bone flap is reattached using titanium plates. **(t)** The suboccipital muscles and fascia are tightly reapproximated.

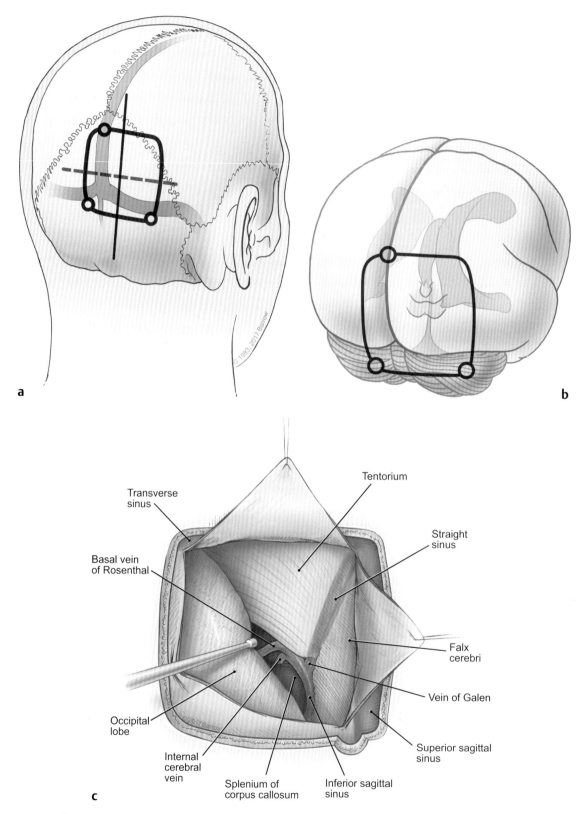

Figure 4.31. Occipital-transtentorial approach. **(a)** The skin incision(s) and craniotomy for a posterior occipital-transtentorial approach. **(b)** The relationship of the craniotomy to the ventricular system and pineal region. **(c)** The splenium of the corpus callosum is visualized after minimal retraction of the occipital lobe. The retraction can often be performed dynamically with the tip of the suction cannula. Care is taken to minimize retraction on the mesial surface of the occipital lobe because visual fibers pass through this region and can be easily damaged.

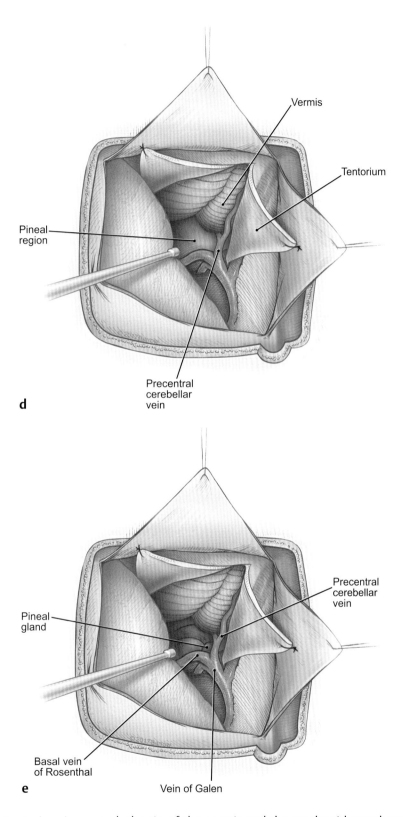

Figure 4.31. (d) After the tentorium is opened, the tip of the vermis and the arachnoid membrane of the pineal region can be seen. **(e)** The pineal gland, precentral cerebellar vein, vein of Galen, and paired basal veins of Rosenthal are visible after the arachnoid planes are opened. The precentral cerebellar vein can be sacrificed to enhance exposure.

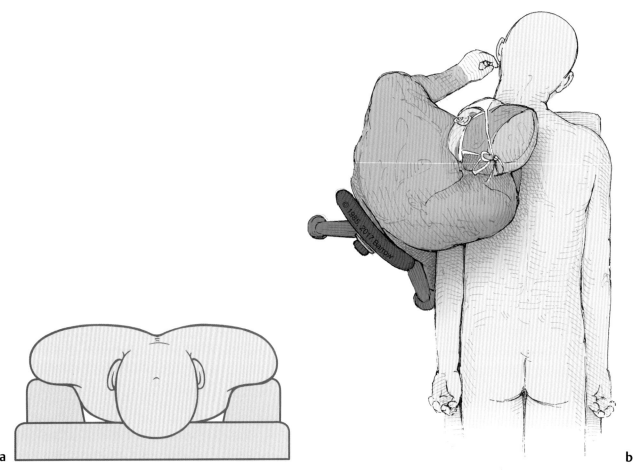

a

b

Figure 4.32. Supracerebellar infratentorial approach. **(a)** The patient is placed in the prone position with the neck flexed to expose the posterior incisura. **(b)** Alternatively, the patient can be placed in a modified Concorde position, prone, and with the head flexed and turned toward the contralateral shoulder. Then the surgeon sits behind the ipsilateral shoulder. With the operating table tilted toward the surgeon, the surgeon can remain comfortably seated for the duration of the operation. For a lateral supracerebellar infratentorial craniotomy, the patient can be placed in a supine position with the ipsilateral shoulder elevated, similar to the positioning for the retrosigmoid approach. Another option for the lateral supracerebellar infratentorial approach is to place the patient in a modified park bench position **(Figure 4.16b)**.

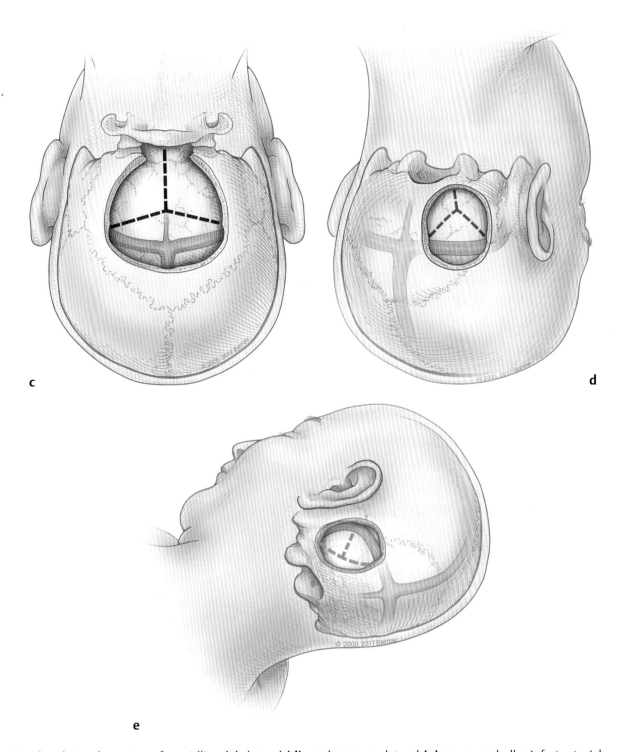

c

d

e

Figure 4.32. (c–e) Dural openings for midline **(c)**, lateral **(d)**, and extreme-lateral **(e)** supracerebellar infratentorial craniotomies (*dashed lines*).

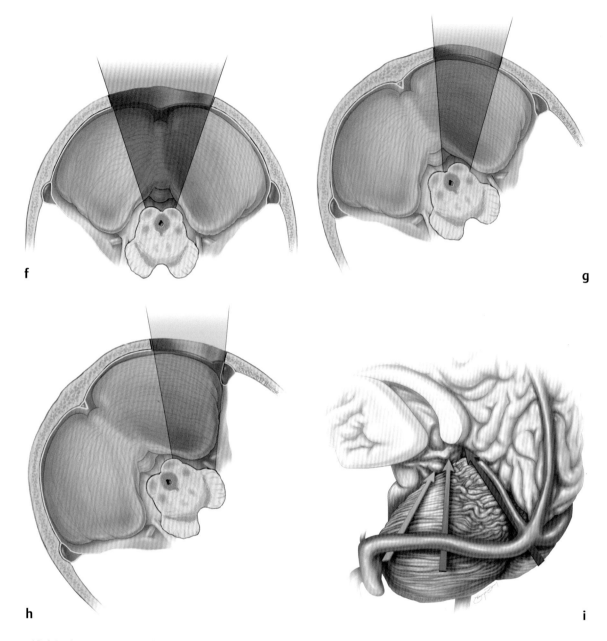

Figure 4.32. (f–h) The exposures through the midline **(f)**, lateral **(g)**, and extreme-lateral **(h)** supracerebellar infratentorial approaches to the brainstem. **(i)** The midline (*dark blue arrow*), lateral (*light blue arrow*), and extreme-lateral (*teal arrow*) supracerebellar infratentorial approaches and the trajectory afforded by each.

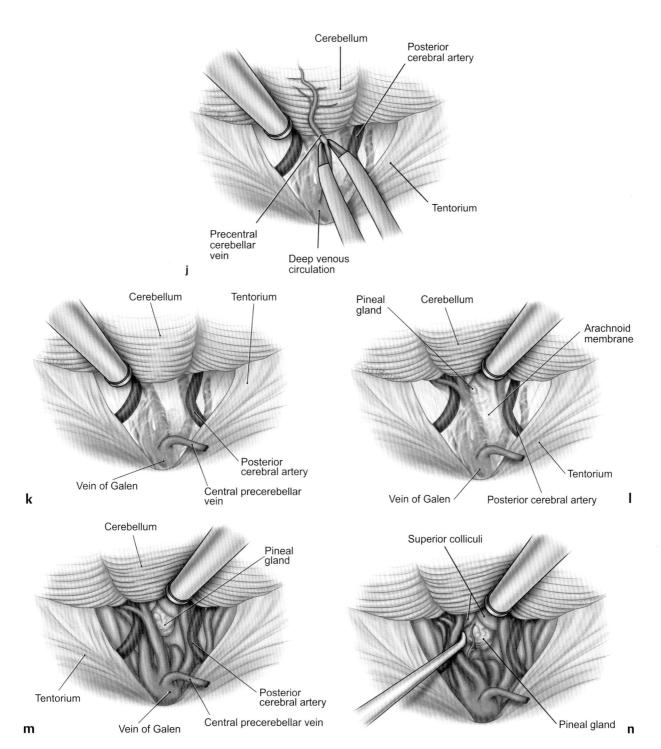

Figure 4.32. **(j)** With the midline supracerebellar infratentorial approach, upon supracerebellar dissection, the surgeon arrives at the dorsal midbrain and pineal region. Exposure to this area may be enhanced by coagulation and cutting of bridging veins to the tentorium. Here the superior vermian vein is coagulated and cut. **(k)** The arachnoid membrane overlying the pineal region and deep venous circulation is visualized. **(l)** The cerebellar hemispheres and vermis are gently retracted to expose the pineal region. When the patient is positioned properly, gravity will retract these structures. The quadrigeminal cistern rests deep in the dissection cavity. The internal cerebral and internal occipital veins, the basal veins of Rosenthal, and the vein of the cerebellomesencephalic fissure reside in the quadrigeminal cistern. **(m)** After dissection of the arachnoid membrane overlying the pineal region, the pineal gland and quadrigeminal plate can be visualized. **(n)** Further inferior dissection reveals the pineal gland and the rich network of veins surrounding it. Inferiorly, the superior colliculi are visible projecting from the quadrigeminal plate.

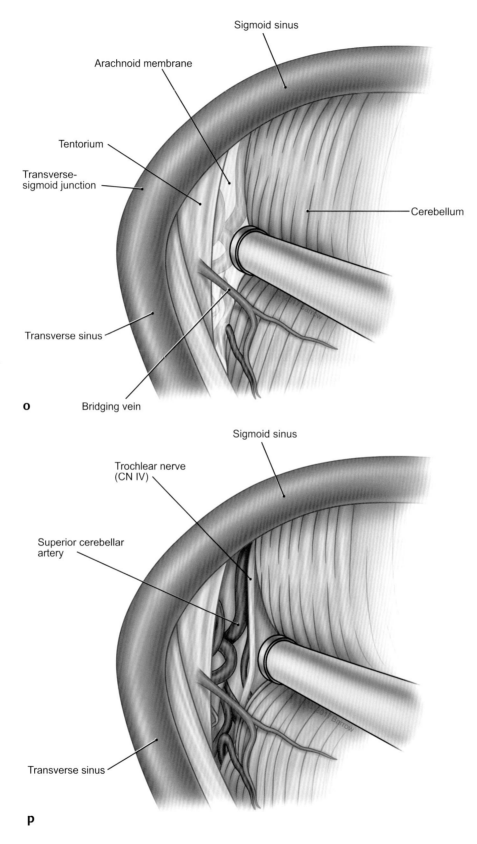

Figure 4.32. (o) In the case of the extreme-lateral supracerebellar infratentorial approach, the exposure is enhanced by cutting the arachnoid membrane along the tentorial surface of the cerebellum and by coagulating as few bridging veins as necessary to reach the cerebellomesencephalic fissure. **(p)** The ambient cistern is then opened, exposing the trochlear nerve (CN IV) running along the posterolateral midbrain, frequently close to the superior cerebellar artery.

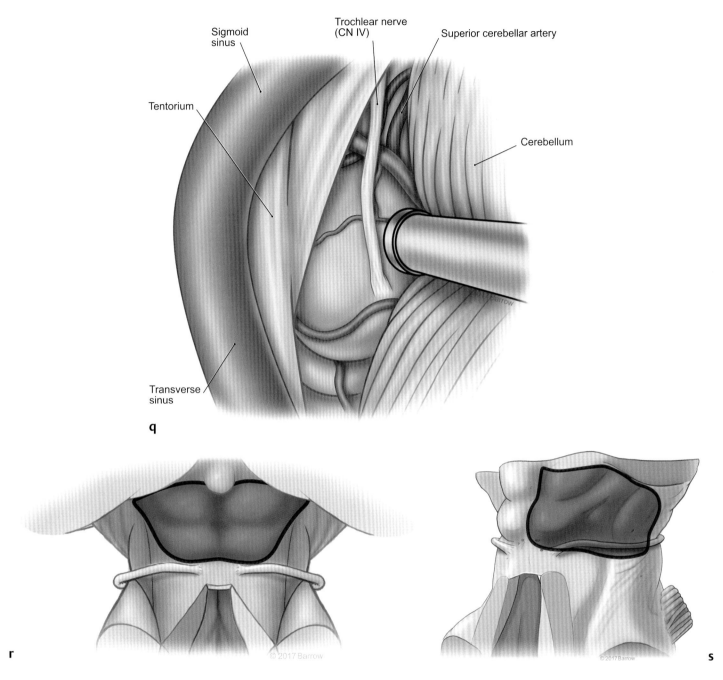

Figure 4.32. (q) Opening the quadrigeminal cistern provides an oblique approach to the collicular region. The trochlear nerve can be traced to its origin laterally, below the inferior colliculus. **(r)** The dorsal anatomy (*shaded area*) exposed by the midline supracerebellar infratentorial approach. **(s)** The dorsolateral anatomy (*shaded area*) exposed by the lateral supracerebellar infratentorial approach and the extreme-lateral supracerebellar infratentorial approach.

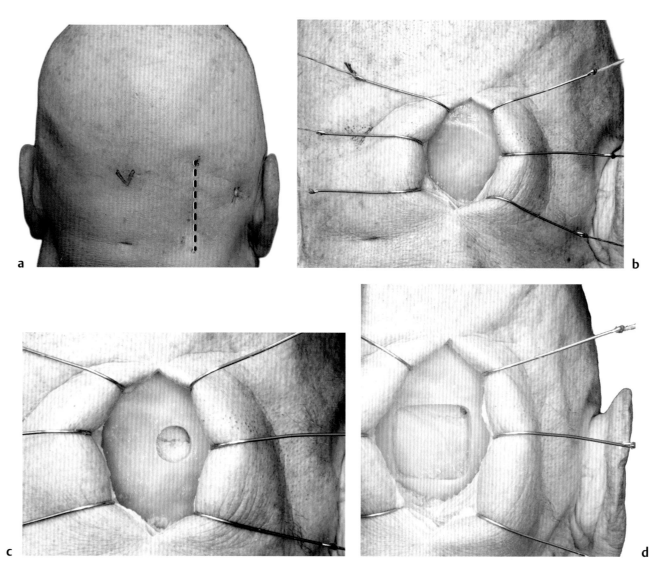

Figure 4.33. Cadaveric dissection demonstrating the supracerebellar infratentorial approach. **(a)** A vertical incision is made midway between the asterion and inion. **(b)** The suboccipital muscles are cut in the same manner as the scalp and retracted laterally with fishhook retractors. **(c)** A bur hole is placed below the superior nuchal line. **(d)** A 3 × 3-cm craniotomy is performed.

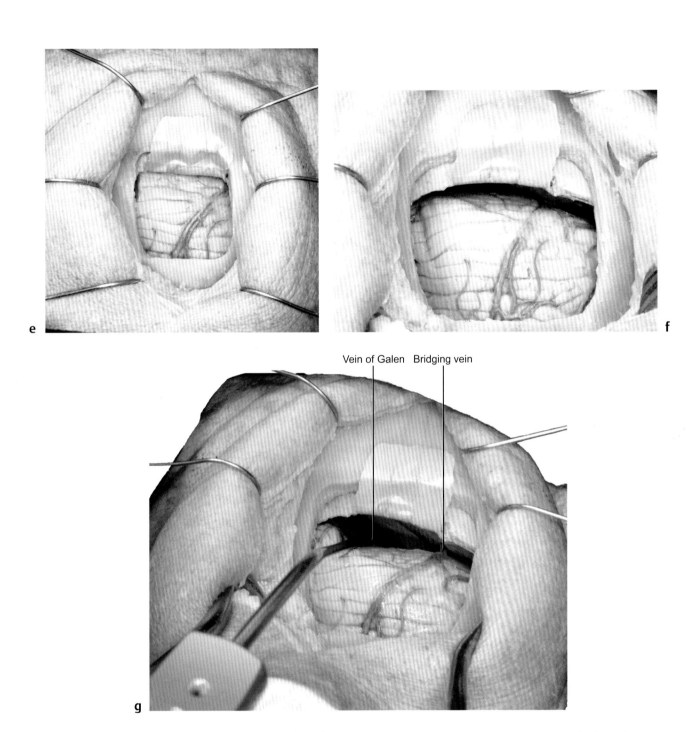

Vein of Galen   Bridging vein

Figure 4.33. **(e)** The dura is incised in a U shape with its base at the transverse sinus. **(f)** The supracerebellar infratentorial space is exposed. **(g)** The pineal region is exposed from the midline supracerebellar infratentorial approach.

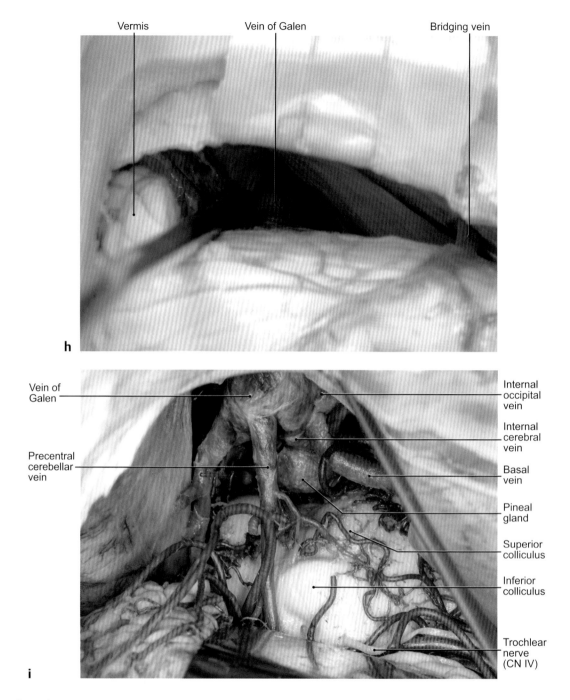

Figure 4.33. (h) Enlarged view of pineal region exposure obtained with midline supracerebellar infratentorial approach shown in **(g)**. **(i)** Magnified view of the anatomy visualized from a midline supracerebellar infratentorial approach. Note the pineal gland and the complex of deep veins intimately associated with it.

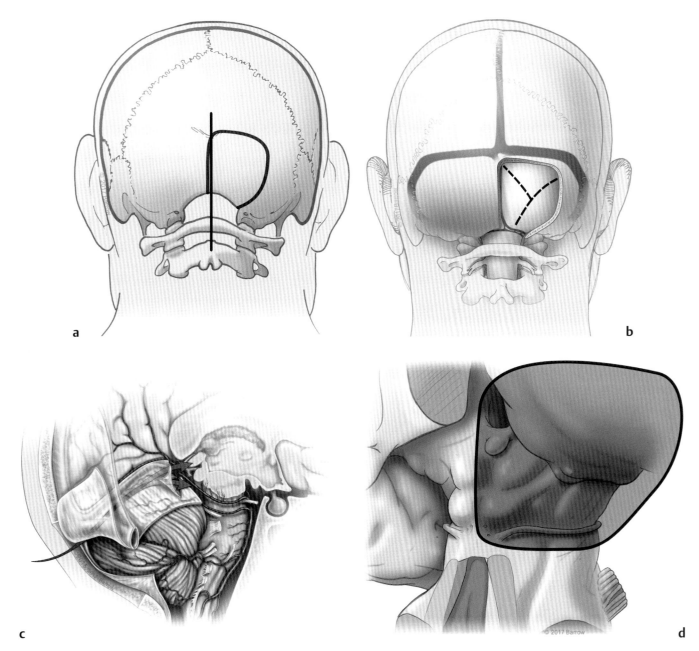

Figure 4.34. Supracerebellar transtentorial approach. **(a)** The planned scalp incision and craniotomy for the paramedian supracerebellar transtentorial approach. **(b)** The craniotomy and dural incision (*dashed lines*) for the supracerebellar transtentorial approach. **(c)** Lateral view. Coagulating and cutting the tentorium provides access to lesions in the mesial temporal lobe and the thalamus as well as the dorsal brainstem. **(d)** The dorsolateral anatomic structures (*shaded area*) exposed upon resection of the tentorium using the supracerebellar transtentorial approach.

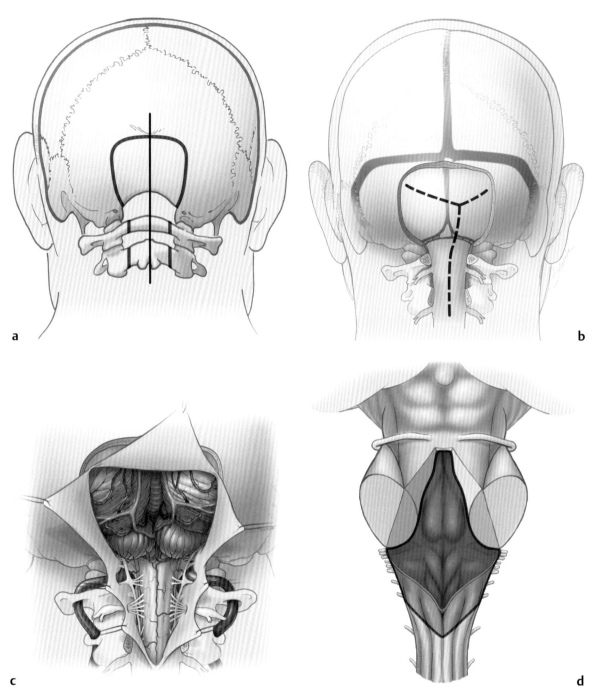

a

b

c

d

Figure 4.35. Suboccipital spinal approach. **(a)** Lesions in the cervicomedullary junction can be approached using a suboccipital spinal approach. The patient is placed prone in a position akin to that used for the standard suboccipital approach. The vertical scalp incision (*line*) overlies the posterior fossa and extends down to the cervical spine. The caudal extent of the incision depends on the extent of the lesion. **(b)** The dural opening (*dashed lines*) used for the suboccipital spinal approach. **(c)** A dorsal view, after the dura is opened, of the cervicomedullary junction and upper cervical spine, with relative orientation of the vertebral artery, spinal nerve roots, and lower cranial nerves. **(d)** The extent of the anatomic exposure (*shaded area*) afforded by the suboccipital spinal approach.

Table 4.1. Approaches to Lesions in Specific Regions of the Brainstem

Lesion Location	Anterior	Lateral	Posterior
Midbrain	• Pterional ± orbitozygomatic osteotomies	• Anterolateral: pterional ± orbitozygomatic osteotomies • Posterolateral: paramedian or extreme-lateral supracerebellar infratentorial	• Median supracerebellar infratentorial
Pons	• Pterional ± orbitozygomatic osteotomies • Subtemporal ± transtentorial extension • Retrolabyrinthine • Retrosigmoid	• Retrosigmoid	• Suboccipital telovelar • Suboccipital
Medulla	• Far-lateral • Retrosigmoid	• Far-lateral • Retrosigmoid	• Suboccipital telovelar • Suboccipital

5 Case Examples

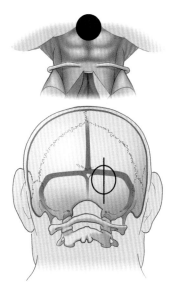

Case 5.1

- Diagnosis: Pineal cyst (related anatomy: pp. **10, 11, 38–47**)

- Preoperative examination: Neurologically intact

- Approach: Right paramedian keyhole endoscopic-assisted supracerebellar infratentorial (related approach: pp. **238–246**)

- Positioning: Sitting

- Monitoring: Somatosensory evoked potentials

- Outcome: Complete removal of the cyst; patient is neurologically intact, with resolution of headaches.

See Video 5.1

Figure 5.1. A 33-year-old woman presented with a long history of migraines.

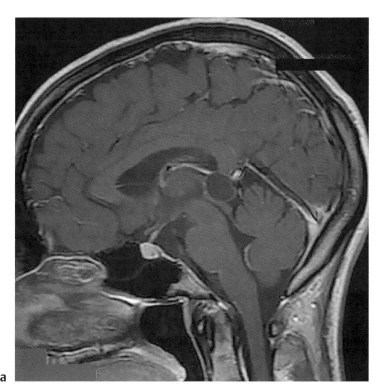
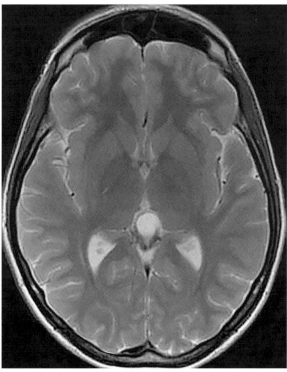

a   b

Figure 5.1. (a) Sagittal T1-weighted magnetic resonance image with contrast and **(b)** axial T2-weighted magnetic resonance image demonstrate a pineal region mass causing tectal compression; imaging characteristics are consistent with a 1.6-cm pineal cyst.

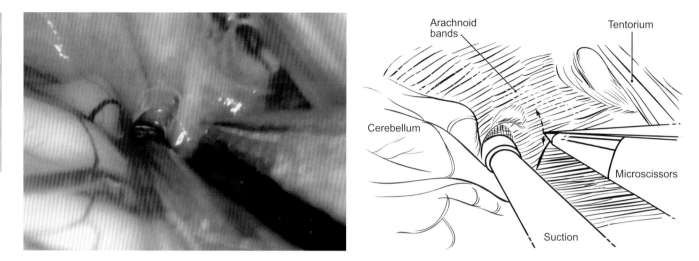

Figure 5.1. (c) The patient is placed in a sitting position, and a right keyhole, endoscopic-assisted, supracerebellar infratentorial craniotomy is performed. The arachnoid bands between the cerebellum and tentorium are sharply cut, and the opening is widened using the microscissors (*dashed line*), enabling the cerebellum to fall away from the tentorium to provide a surgical corridor to the pineal region.

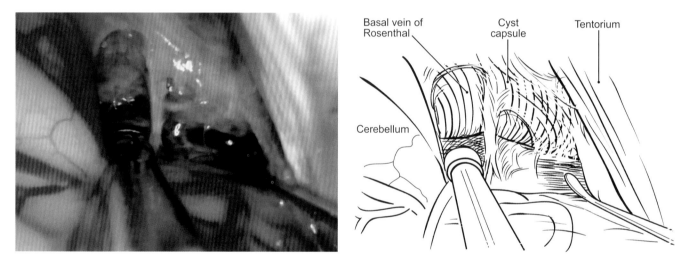

Figure 5.1. (d) Further dissection exposes the pineal region and the complex of deep veins.

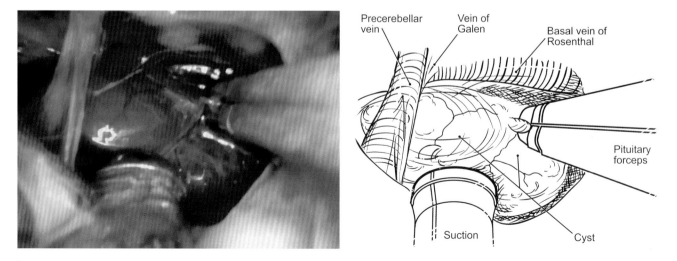

Figure 5.1. (e) Mobilization of the veins exposes the pineal cyst, containing hemosiderin-stained cystic fluid. With the endoscope held by an assistant, four-handed endoscopy is performed, and the lesion is dissected circumferentially. The suction cannula provides countertraction while the pituitary forceps are used to roll the lesion away from adjacent points of connection.

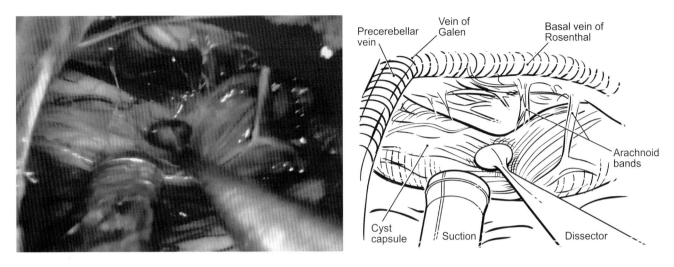

Figure 5.1. (f) The cyst is mobilized off the arachnoid bands connecting it to the tectum and brainstem.

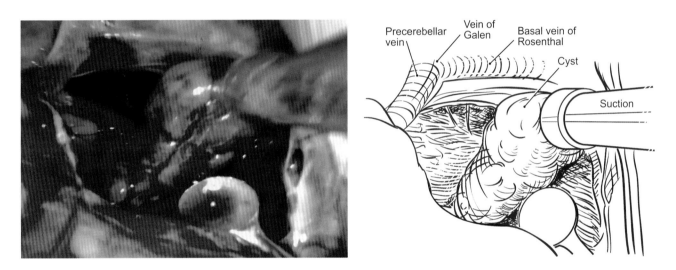

Figure 5.1. (g) After being freed circumferentially, the lesion is removed.

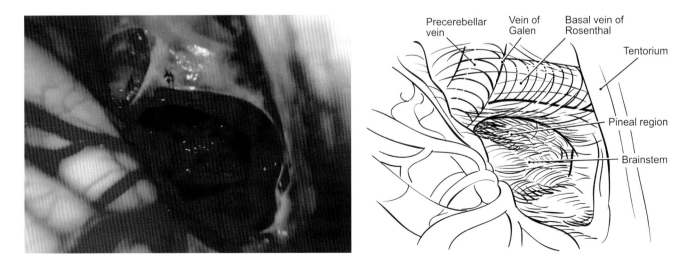

Figure 5.1. (h) Final view of the resection cavity shows complete removal of the tumor.

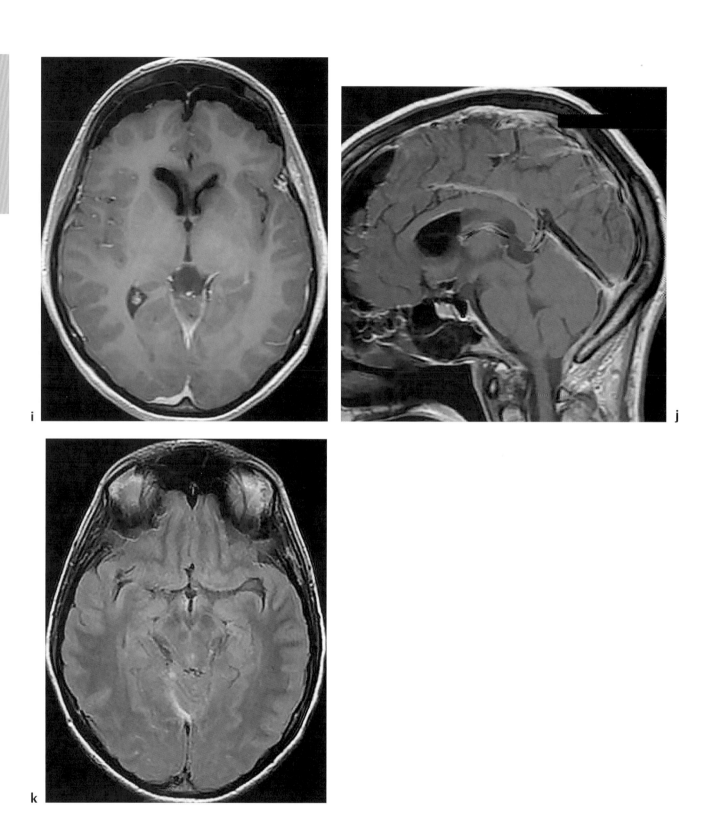

Figure 5.1. Postoperative **(i)** axial and **(j)** sagittal T1-weighted magnetic resonance images with contrast and **(k)** axial fluid-attenuated inversion recovery (FLAIR) magnetic resonance image confirm gross-total removal of the pineal cyst.

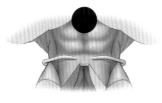

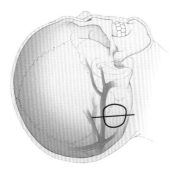

Case 5.2

- Diagnosis: Pineal cyst (related anatomy: pp. **10, 11, 38–47**)
- Preoperative examination: Neurologically intact
- Approach: Right paramedian keyhole supracerebellar infratentorial (related approach: pp. **238–246**)
- Positioning: Left-sided park bench position
- Monitoring: Somatosensory evoked potentials
- Outcome: Complete removal of the cyst; patient has resolution of symptoms and is neurologically intact.

See Video 5.2

Figure 5.2. A 42-year-old woman presented with headaches, visual disturbance, and diplopia.

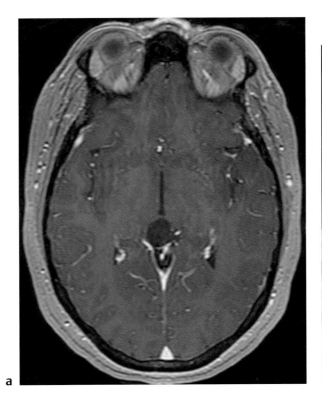

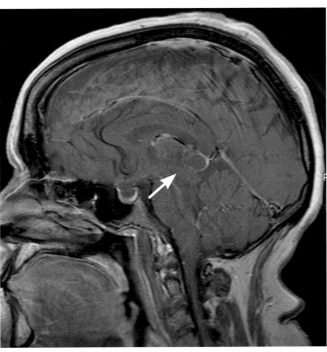

a   b

Figure 5.2. (a) Axial and **(b)** sagittal T1-weighted magnetic resonance images with contrast demonstrate a pineal region cyst with compression of the tectum (**b,** *arrow*).

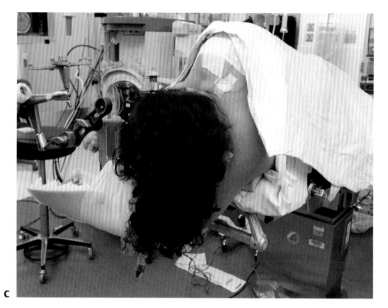

c

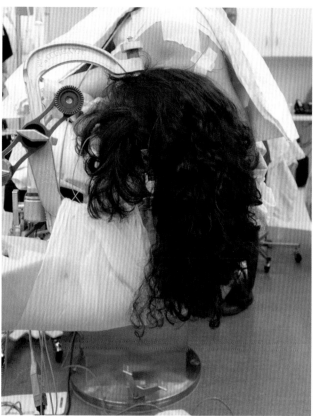

d

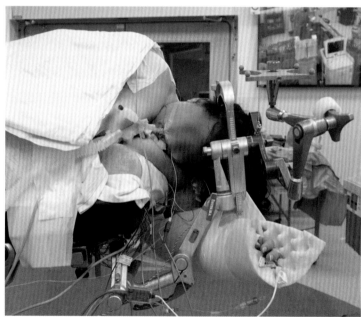

e

Figure 5.2. **(c–e)** Intraoperative photographs demonstrate patient positioning for this lateral supracerebellar infratentorial approach. The patient can be placed supine with the shoulder elevated or can be placed in the park bench position (as depicted). **(d)** The patient's head is flexed slightly to the left to enable gravity retraction of the cerebellum. **(e)** For patients with large breasts or a barrel chest, the park bench position enables the surgeon to optimize the opening of the angle between the head and the shoulder, which facilitates surgeon comfort during the operation. The subtle flexion of the neck toward the floor enables the cerebellum to fall away from the tentorium upon the disconnection of the arachnoid membrane and the release of cerebrospinal fluid.

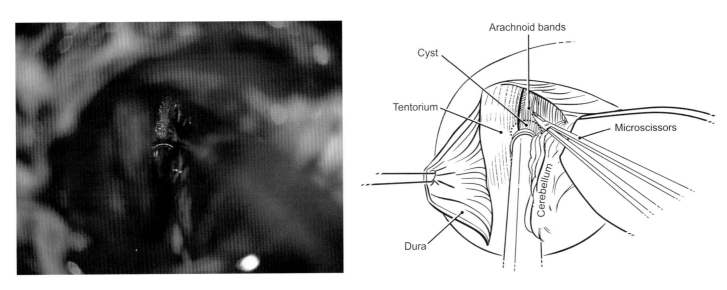

Figure 5.2. (f) After the right supracerebellar infratentorial craniotomy is performed, the arachnoid bands connecting the cerebellum to the tentorium are sharply cut to expand the space above the cerebellum and to arrive at the deep venous complex and the pineal region where the cyst (*dotted line*) is located.

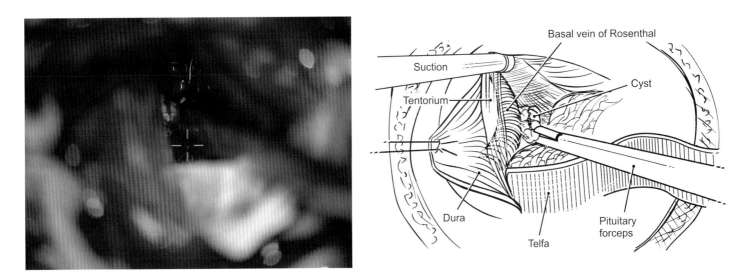

Figure 5.2. (g) The cyst is debulked and resected piecemeal to avoid damaging the deep venous circulation.

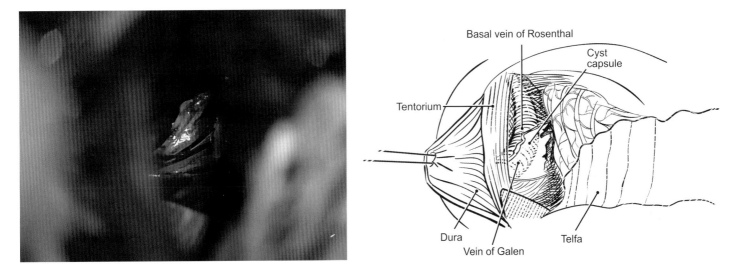

Figure 5.2. (h) Resecting the cyst often requires sharp dissection of the cyst capsule from the deep veins. After removal of the cyst contents, the remnant can be sharply resected from the veins.

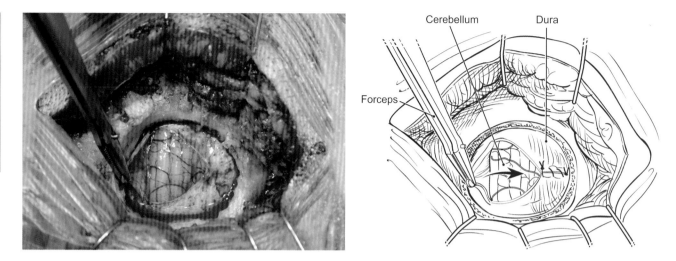

Figure 5.2. (i) Intraoperative photograph and illustration show the size of the opening and the stepwise closure of the dura.

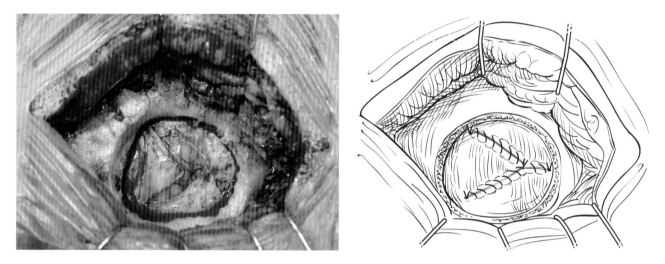

Figure 5.2. (j) Watertight closure of the dura is essential to prevent leakage of cerebrospinal fluid after operations in the posterior fossa. When the dura is damaged, graft material should be used to complete the dural closure.

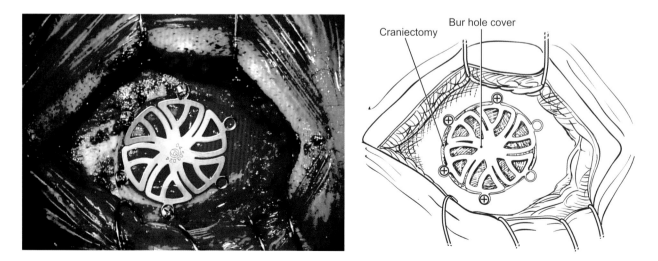

Figure 5.2. (k) Intraoperative photograph and illustration show how a single large bur hole cover can be used to repair a skull defect.

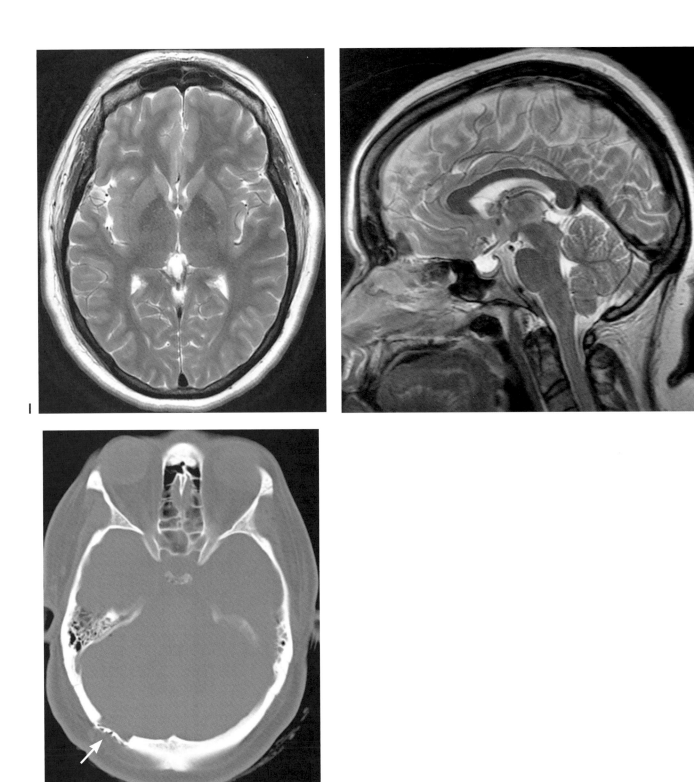

Figure 5.2. Postoperative **(l)** axial and **(m)** sagittal T2-weighted magnetic resonance images demonstrate complete resection of the lesion and decompression of the tectum. **(n)** Postoperative axial computed tomogram demonstrates the size and location of the craniotomy (*arrow*) needed to approach this lesion using the lateral supracerebellar infratentorial approach.

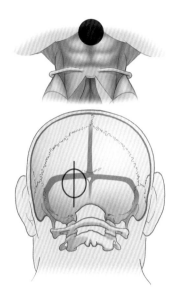

Case 5.3

- Diagnosis: Pineal parenchymal tumor (related anatomy: pp. **10, 11, 38–47**)
- Preoperative examination: Neurologically intact
- Approach: Left lateral keyhole endoscopic-assisted supracerebellar infratentorial (related approach: pp. **238–246**)
- Positioning: Sitting
- Monitoring: Somatosensory evoked potentials
- Outcome: Complete resection of tumor; patient is neurologically intact but later required shunting.

See Video 5.3

Figure 5.3. A 24-year-old woman presented with headaches.

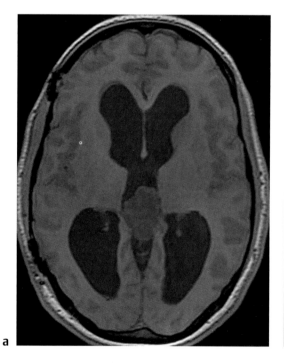
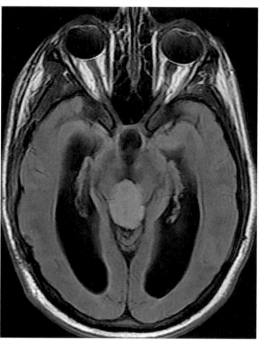

a   b

Figure 5.3. Axial T1-weighted magnetic resonance images **(a)** without and **(b)** with contrast and **(c)** sagittal T2-weighted magnetic resonance image demonstrate a large pineal mass with significant compression of the tectum. The lesion is accessed using a left lateral keyhole endoscopic-assisted, supracerebellar infratentorial approach with the patient in the sitting position.

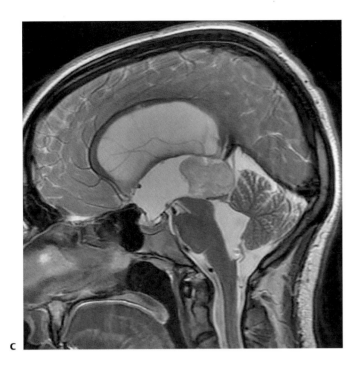

c

Figure 5.3. (*Continued*)

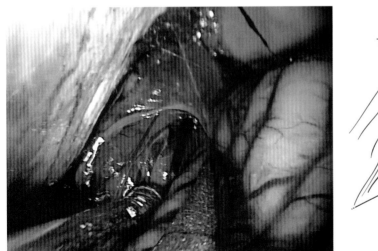

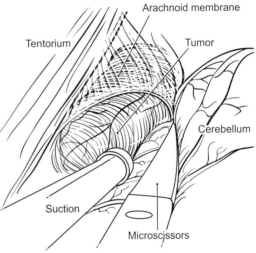

Figure 5.3. (**d**) Dissection of the arachnoid membrane develops the supracerebellar infratentorial path to the pineal region. The pineal tumor is visible beneath the arachnoid membrane. In this four-handed endoscopic resection, the surgeon uses microscissors and suction to perform dissection of the arachnoid bands, while the assistant maneuvers the endoscope.

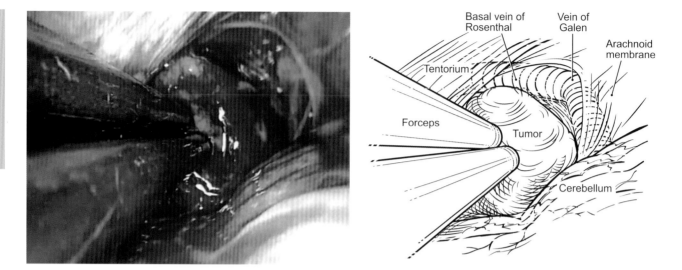

Figure 5.3. (e) The tumor is visualized, and a biopsy specimen is obtained. Long angled instruments are essential for carrying out dissection at this depth. The tumor is debulked internally and mobilized from adjacent deep veins.

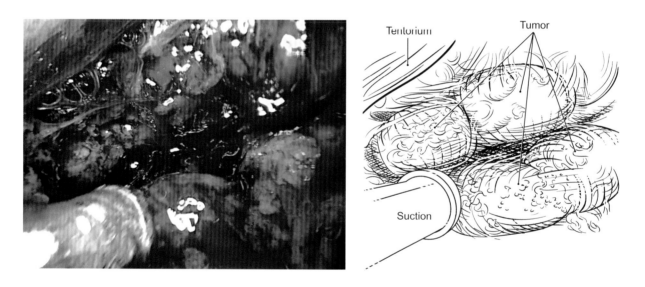

Figure 5.3. (f) Suction is used to keep the operative field clear and to provide countertraction on the tumor.

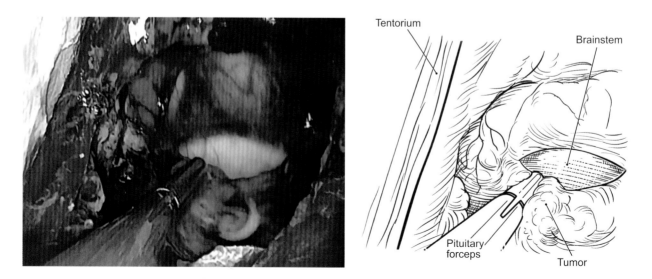

Figure 5.3. (g) Pituitary forceps are used to remove the tumor piecemeal, gradually exposing the brainstem beyond the tumor.

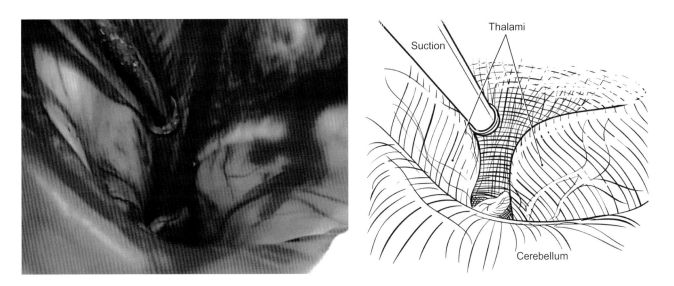

Figure 5.3. **(h)** The final tumor cavity is inspected, and hemostasis is obtained.

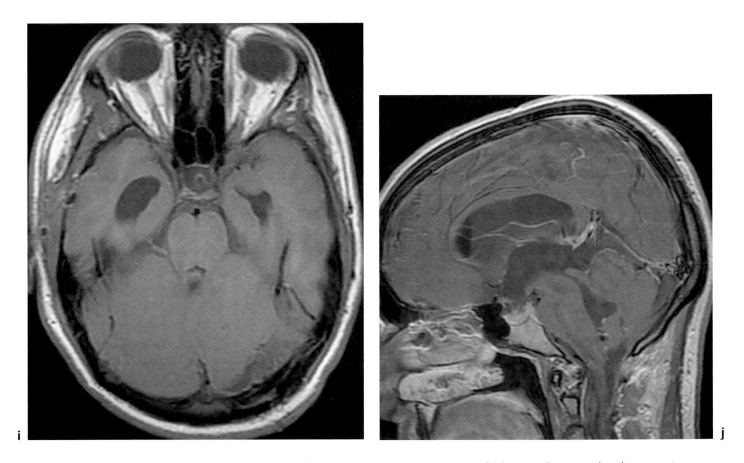

Figure 5.3. (i,j) Postoperative **(i)** axial T1-weighted magnetic resonance image and **(j)** sagittal T1-weighted magnetic resonance image with contrast confirm gross-total resection of the tumor.

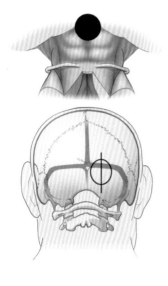

Case 5.4

- Diagnosis: Pineal cavernous malformation (related anatomy: pp. **10, 11, 38–47**)

- Preoperative examination: Neurologically intact

- Approach: Right paramedian endoscopic-assisted supracerebellar infratentorial (related approach: pp. **238–246**)

- Positioning: Sitting

- Monitoring: Somatosensory evoked potentials

- Outcome: Complete removal of the lesion; patient is at neurologic baseline, with persistent diplopia that gradually resolved.

See Video 5.4 and Animation 5.1

Figure 5.4. A 31-year-old man presented with a history of headaches and difficulty with eye movement.

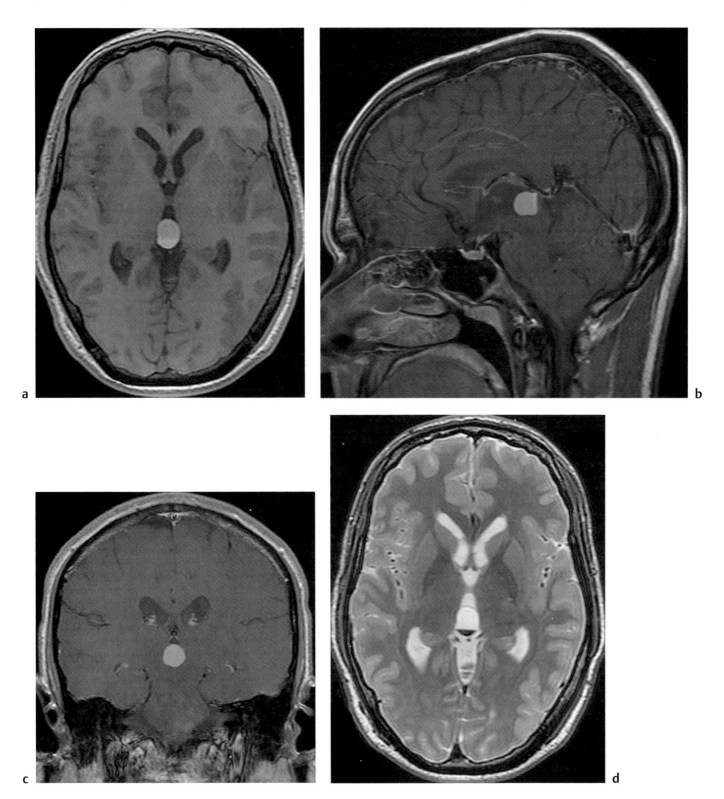

Figure 5.4. **(a)** Axial, **(b)** sagittal, and **(c)** coronal T1-weighted and **(d)** axial T2-weighted magnetic resonance images demonstrate a pineal region mass with layers of liquid contents of different densities in a cyst capsule and evidence of hemorrhage. The differential diagnosis was a pineal region cyst or a pineal tumor.

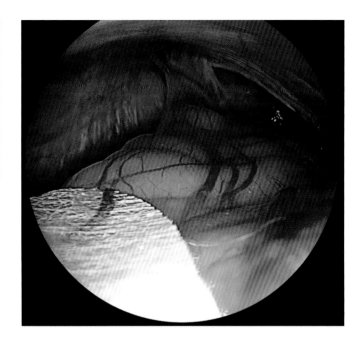

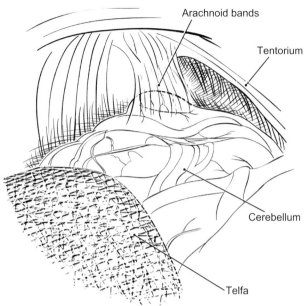

Figure 5.4. (e) The lesion was accessed using a right paramedian endoscopic-assisted, supracerebellar infratentorial approach with the patient in the sitting position. The lesion was approached a few centimeters off the midline to maximize the use of the slope of the tentorium to arrive at the pineal region while minimizing retraction of the cerebellum. A small piece of Telfa is placed on the cerebellum to keep it moist, and gravity retraction is used to develop the potential space between the cerebellum and the tentorium by disconnecting the arachnoid bands, mobilizing veins draining to the tentorium, and releasing cerebrospinal fluid.

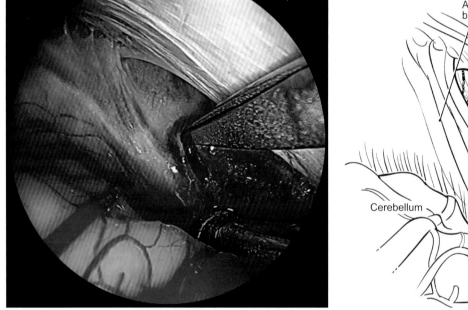

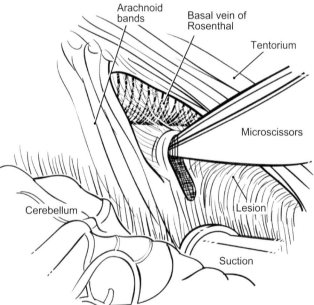

Figure 5.4. (f) Sharp dissection is used to release the arachnoid bands overlying the pineal region.

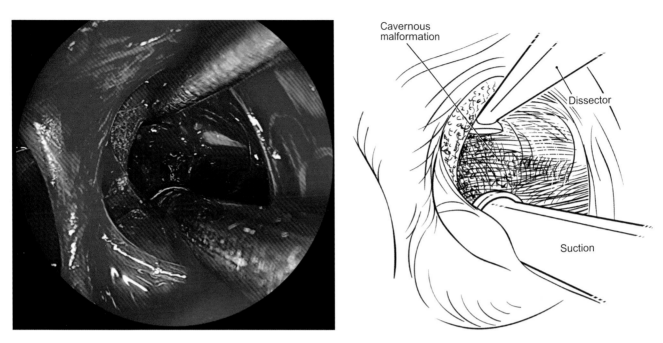

Figure 5.4. (g) This maneuver exposes the pineal region and enables the surgeon to obtain a biopsy of the lesion. In this case, histological analysis of the biopsy specimen identified the lesion as a cavernous malformation.

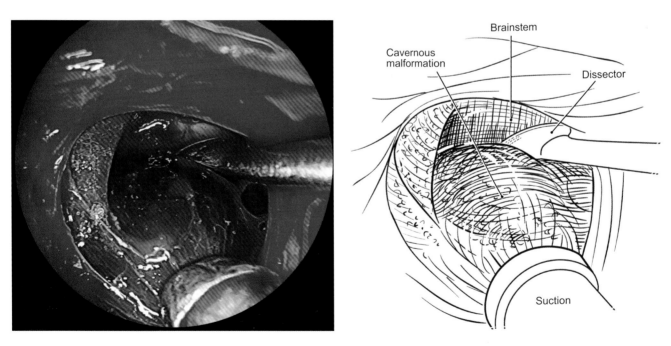

Figure 5.4. (h) The lesion is mobilized with a microdissector and removed piecemeal. Suction is used to mobilize the lesion while the microdissector is used to peel the lesion from the brainstem.

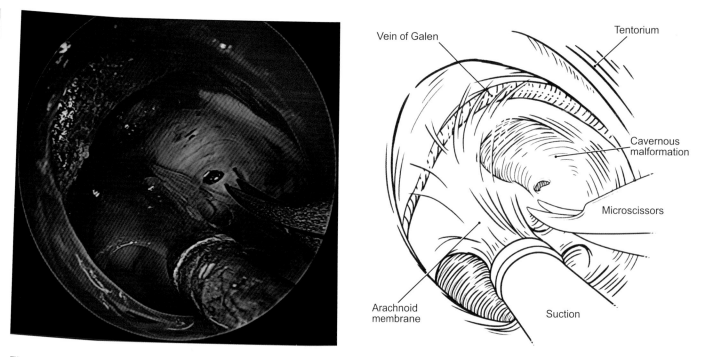

Figure 5.4. (i) Arachnoid bands are sharply cut with microscissors.

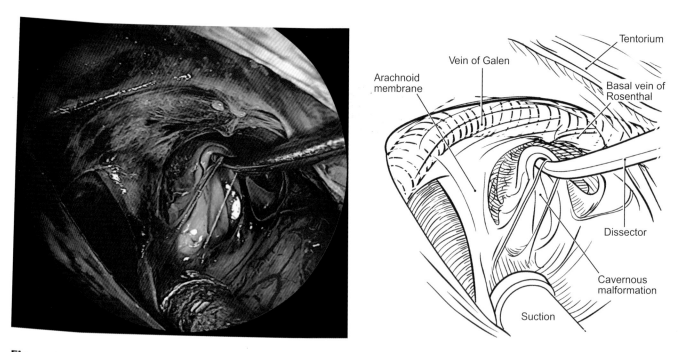

Figure 5.4. (j) The cavernous malformation adherent to the deep venous circulation is sharply mobilized using microdissectors and is ultimately removed using pituitary forceps.

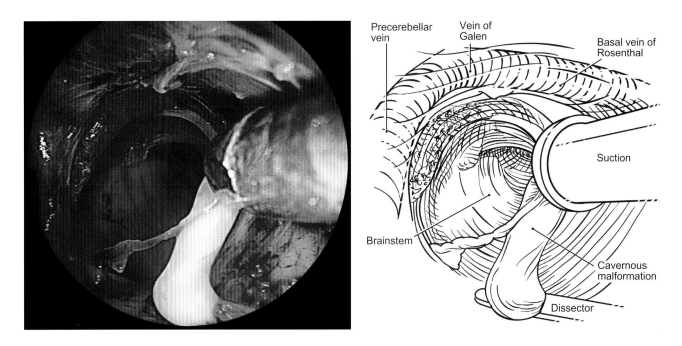

Labels: Precerebellar vein, Vein of Galen, Basal vein of Rosenthal, Suction, Brainstem, Cavernous malformation, Dissector

Figure 5.4. (k) Any remnant of the cavernous malformation is peeled from the cavity and removed.

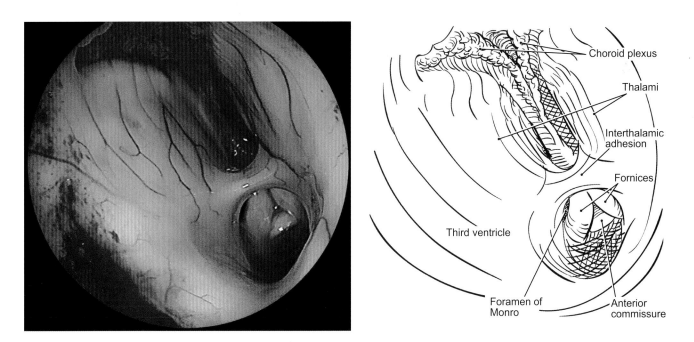

Labels: Choroid plexus, Thalami, Interthalamic adhesion, Fornices, Third ventricle, Foramen of Monro, Anterior commissure

Figure 5.4. (l) The removal of the lesion and the use of an angled endoscope make possible better views of the ventricular system as it narrows to the aqueduct of Sylvius.

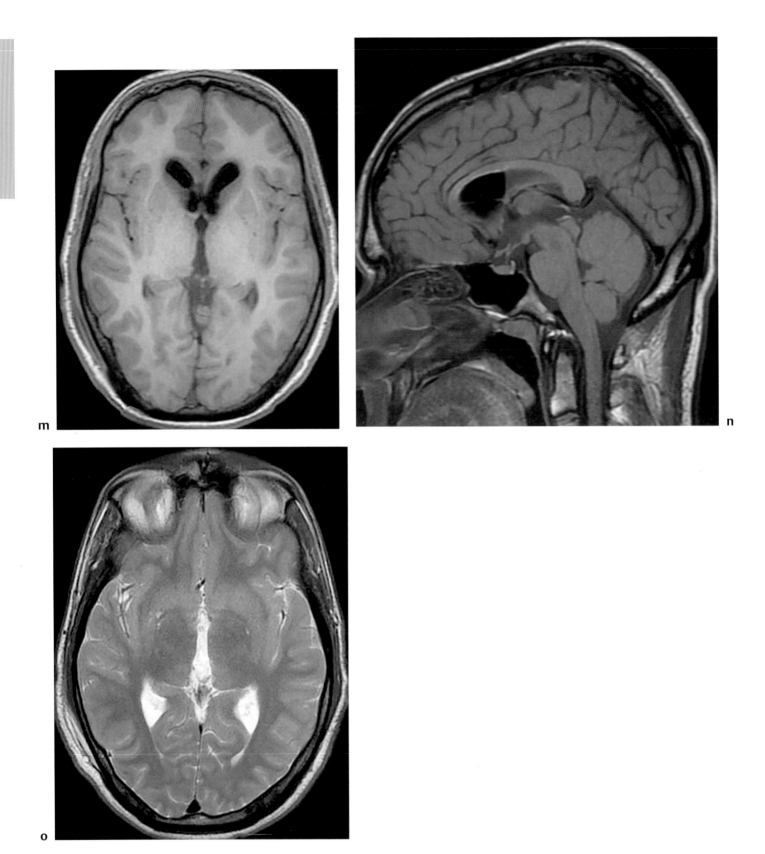

Figure 5.4. Postoperative **(m)** axial and **(n)** sagittal T1-weighted and **(o)** axial T2-weighted magnetic resonance images demonstrate complete removal of the cavernous malformation.

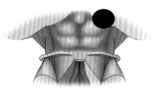
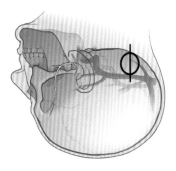

Case 5.5

- Diagnosis: Right posterior thalamic cavernous malformation (related anatomy: pp. **9–12, 14–16**)
- Preoperative examination: Neurologically intact
- Approach: Right lateral supracerebellar transtentorial (related approach: p. **247**)
- Positioning: Prone
- Monitoring: Somatosensory evoked potentials
- Outcome: Complete removal of the lesion; patient is neurologically intact.

See Video 5.5

Figure 5.5. A 10-year-old girl with a family history of cavernous malformations presented with a recent history of headaches and diplopia.

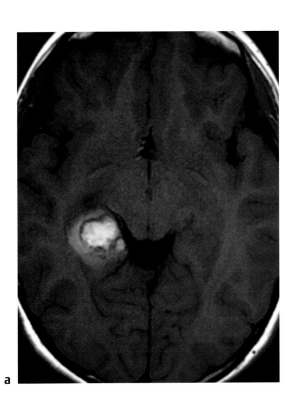
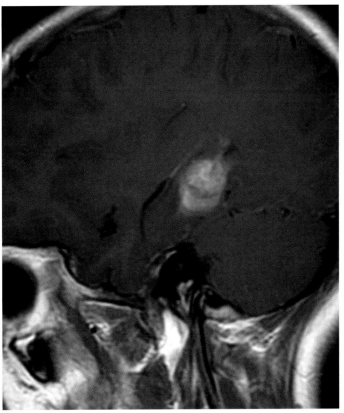

a   b

Figure 5.5. **(a)** Axial and **(b)** sagittal T1-weighted magnetic resonance images and **(c)** coronal gradient-echo magnetic resonance image show a right posterior thalamic cavernous malformation with evidence of hemorrhage.

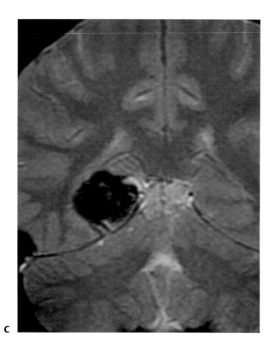

c

Figure 5.5 (*Continued*)

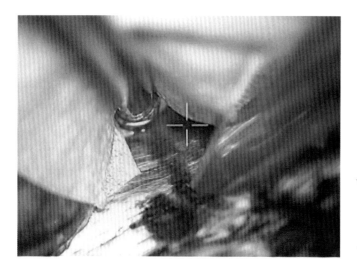

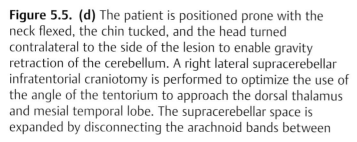

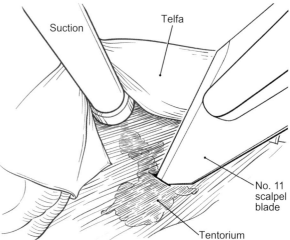

Figure 5.5. (d) The patient is positioned prone with the neck flexed, the chin tucked, and the head turned contralateral to the side of the lesion to enable gravity retraction of the cerebellum. A right lateral supracerebellar infratentorial craniotomy is performed to optimize the use of the angle of the tentorium to approach the dorsal thalamus and mesial temporal lobe. The supracerebellar space is expanded by disconnecting the arachnoid bands between the cerebellum and the tentorium. The tentorium is then coagulated and cut to expose the supratentorial compartment. It is important not to incise the entire tentorium and to coagulate and cut only the tentorium immediately adjacent to the lesion. Care must also be exercised to prevent injury to the trochlear nerve (CN IV), which abuts the tentorial edge.

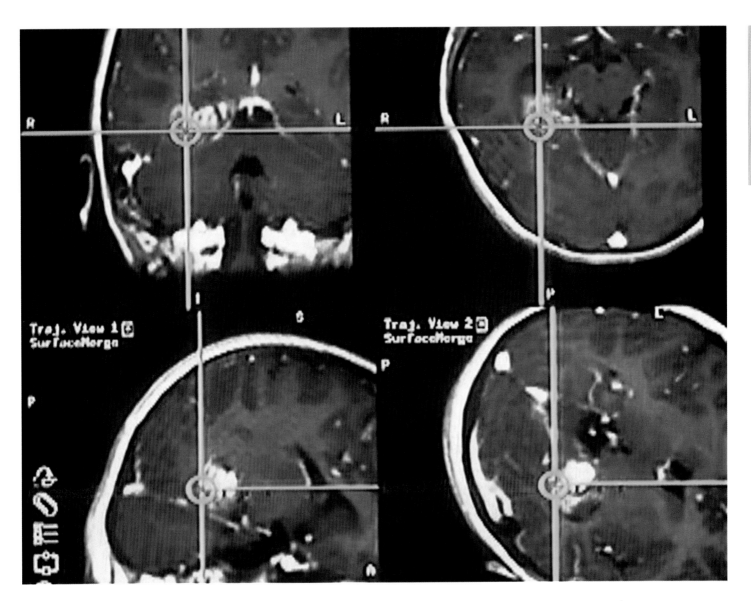

Figure 5.5. (e) Neuronavigation greatly assists with the planning of the craniotomy and the incision into the tentorium. Neuronavigation images show the additional exposure afforded by cutting the tentorium and help to pinpoint the location of the cavernous malformation.

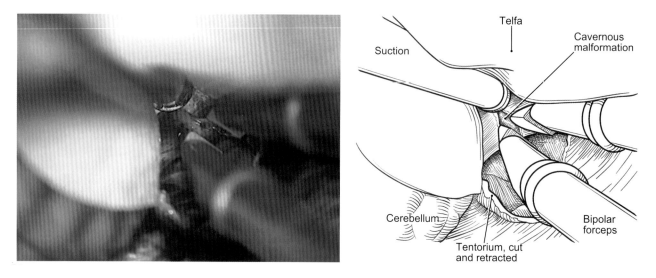

Figure 5.5. (f) Cutting the tentorium provides additional exposure. A corticectomy is performed after neuronavigation is used to identify the optimal point of entry into the cavernous malformation.

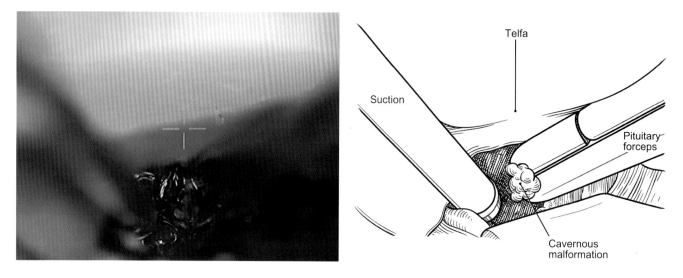

Figure 5.5. (g) The cavernous malformation is entered, releasing blood of various ages. The lesion is then dissected circumferentially using microdissectors, toothed forceps, and pituitary forceps.

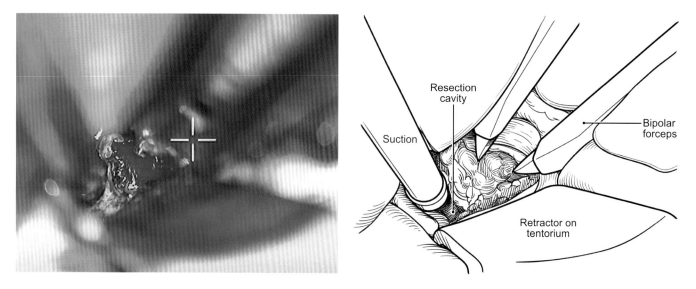

Figure 5.5. (h) The resection cavity is inspected, and hemostasis is obtained.

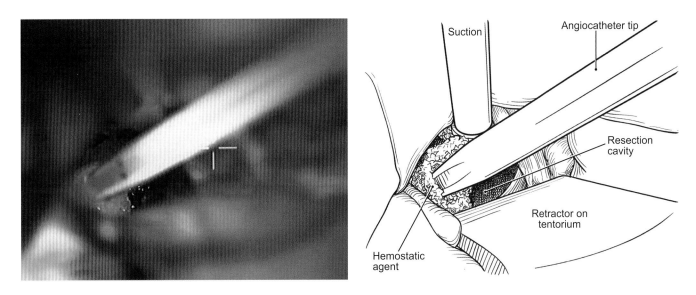

Figure 5.5. (i) In some cases, a small amount of hemostatic agent is placed in the resection cavity to stop venous bleeding. The hemostatic agent is subsequently washed out before closure.

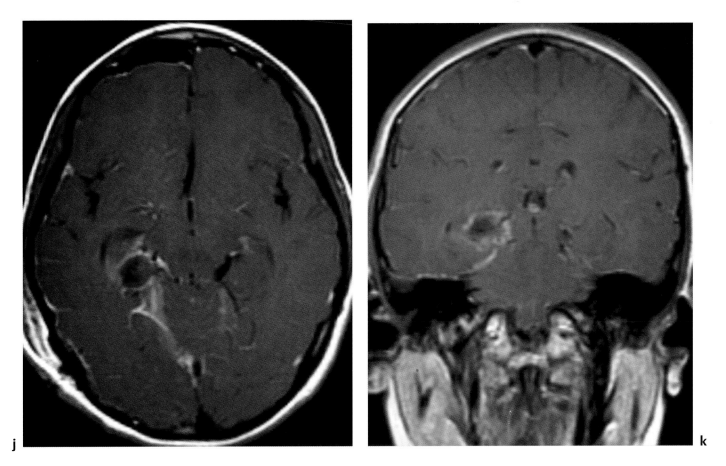

j   k

Figure 5.5. Postoperative **(j)** axial and **(k)** coronal T1-weighted magnetic resonance images confirm complete removal of the lesion. The supracerebellar transtentorial approach enables resection of the lesion with minimal violation of overlying brain tissue.

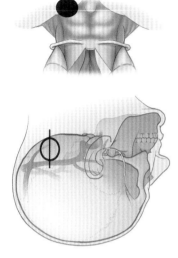

Case 5.6

- Diagnosis: Thalamic cavernous malformation (related anatomy: pp. **9–12, 14–16**)
- Preoperative examination: Left oculomotor nerve palsy, upward gaze paresis, and mild right arm weakness
- Approach: Left lateral supracerebellar transtentorial (related approach: p. **247**)
- Positioning: Modified park bench
- Monitoring: Somatosensory evoked potentials
- Outcome: Complete removal of the lesion; patient is at neurologic baseline.

See Video 5.6

Figure 5.6. A 15-year-old girl, who had undergone a previous craniotomy and shunting, presented with left oculomotor nerve (CN III) palsy, upward gaze paresis, and mild right arm weakness.

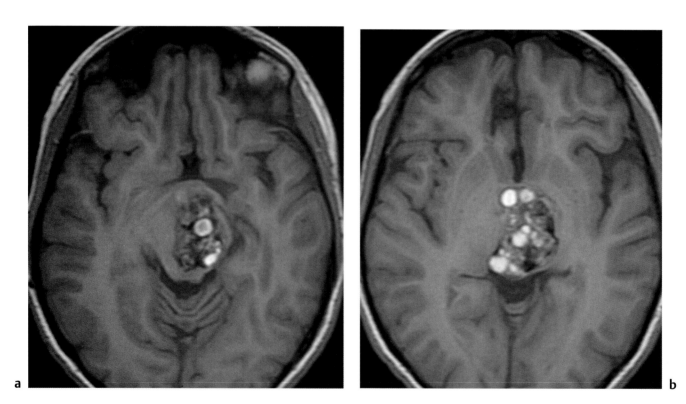

a   b

Figure 5.6. Axial T1-weighted magnetic resonance images at two levels **(a,b)** demonstrate a complex cavernous malformation involving the left thalamus and mesencephalon.

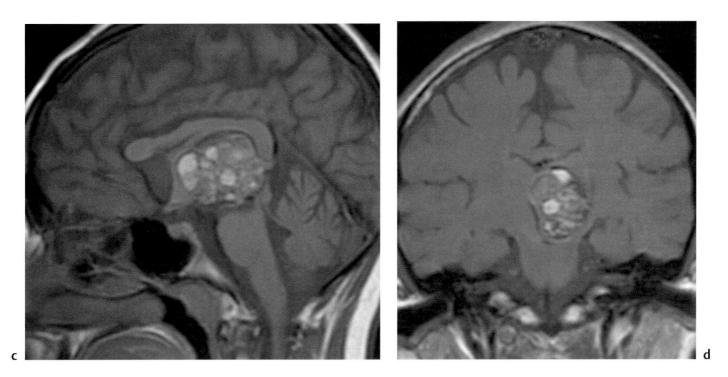

Figure 5.6. (c) Sagittal and **(d)** coronal T1-weighted magnetic resonance images demonstrate the extent of this well-encapsulated lesion.

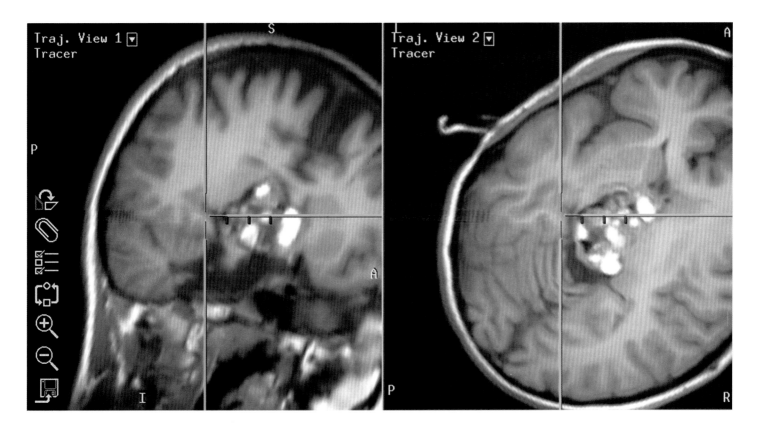

Figure 5.6. (e) Intraoperative neuronavigation images show the trajectory used during the procedure to address this large, complex cavernous malformation involving the midbrain and thalamus. The lesion is accessed using a left lateral supracerebellar infratentorial approach with the patient in a modified park bench position. This approach facilitates entry into the brainstem with minimal transgression of normal tissue and places the surgeon down the long axis of the cavernous malformation. The dorsolateral surface of the midbrain can be accessed using the lateral mesencephalic sulcus safe entry zone or, for lesions that abut a pial plane, it can be accessed directly through the lesion. Disconnection of the tentorium affords the additional view and access necessary to remove the thalamic component of this lesion.

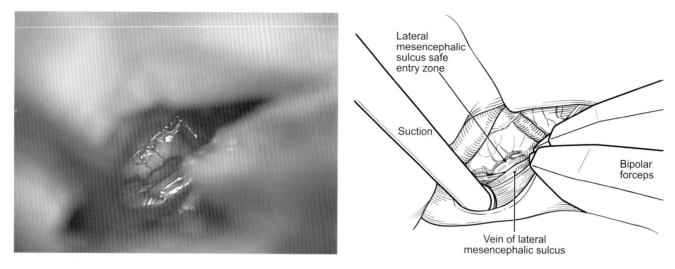

Figure 5.6. (f) The lesion is entered using the lateral mesencephalic sulcus safe entry zone (*dashed line*). The cavernous malformation can often be identified by discoloration of the brainstem surface. When obvious discoloration is not readily apparent, neuronavigation images can be used to plan the optimal point of entry that minimizes transgression of critical pathways.

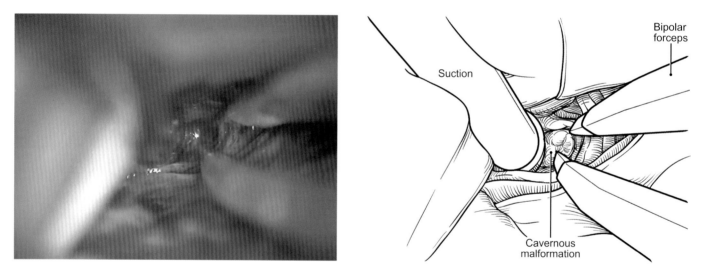

Figure 5.6. (g) The cavernous malformation is dissected from the adjacent brainstem. Coagulation is used sparingly to avoid thermal injury to critical tracts.

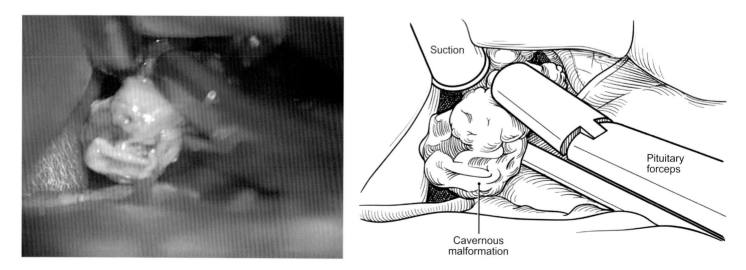

Figure 5.6. (h) The cavernous malformation is removed piecemeal.

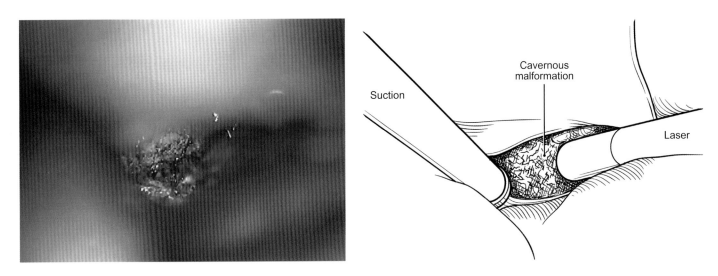

Figure 5.6. (i) In this case, a large cavernous malformation that was too big to be removed through the small opening required the use of a CO_2 laser for devascularization before its piecemeal removal. The use of a laser is not routine.

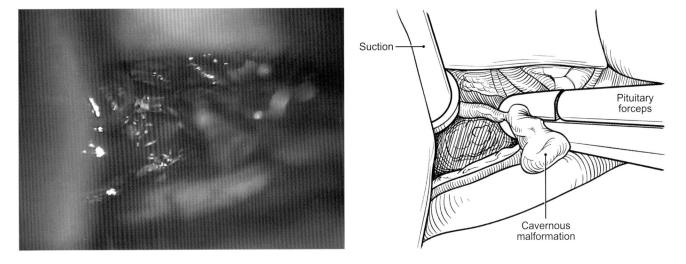

Figure 5.6. (j) Remnants of the cavernous malformation are mobilized off the adjacent brainstem and removed.

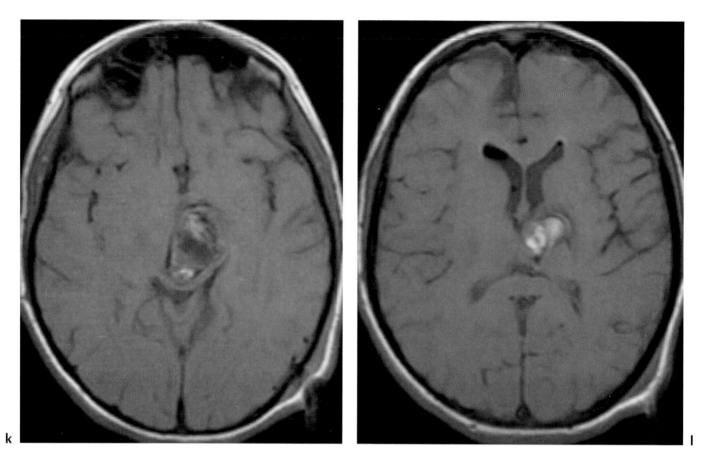

k

l

Figure 5.6. Axial T1-weighted magnetic resonance images at two levels **(k,l)** confirm the removal of that portion of the cavernous malformation involving the midbrain. As expected, remnants are seen in the thalamus. Visualization of the thalamic portion of the cavernous malformation (near the foramen of Monro) was obscured by the collapse of the cavity after removal of the large cavernous malformation shown in **(i)**. This large remnant required a second surgery.

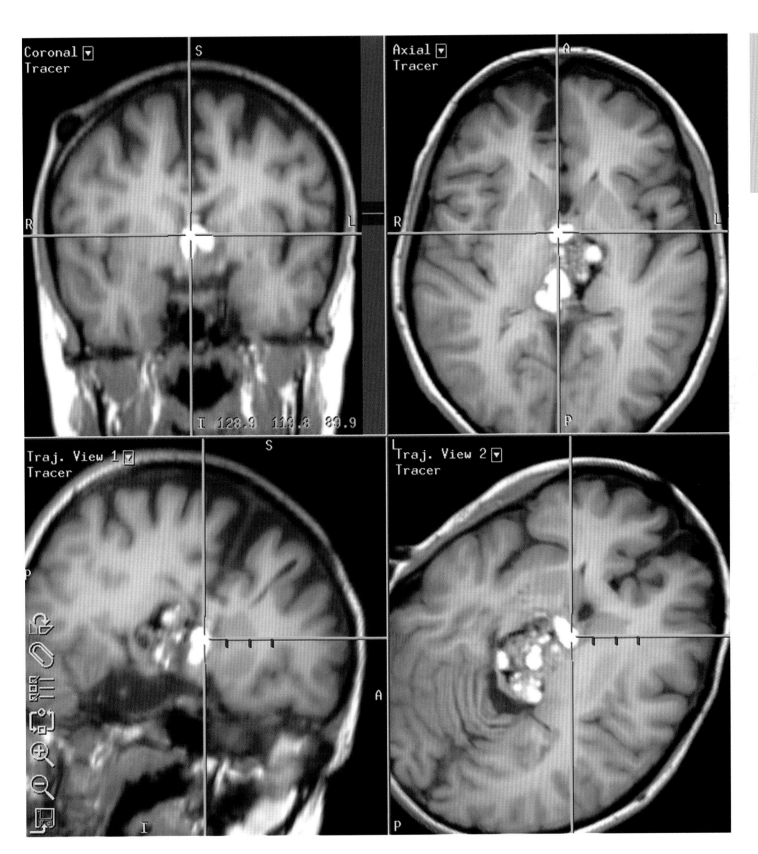

Figure 5.6. (m) Intraoperative neuronavigation images show the trajectory used to resect the remnants of the malformation within the thalamus after disconnecting the tentorium overlying the lesion.

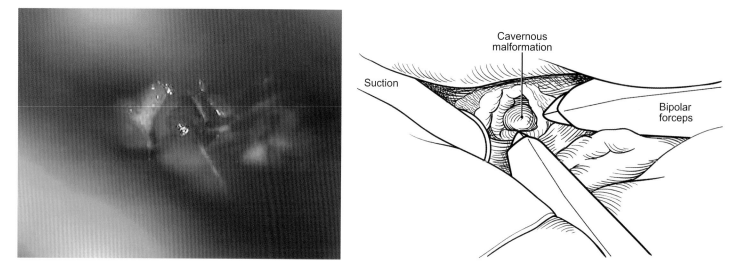

Figure 5.6. (n) The patient is placed in a modified park bench position. This approach made use of the previous surgical corridor, with additional exposure afforded by the previously cut tentorium to expose the residual thalamic cavernous malformation.

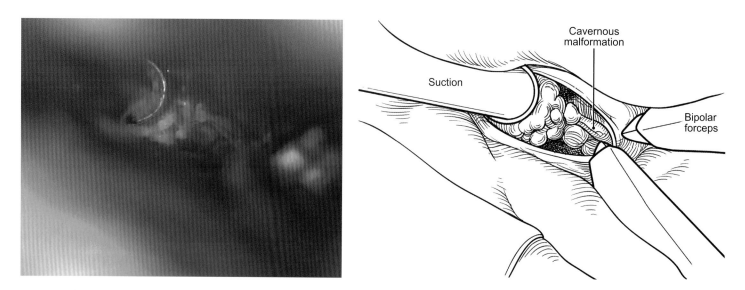

Figure 5.6. (o) The lesion is dissected free and removed piecemeal. The addition of lighted bipolar forceps and lighted suction improves visualization at the depths of such deep approaches.

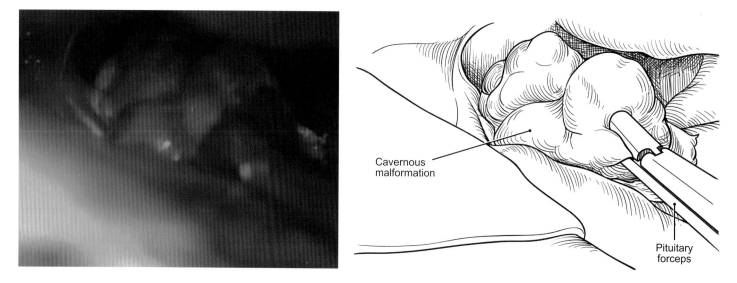

Figure 5.6. (p) Once mobilized, the cavernous malformation is removed using toothed forceps or pituitary forceps. Care must be taken to preserve the developmental venous anomaly associated with these lesions.

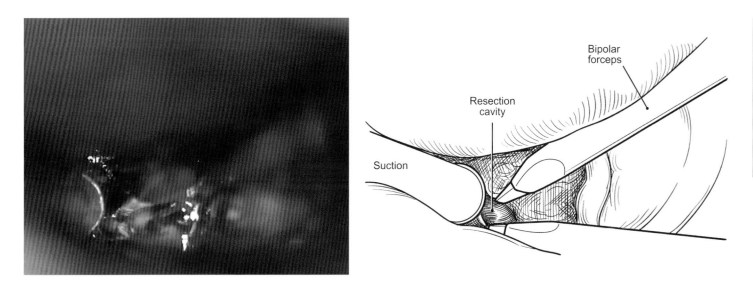

Figure 5.6. **(q)** The resection cavity is inspected, and hemostasis is obtained by judicious use of bipolar cautery on a low setting.

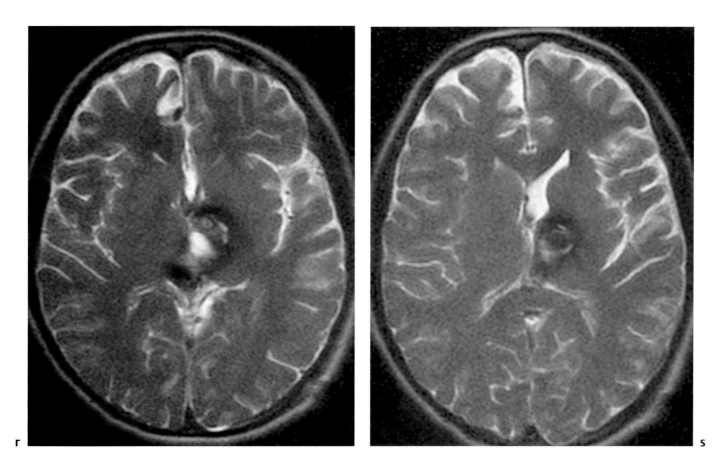

Figure 5.6. Postoperative **(r,s)** axial T2-weighted magnetic resonance images confirm complete removal of the cavernous malformation after the second procedure.

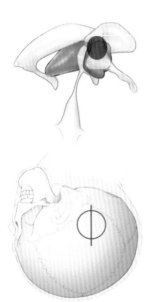

Case 5.7

- Diagnosis: Posterior thalamic cavernous malformation (related anatomy: pp. **9–12, 14–16**)

- Preoperative examination: 4–/5 in left arm and leg

- Approach: Right parieto-occipital transcortical transventricular approach (related approach: p. **185**)

- Positioning: Supine

- Monitoring: Somatosensory evoked potentials

- Outcome: Complete removal of the lesion; patient is at neurologic baseline.

See Video 5.7

Figure 5.7. A 25-year-old woman presented with sudden-onset left-sided weakness.

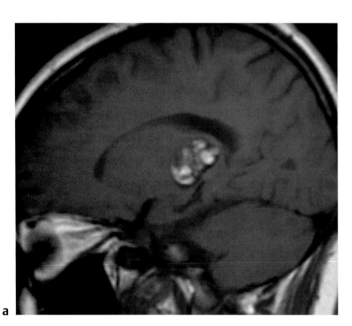
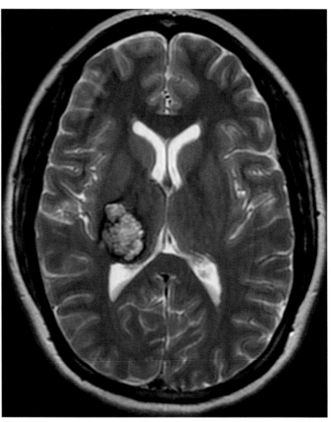

a   b

Figure 5.7. **(a)** Sagittal T1-weighted and **(b)** axial T2-weighted magnetic resonance images demonstrate a posterior thalamic cavernous malformation.

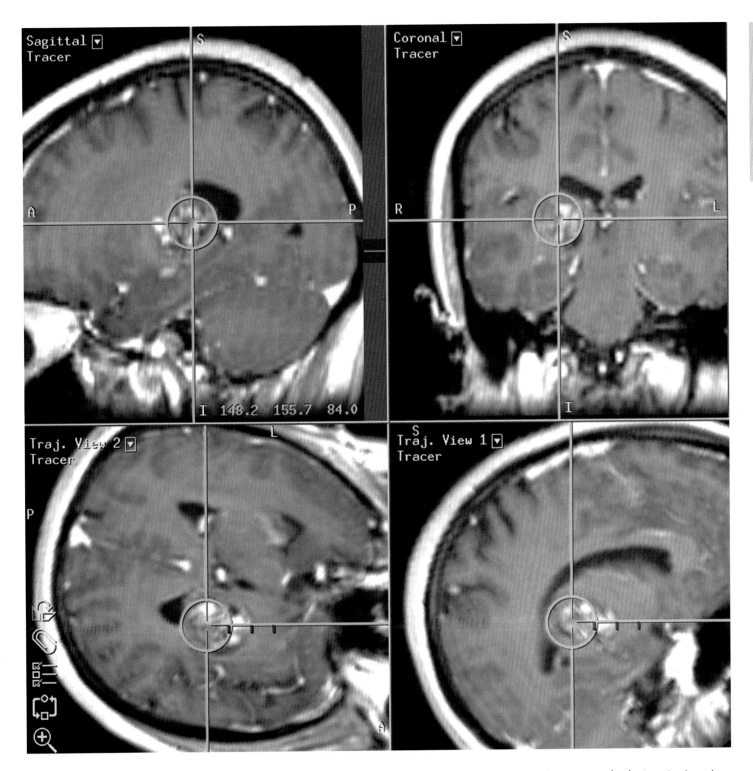

Figure 5.7. (c) Intraoperative neuronavigation images show the transcortical trajectory used to access the lesion. Lesions in the posterior thalamus may be accessed through the pulvinar via a parieto-occipital transventricular approach. The patient is placed supine, with a large shoulder wedge under the ipsilateral shoulder and the head turned contralaterally. The chin should be tucked and the head should be slightly flexed toward the floor to optimize the use of gravity retraction.

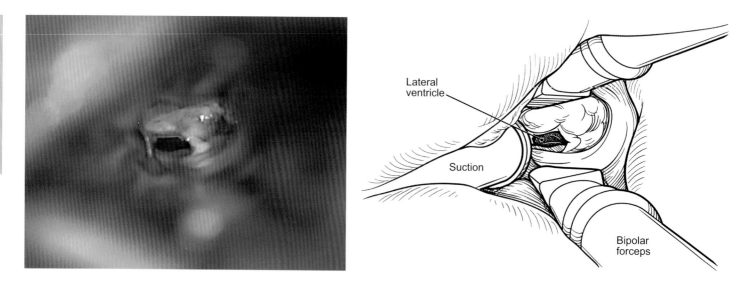

Figure 5.7. (d) The craniotomy is placed using neuronavigation to avoid visual fibers and to enable the surgeon to access the ventricle. Cerebrospinal fluid is released.

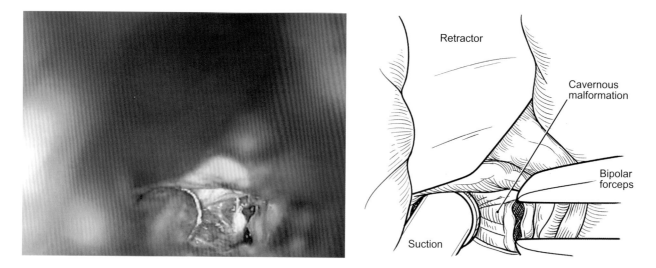

Figure 5.7. (e) The pulvinar is then used to gain access to the cavernous malformation. The pulvinar tolerates manipulation and can be safely used to gain access to the thalamus via a transcortical parieto-occipital approach. Although not essential, the use of a minimally invasive port or a retractor can improve visualization of the ventricle and beyond.

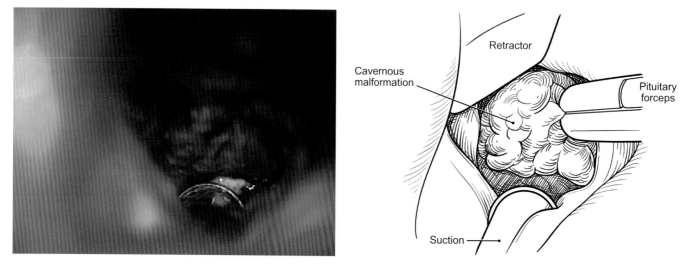

Figure 5.7. (f) After dissection from adjacent tissues, the cavernous malformation is removed piecemeal.

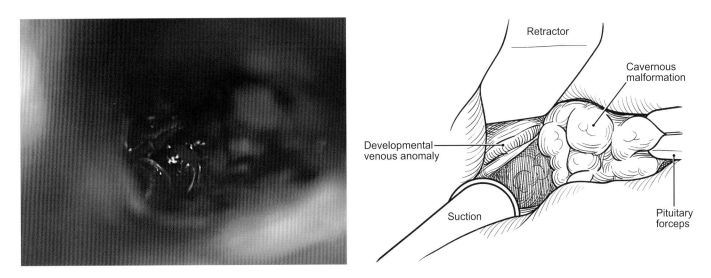

Figure 5.7. (g) A developmental venous anomaly is commonly associated with cavernous malformations and can often be identified. Such lesions should be preserved to avoid venous infarction. In this case, a developmental venous anomaly can be seen deep in the resection cavity.

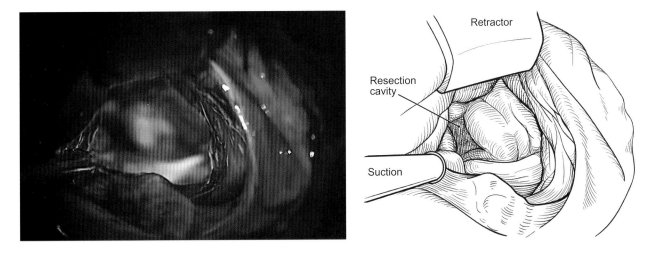

Figure 5.7. (h) Final inspection of the resection cavity is performed, and hemostasis is obtained.

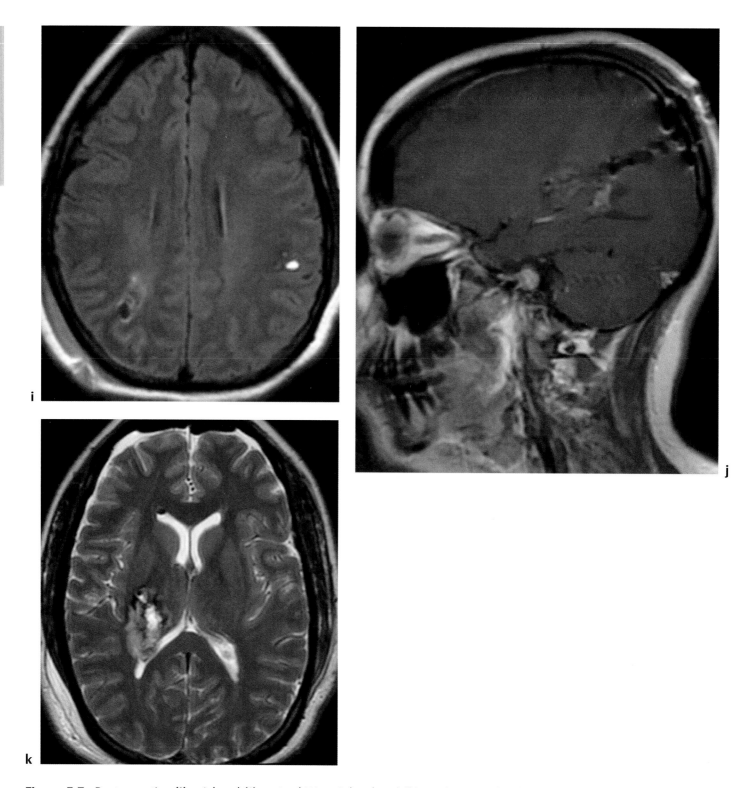

Figure 5.7. Postoperative **(i)** axial and **(j)** sagittal T1-weighted and **(k)** axial T2-weighted magnetic resonance images show the tract used to access the lesion, which was removed in a gross-total fashion.

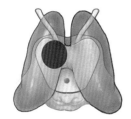

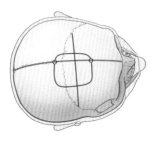

Case 5.8

- Diagnosis: Thalamic cavernous malformation (related anatomy: pp. **9–12, 14–16**)
- Preoperative examination: Sudden-onset, progressive, right hemiparesis in arm and leg
- Approach: Anterior interhemispheric transcallosal transchoroidal fissure (related approach: pp. **186–194**)
- Positioning: Supine, with head turned to place lesion up
- Monitoring: Somatosensory evoked potentials
- Outcome: Complete removal of the lesion; patient is at neurologic baseline.

See Video 5.8

Figure 5.8. A 26-year-old man presented with sudden-onset right-sided weakness.

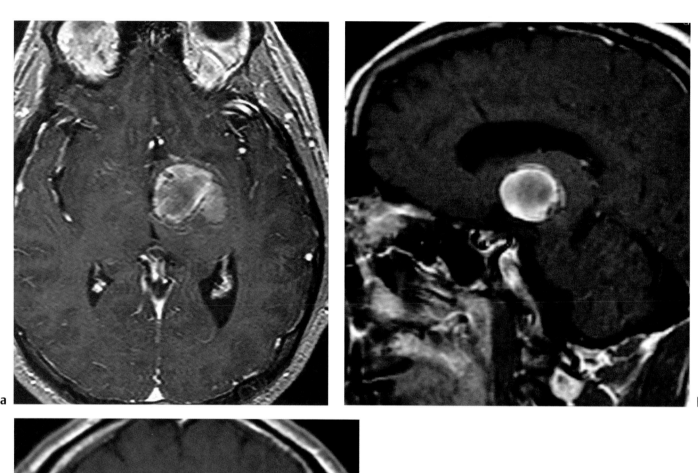

a   b

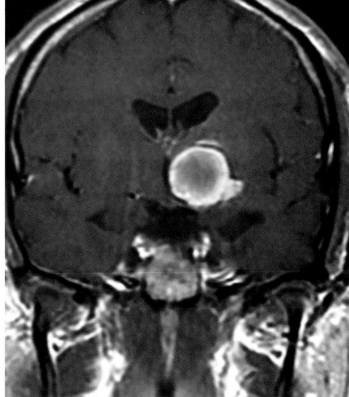

c

Figure 5.8. (a) Axial, (b) sagittal, and (c) coronal T1-weighted magnetic resonance images demonstrate a large hemorrhage with an associated left thalamic cavernous malformation. The lesion was accessed using an anterior interhemispheric transcallosal transchoroidal fissure approach. The patient is placed supine, with the head turned to place the lesion up to minimize retraction of the dominant left frontal lobe and to use gravity to retract the right frontal lobe, thereby improving surgical visualization and the corridor necessary to remove the lesion. This position minimizes trauma to the dominant hemisphere while using the falx to retract the left frontal lobe. The craniotomy is placed two-thirds in front and one-third behind the coronal suture on the right side. The contralateral approach also places the surgeon down the longest axis of the lesion. A wedge can be placed under the left shoulder of the patient with a rigid, inflexible neck to help position the patient. The head should be elevated above the heart to assist with venous drainage.

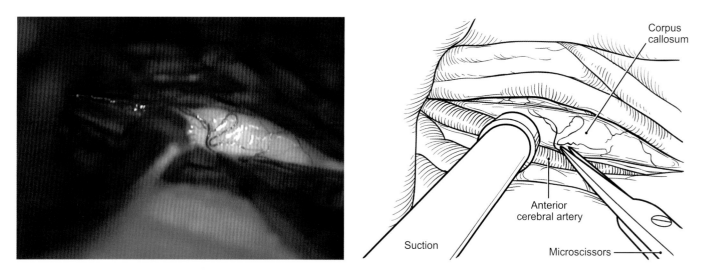

Figure 5.8. (d) A small callosotomy is performed and expanded to gain access to the ventricular system. The craniotomy should be placed to enter the ventricle of interest and to avoid opening the corpus callosum into both ventricles, unless doing so is necessary for the operation.

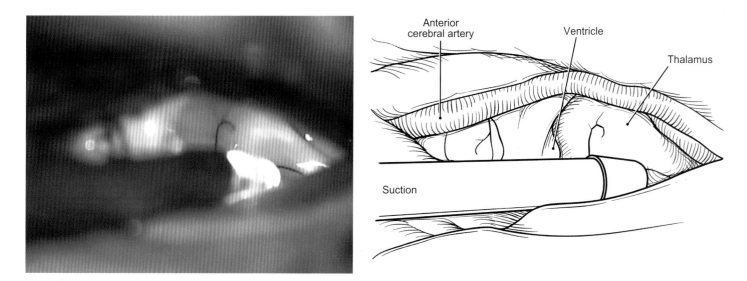

Figure 5.8. (e) The use of a lighted suction cannula and/or lighted bipolar forceps greatly assists with illumination at this depth.

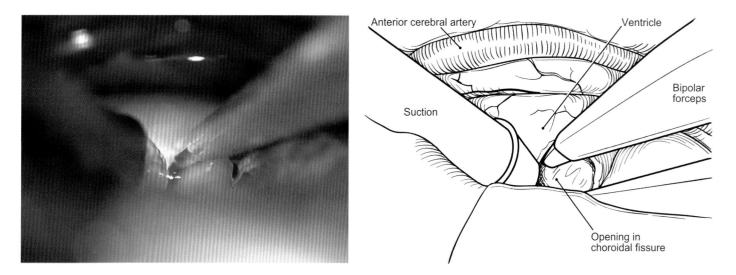

Figure 5.8. (f) The choroidal fissure is opened to gain access to the lesion, which was exophytic into the third ventricle in this patient. The choroidal fissure can be opened either on the forniceal side or on the thalamic side of the fissure. Although there are merits and drawbacks to each approach, opening the fissure on the thalamic side can avoid retraction injury to the fornices. The choroid plexus can also be used as a cushion during retraction of the fornix.

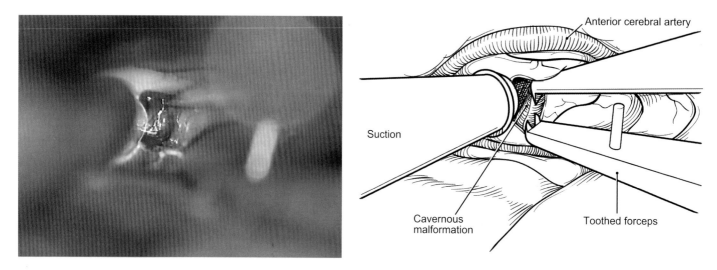

Figure 5.8. (g) A small cortical opening is made to arrive at the cavernous malformation. In cases where the lesion abuts a pial plane, hemorrhage may have led to hemosiderin deposition, leading to discoloration of the brain surface, which simplifies the point of entry. In other cases, when the lesion does not arrive at a pial surface, neuronavigation may assist with selection of the trajectory and the ideal entry point.

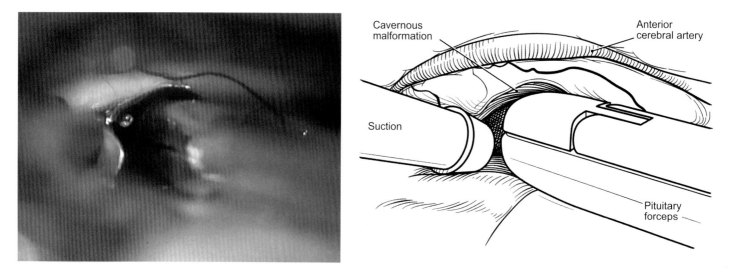

Figure 5.8. (h) The opening is expanded to facilitate suction and to accommodate a second microinstrument to mobilize and resect the lesion. In this case, pituitary forceps are used to debulk the cavernous malformation piecemeal.

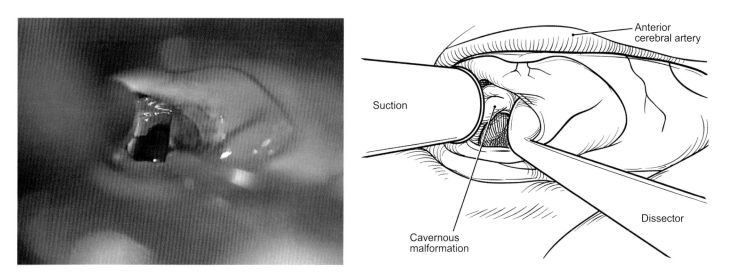

Figure 5.8. (i) A microdissector is then used to mobilize the lesion from the thalamus. When the lesion is a cavernous malformation, there is usually an identifiable plane to perform this separation.

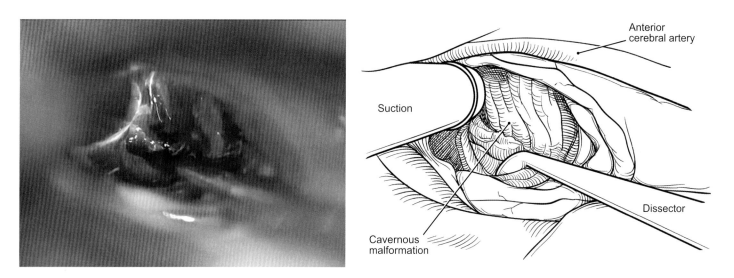

Figure 5.8. (j) Once mobilized, the cavernous malformation is removed by peeling it from adjacent structures.

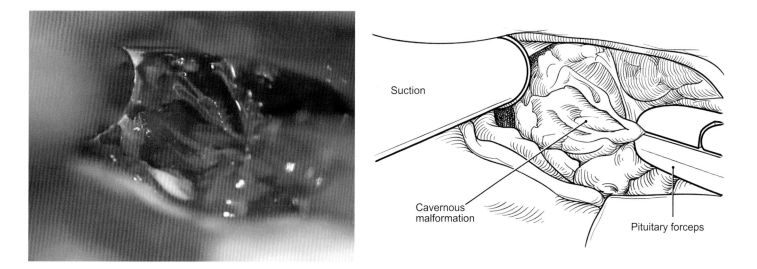

Figure 5.8. (k) Pituitary forceps are used to peel away bands of cavernous malformation adherent to adjacent brain tissue.

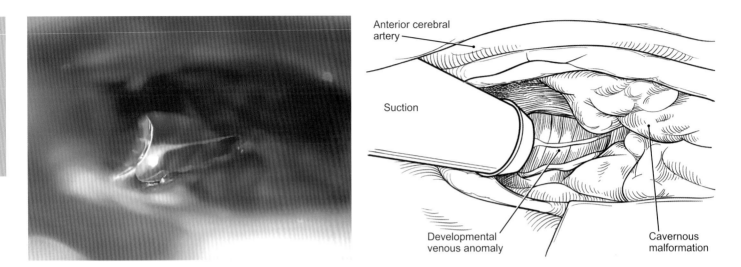

Figure 5.8. (l) A developmental venous anomaly is often associated with these lesions. This structure should be identified and preserved to avoid venous infarction.

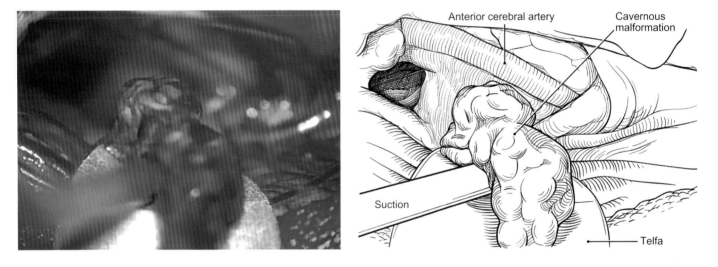

Figure 5.8. (m) After removal of the cavernous malformation, the depth of the surgical cavity can be appreciated.

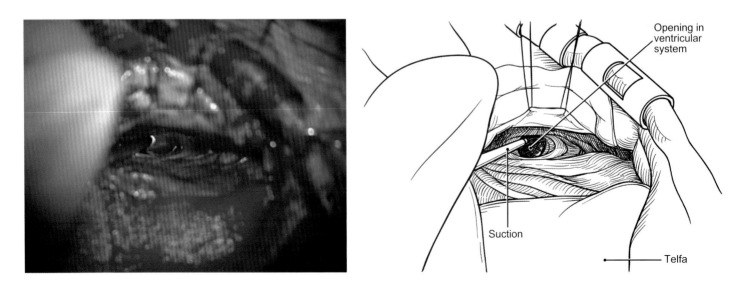

Figure 5.8. (n) Final inspection of the resection cavity is performed, and hemostasis is obtained before closure.

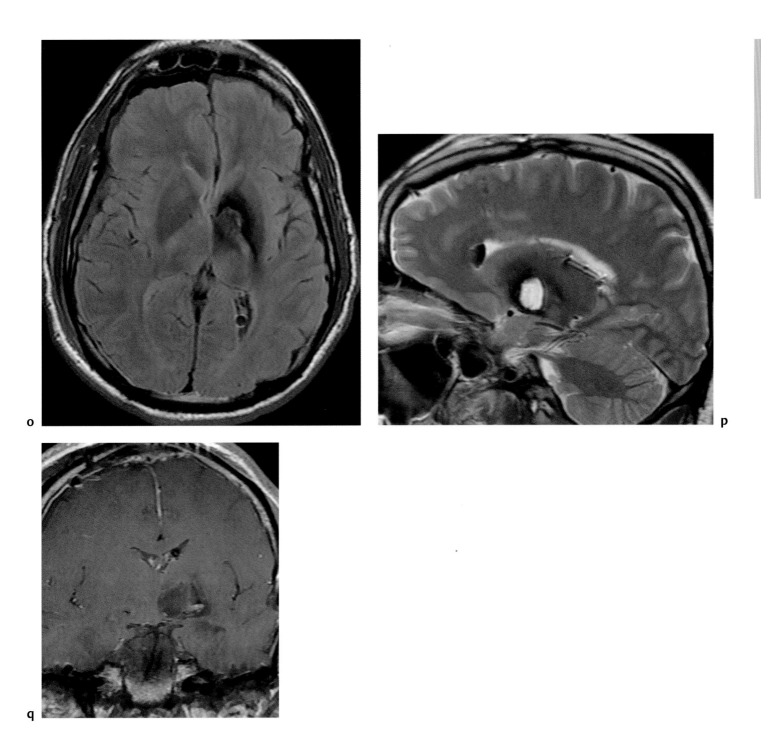

Figure 5.8. Postoperative **(o)** axial, **(p)** sagittal, and **(q)** coronal T1-weighted magnetic resonance images show complete removal of the lesion.

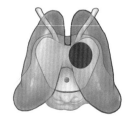

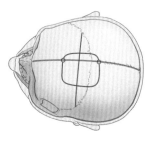

Case 5.9

- Diagnosis: Third ventricular/thalamic cavernous malformation (related anatomy: pp. **9–12, 14–16**)
- Preoperative examination: Left hemiparesis in arm and leg
- Approach: Anterior interhemispheric transcallosal transchoroidal fissure (related approach: pp. **186–194**)
- Positioning: Supine, with head turned to place lesion up
- Monitoring: Somatosensory evoked potentials
- Outcome: Complete removal of the lesion; patient is at neurologic baseline.

See Video 5.9

Figure 5.9. A 35-year-old man presented with sudden-onset left-sided weakness.

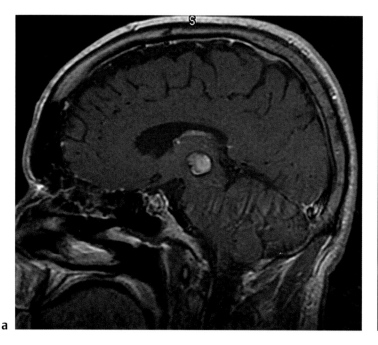

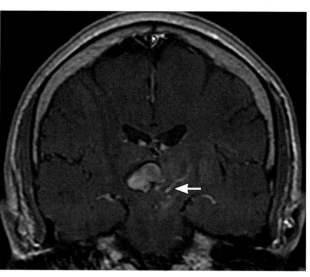

a   b

Figure 5.9. **(a)** Sagittal and **(b)** coronal T1-weighted magnetic resonance images demonstrate a right thalamic cavernous malformation. **(b)** Coronal image shows a developmental venous anomaly (*arrow*) associated with the cavernous malformation. For the optimal trajectory to the lesion, the anterior interhemispheric craniotomy should be placed two-thirds in front of and one-third behind the coronal suture.

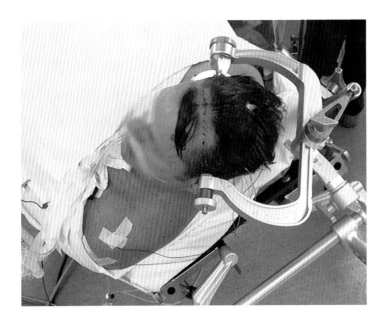

Figure 5.9. (c) The patient is positioned supine with the ipsilateral shoulder elevated and the head turned horizontally to be parallel to the floor so that the lesion is positioned superiorly. The neck is slightly extended. This simple maneuver facilitates visualization of the posterior lesions and of lesions located in the body of the corpus callosum. The falx cerebri can be used to retract the right frontal lobe while the left frontal lobe is retracted by gravity. Opening the choroidal fissure provides a direct trajectory to the lesion. For lesions in the anterior body of the corpus callosum or adjacent to the rostrum of the corpus callosum, the neck should be flexed toward the chest to optimize the trajectory and to maximize the view of these more anterior lesions. The craniotomy is placed eccentrically to the left side.

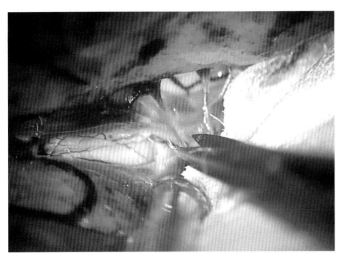
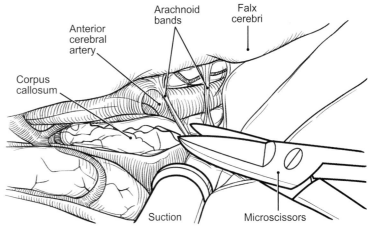

Figure 5.9. (d) The interhemispheric fissure is opened to release the frontal lobes and to provide a direct path to the corpus callosum. The anterior cerebral arteries, which course over the corpus callosum, can be dissected and mobilized to perform the callosotomy.

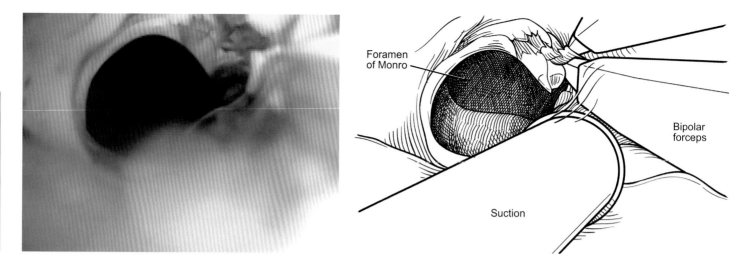

Figure 5.9. (e) The choroidal fissure is opened to gain access to the third ventricle. Care must be taken to avoid traction injury to the thalami and fornices, because damage to these structures can greatly influence the outcome and result in reduced quality of life for the patient. Select lesions can be easily accessed via the foramen of Monro and do not require opening of the choroidal fissure.

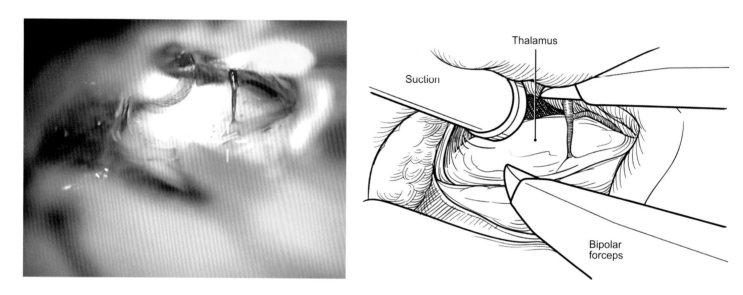

Figure 5.9. (f) The opening into the thalamus is expanded to arrive at the lesion.

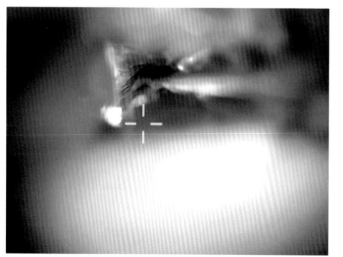

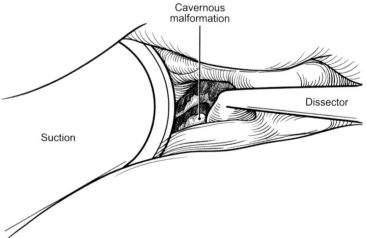

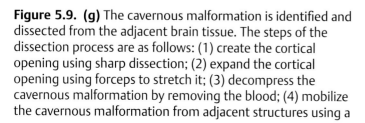

Figure 5.9. (g) The cavernous malformation is identified and dissected from the adjacent brain tissue. The steps of the dissection process are as follows: (1) create the cortical opening using sharp dissection; (2) expand the cortical opening using forceps to stretch it; (3) decompress the cavernous malformation by removing the blood; (4) mobilize the cavernous malformation from adjacent structures using a combination of microdissectors, microforceps, and microscissors; (5) remove the cavernous malformation piecemeal while taking care to preserve the developmental venous anomaly associated with it; (6) peel and remove the remnants of the cavernous malformation from the resection cavity; (7) inspect the resection cavity and obtain hemostasis; and (8) perform a final check of the resection cavity.

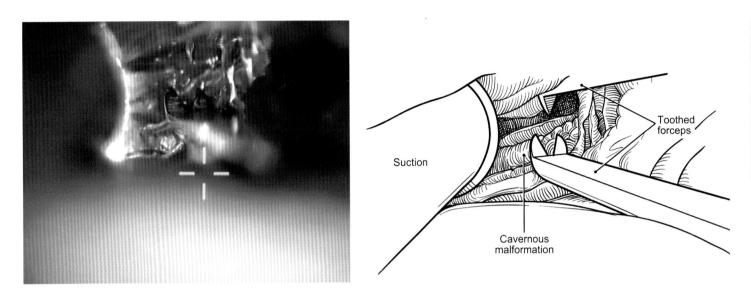

Figure 5.9. (h) Toothed forceps are used to peel away the remnants of the cavernous malformation adherent to the thalamus.

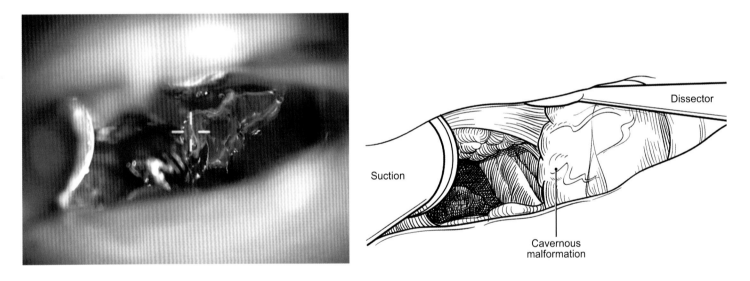

Figure 5.9. (i) Lighted microinstruments illuminate the depth of deep surgical corridors. The lighted suction provides illumination, keeps the operative bed dry, and provides countertraction during dissection.

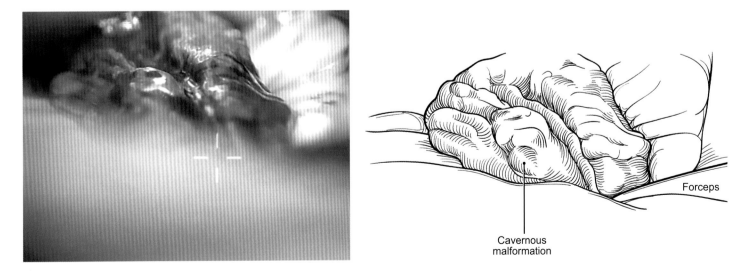

Figure 5.9. (j) After the lesion is fully mobilized, it is resected piecemeal.

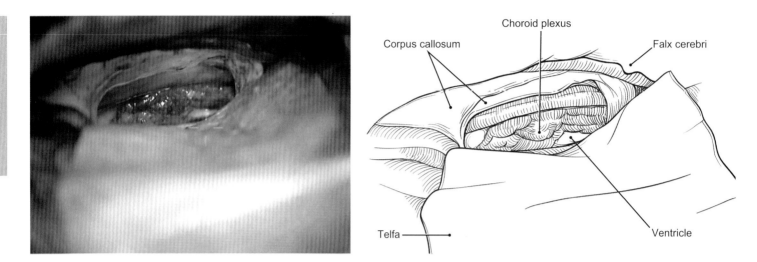

Figure 5.9. (k) Final inspection of the resection bed demonstrates excellent hemostasis. The depth of the surgical corridor can be better appreciated at this lower magnification.

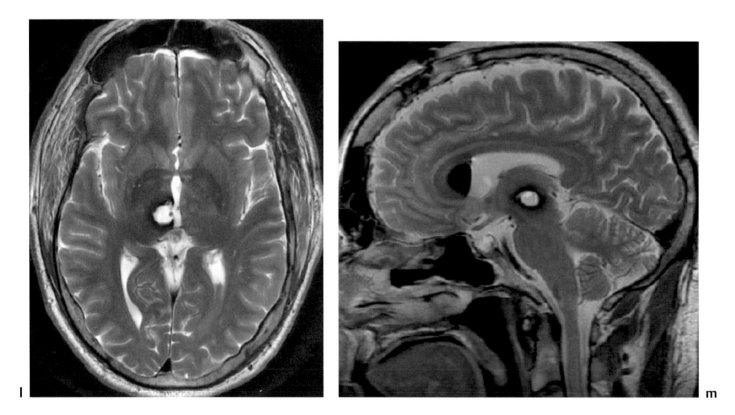

Figure 5.9. Postoperative **(l)** axial and **(m)** sagittal T2-weighted magnetic resonance images confirm complete removal of the cavernous malformation.

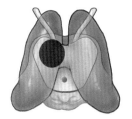
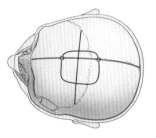

Case 5.10

- Diagnosis: Thalamic cavernous malformation (related anatomy: pp. **9–12, 14–16**)
- Preoperative examination: Right hemiparesis in arm and leg
- Approach: Anterior interhemispheric (related approach: pp. **186–194**)
- Positioning: Supine, with head turned to place lesion down; craniotomy on side of lesion
- Monitoring: Somatosensory evoked potentials
- Outcome: Complete removal of lesion; patient is at neurologic baseline.

See Video 5.10

Figure 5.10. A preteen girl presented with sudden-onset right-sided weakness.

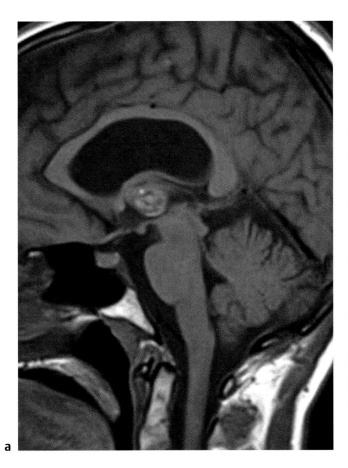
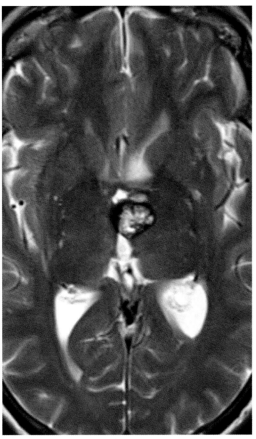

a
b

Figure 5.10. **(a)** Sagittal T1-weighted and **(b)** axial T2-weighted magnetic resonance images demonstrate an exophytic thalamic cavernous malformation. Because the lesion extends almost exclusively into the ventricular system, a left anterior interhemispheric craniotomy is performed to remove it. The head is turned horizontally to be parallel to the floor, with the lesion side down.

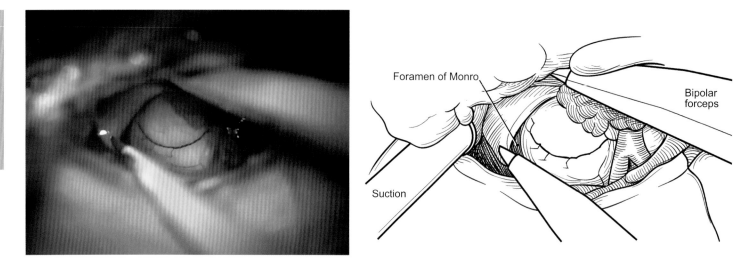

Figure 5.10. (c) Dissection is performed to arrive in the ventricle on the left side. The choroidal fissure is opened on the thalamic side to protect the fornix from retraction injury.

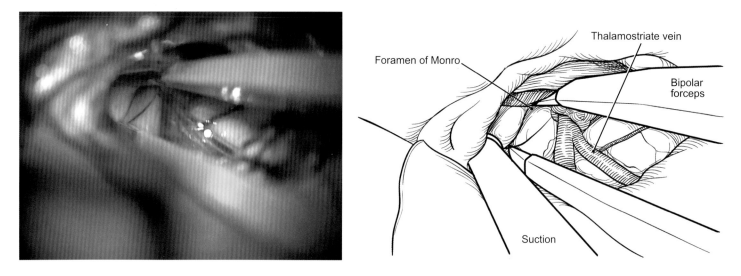

Figure 5.10. (d) Intraoperative photograph and illustration show the opening of the choroidal fissure. Opening the fissure on the thalamic side minimizes injury to the fornix. Placing the choroid plexus as a buttress between the surgeon and the fornix helps minimize retraction injury to the fornix.

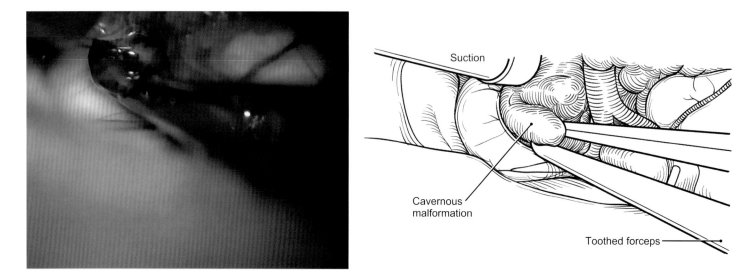

Figure 5.10. (e) The cavernous malformation, which protrudes into the ventricle, is readily identified.

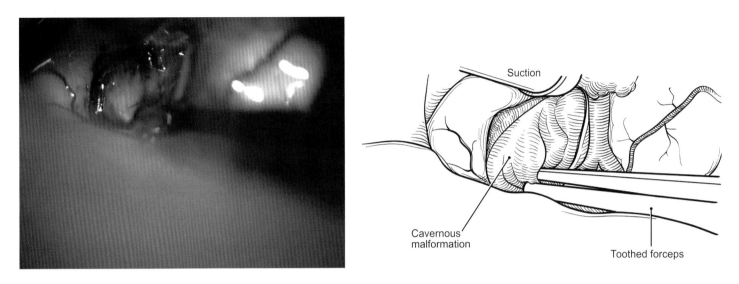

Figure 5.10. (f) The lesion is mobilized and resected piecemeal.

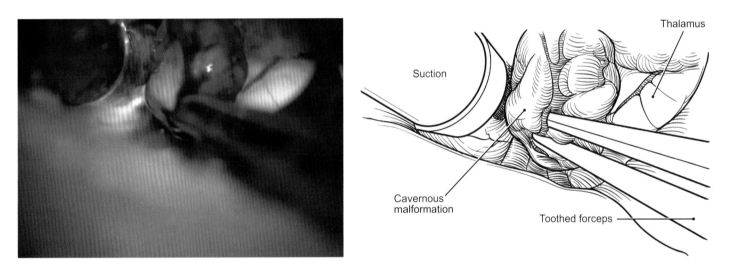

Figure 5.10. (g) The lesion is removed from the cavity.

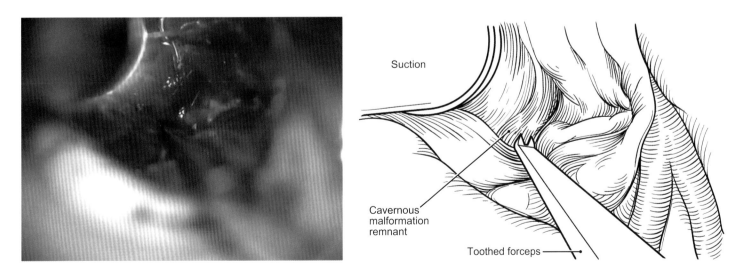

Figure 5.10. (h) Final inspection of the cavity demonstrates cavernous malformation remnants adherent to the thalamus. These strands are carefully peeled from the thalamus using toothed forceps. It is often difficult to distinguish between cavernous malformation remnants and hemosiderin-stained brain indicative of a prior hemorrhage. Care must be exercised, especially when removing lesions from eloquent areas, to avoid removing normal hemosiderin-stained brain.

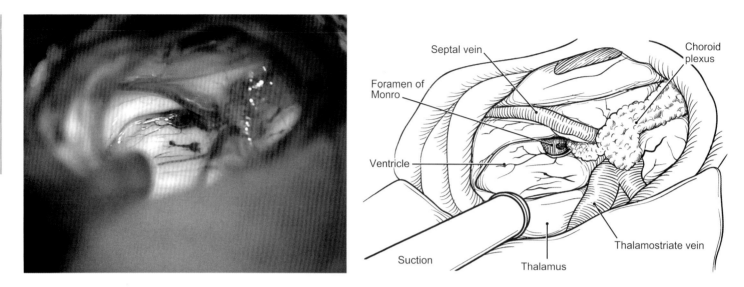

Labels on illustration: Septal vein, Choroid plexus, Foramen of Monro, Ventricle, Suction, Thalamus, Thalamostriate vein

Figure 5.10. (i) Final inspection of the cavity demonstrates excellent hemostasis and no cavernous malformation remnants.

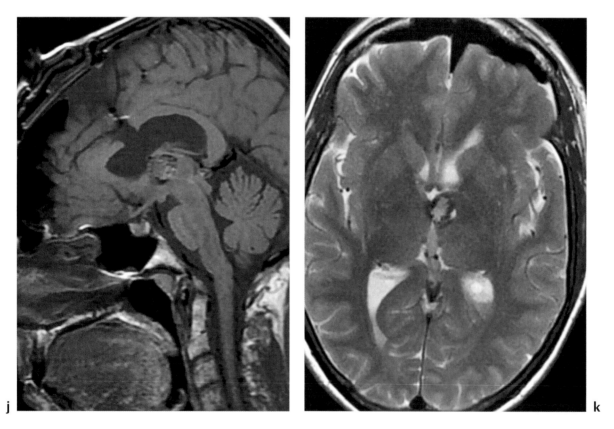

j   k

Figure 5.10. Postoperative **(j)** sagittal T1-weighted and **(k)** axial T2-weighted magnetic resonance images confirm the complete removal of the cavernous malformation.

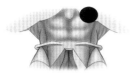

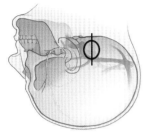

Case 5.11

- Diagnosis: Thalamic cavernous malformation (related anatomy: pp. **9–12, 14–16**)
- Preoperative examination: Left hemiparesis in hand and diminished left upper-extremity sensation
- Approach: Right supracerebellar transtentorial (related approach: p. **247**)
- Positioning: Prone
- Monitoring: Somatosensory evoked potentials
- Outcome: Complete removal of the lesion; patient is at neurologic baseline.

See Video 5.11

Figure 5.11. A 5-year-old girl presented with a history of sudden-onset left hemiparesis that had improved significantly by 4 months after the ictus.

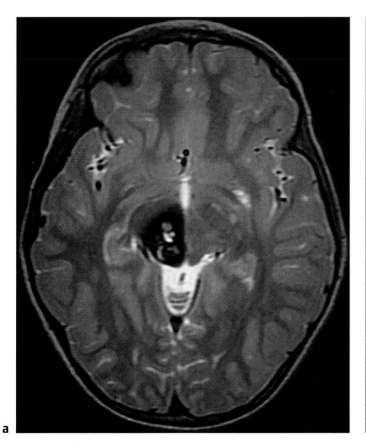

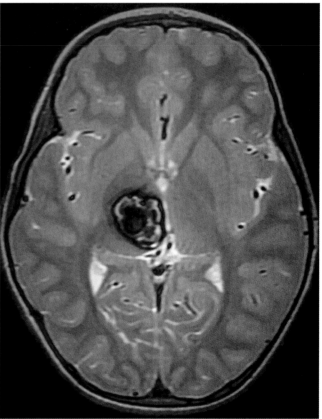

a

b

Figure 5.11. Axial T2-weighted magnetic resonance images at multiple levels **(a–c)** demonstrate a complex right thalamic lesion consistent with a cavernous malformation.

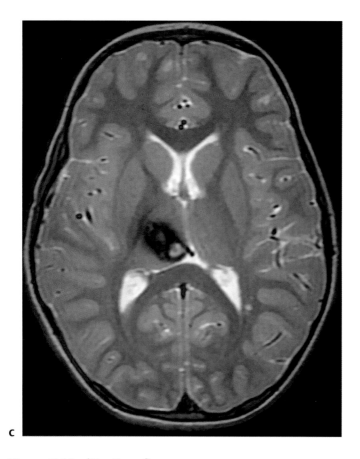

c

Figure 5.11. (*Continued*)

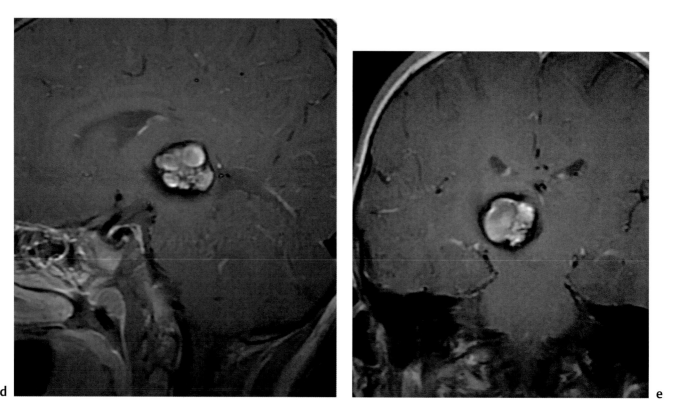

d

e

Figure 5.11. **(d)** Sagittal and **(e)** coronal T1-weighted magnetic resonance images pinpoint the location of the cavernous malformation and its proximity to the tentorium. The lesion is approached using a supracerebellar transtentorial route, with the patient placed prone. The head of the patient is turned to the contralateral side and flexed, and the chin is tucked. These maneuvers optimize surgeon comfort and ease of approach.

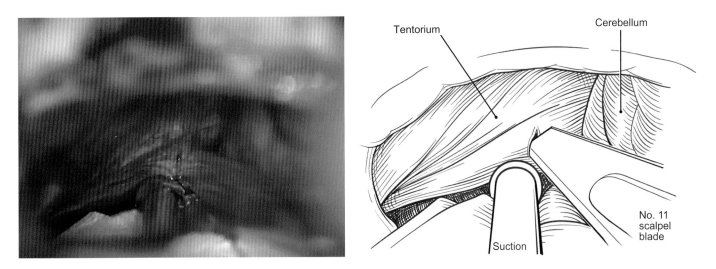

Figure 5.11. (f) The tentorium is coagulated and cut to provide both a supratentorial view and an infratentorial view of the cavernous malformation.

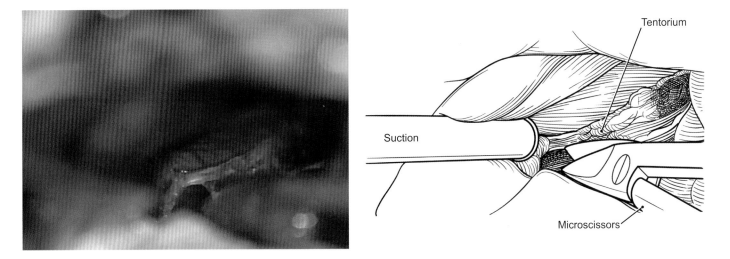

Figure 5.11. (g) This approach readily exposes the thalamus and the entire mesial temporal lobe. Opening the tentorium demonstrates hemosiderin-stained brain tissue, which neuronavigation images show corresponds to the cavernous malformation.

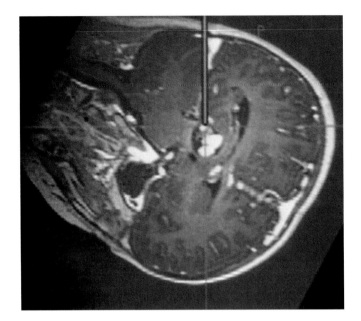

Figure 5.11. (h) Neuronavigation image demonstrates the trajectory to the lesion.

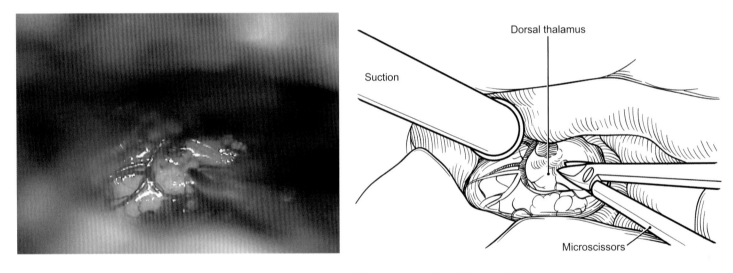

Figure 5.11. (i) The brain tissue overlying the cavernous malformation is sharply incised using microscissors.

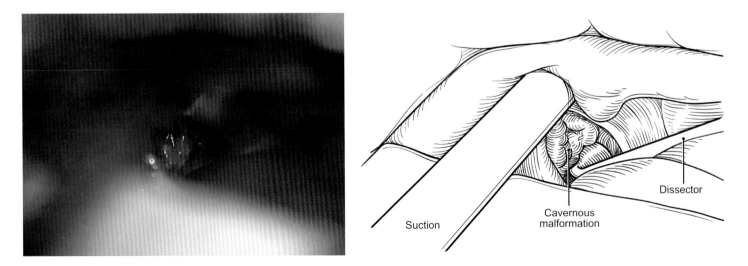

Figure 5.11. (j) The lesion is removed piecemeal using microdissectors and forceps.

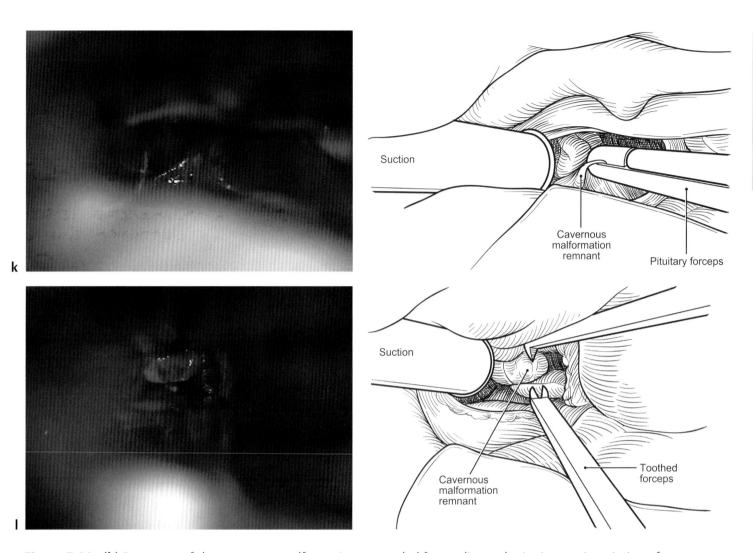

Figure 5.11. (k) Remnants of the cavernous malformation are peeled from adjacent brain tissue using pituitary forceps or **(l)** toothed forceps, with care taken to preserve the developmental venous anomaly associated with the lesion.

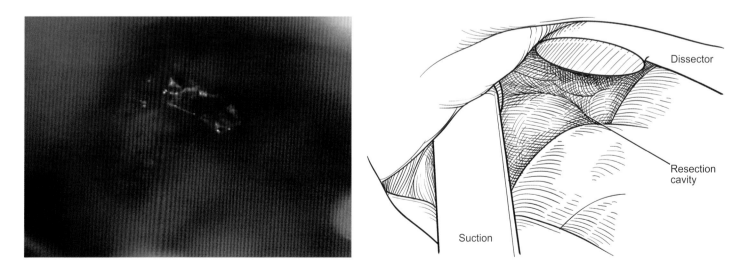

Figure 5.11. (m) The resection cavity is inspected, and hemostasis is obtained.

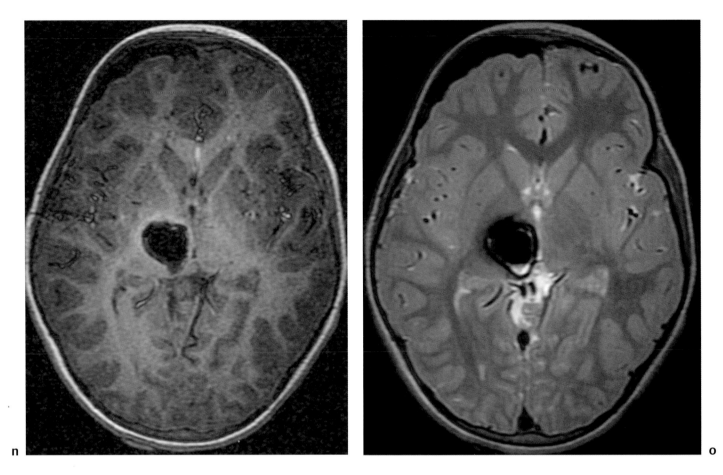

n

o

Figure 5.11. Postoperative axial **(n)** T1-weighted and **(o)** T2-weighted magnetic resonance images demonstrate complete removal of the lesion. Hemosiderin-stained brain tissue, which may cause a susceptibility artifact on some magnetic resonance imaging sequences, is not resected when lesions are located in critical regions (e.g., brainstem and thalamus).

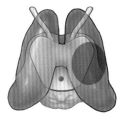
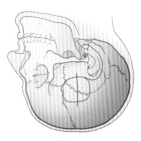

Case 5.12

- Diagnosis: Ruptured grade V thalamic arteriovenous malformation (related anatomy: pp. **9–12, 14–16**)
- Preoperative examination: Left hemiparesis; 2/5 in strength
- Approach: Right transcortical
- Positioning: Prone
- Monitoring: Somatosensory evoked potentials and motor evoked potentials
- Outcome: Obliteration of arteriovenous malformation; patient is at neurologic baseline.

See Video 5.12

Figure 5.12. A 13-year-old boy presented with severe headache and progressive left weakness due to a ruptured grade V thalamic arteriovenous malformation. His history was significant for a prior hemorrhage at age 8 that required a decompressive hemicraniectomy and a ventriculoperitoneal shunt. With rehabilitation after the first operation, he had improved neurologic examination results (4+/5 on the left side), but the family did not follow up with a recommendation for gamma knife radiosurgery.

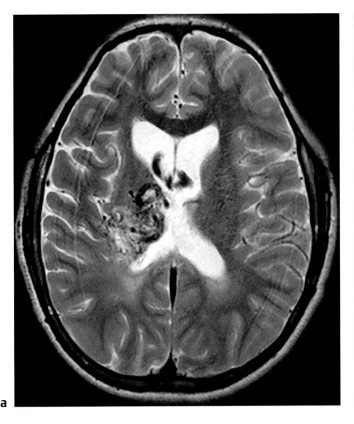
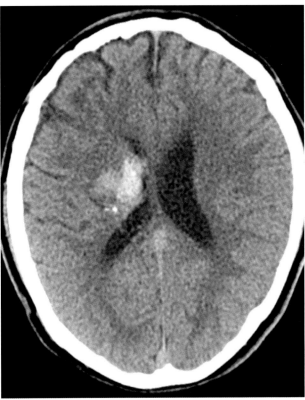

a   b

Figure 5.12. (a) Axial T2-weighted magnetic resonance image demonstrates flow voids in the right thalamus of a 13-year-old patient consistent with a history of a thalamic arteriovenous malformation and a hemorrhage at the age of 8 years. **(b)** Axial computed tomogram demonstrates evidence of a new hemorrhage.

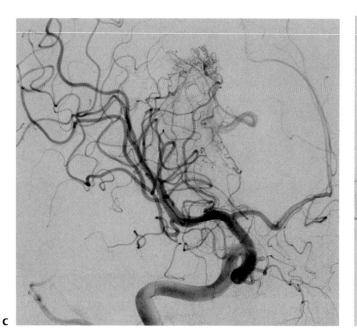
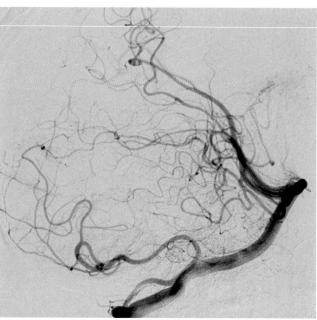

c

d

Figure 5.12. (c) Anteroposterior internal carotid artery and **(d)** lateral vertebral artery angiograms at the time of initial diagnosis of the thalamic arteriovenous malformation.

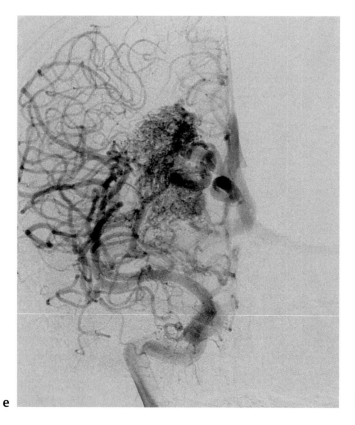
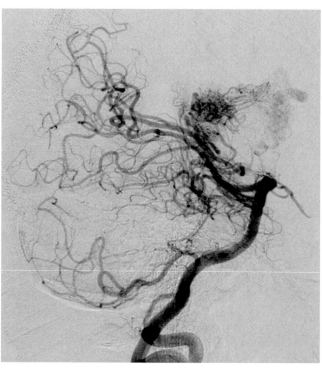

e

f

Figure 5.12. (e) Anteroposterior internal carotid artery and **(f)** lateral vertebral artery angiograms at the time of the second hemorrhage when the patient was 13 years old, 5 years after the initial hemorrhage, document significant interval growth of the arteriovenous malformation. *Stage 1 embolization:* In anticipation of surgical resection, the patient underwent staged embolization of this complex arteriovenous malformation.

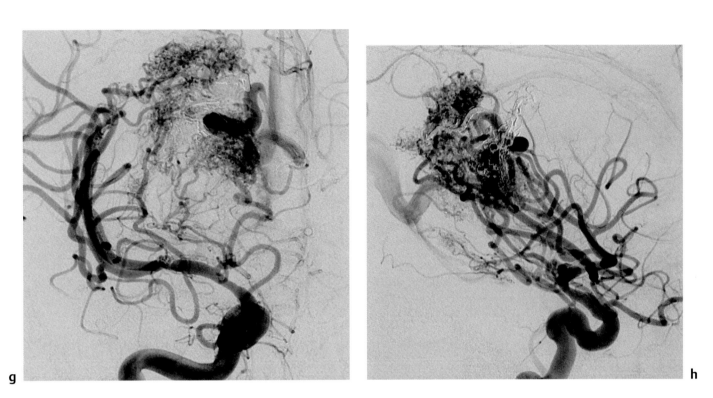

Figure 5.12. (g) Anteroposterior and **(h)** lateral right internal carotid artery angiograms after stage 1 embolization demonstrate significant reduction of middle cerebral artery feeders to the malformation.

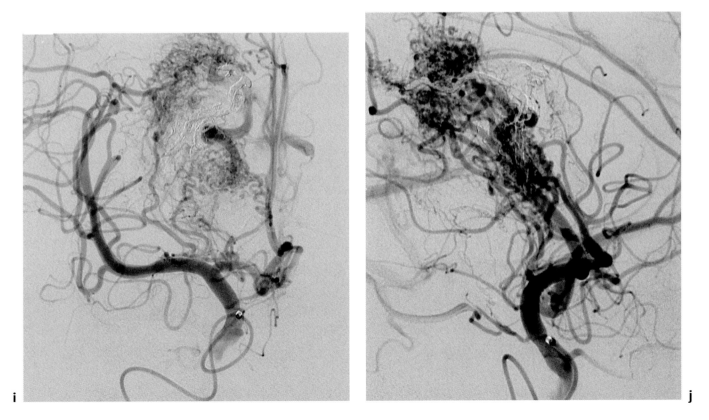

Figure 5.12. *Stage 2 embolization:* **(i)** Anteroposterior and **(j)** lateral right internal carotid artery angiograms demonstrate significant reduction after embolization of a second middle cerebral artery branch to the malformation that resulted in further devascularization of the lesion.

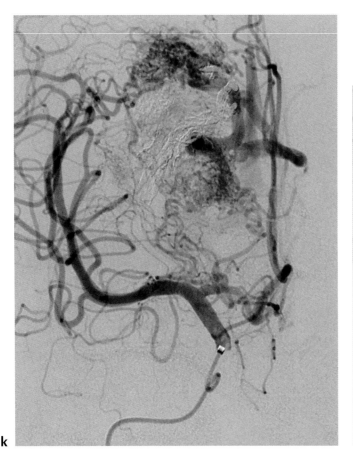
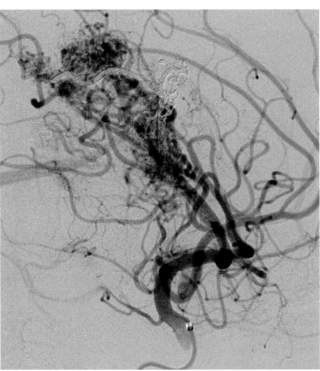

k

l

Figure 5.12. *Stage 3 embolization:* **(k)** Anteroposterior and **(l)** lateral right internal cerebral artery angiograms show further reduction after embolization of a third vascular pedicle feeding the malformation.

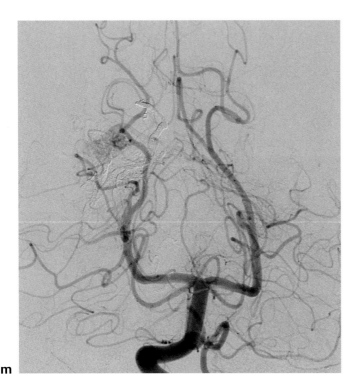
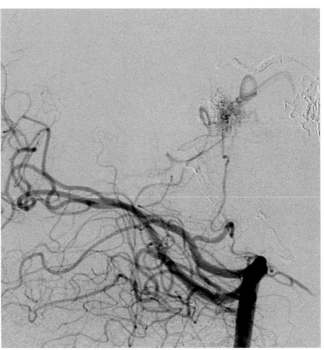

m

n

Figure 5.12. *Stage 4 embolization:* **(m)** Towne and **(n)** lateral right vertebral artery angiograms after stage 4 embolization of right posterior cerebral artery feeders to the malformation.

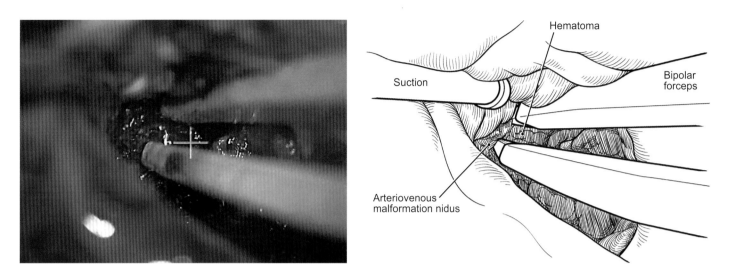

Figure 5.12. (o) The lesion was accessed using a transcortical approach via the cavity created by the multiple hemorrhages.

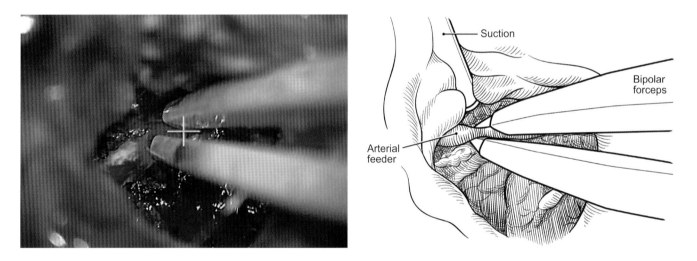

Figure 5.12. (p) Arterial pedicles to the malformation are identified and coagulated. Two different non-stick bipolar forceps are used for large complex lesions. The bipolar forceps are kept in an ice-cold bath and their use is alternated. Cold irrigation is generously used throughout the dissection and devascularization of the arteriovenous malformation.

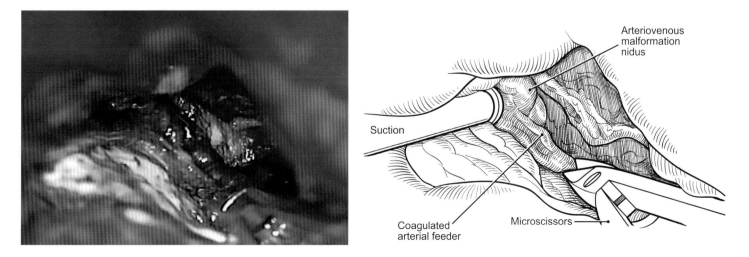

Figure 5.12. (q) The coagulated vessels are sharply cut close to the nidus of the arteriovenous malformation.

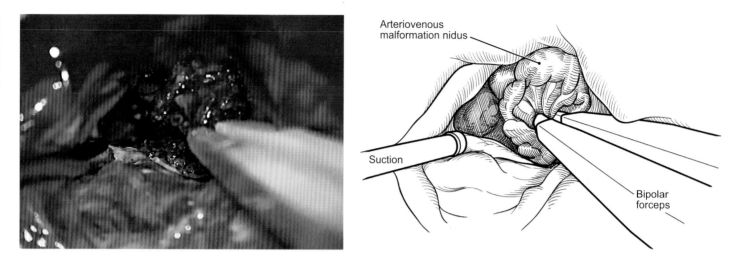

Figure 5.12. **(r)** Circumferential dissection is performed to fully devascularize the malformation.

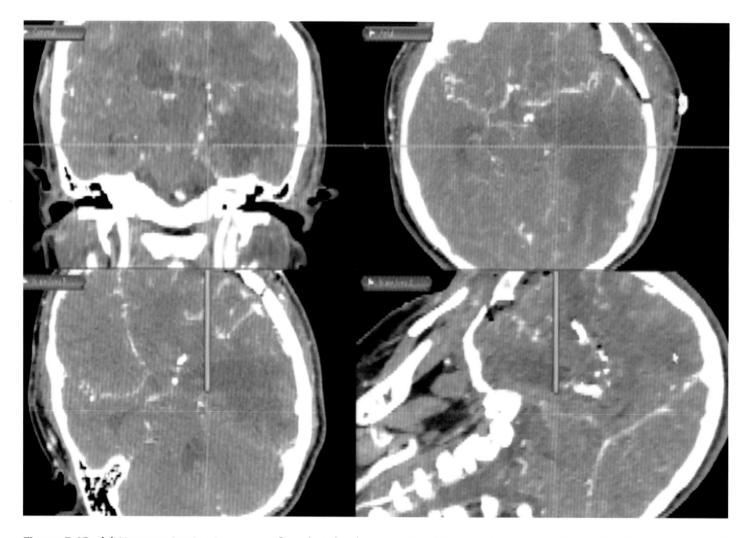

Figure 5.12. **(s)** Neuronavigation images confirm that the deep margin of the arteriovenous malformation has been reached.

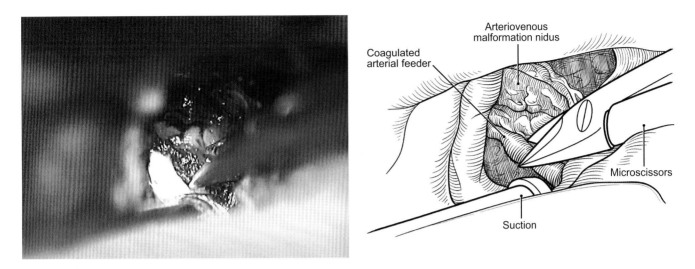

Figure 5.12. **(t)** The deep feeders are coagulated before being sharply cut.

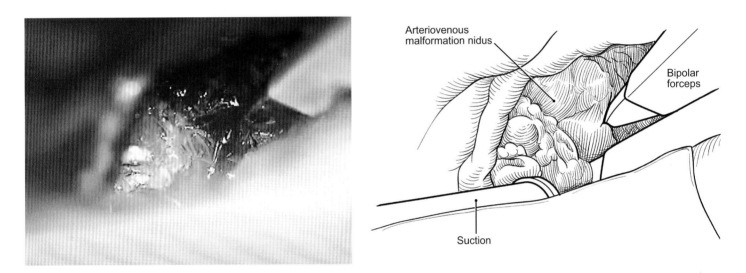

Figure 5.12. **(u)** Small arterial feeders at the depth of the resection cavity are identified and coagulated before being cut. The use of arteriovenous malformation clips may be necessary to control bleeding from these deep feeders, which can retract into the brain parenchyma and be a nuisance cause of bleeding.

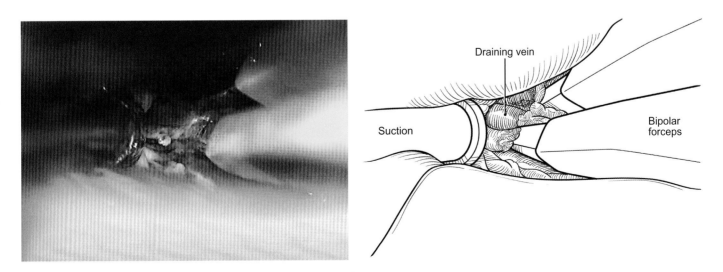

Figure 5.12. **(v)** Once fully devascularized, the deep draining vein is coagulated before being cut.

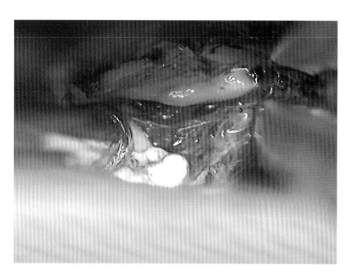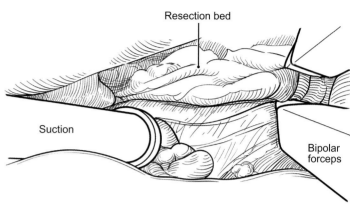

Figure 5.12. (w) The resection bed is inspected, and hemostasis is obtained.

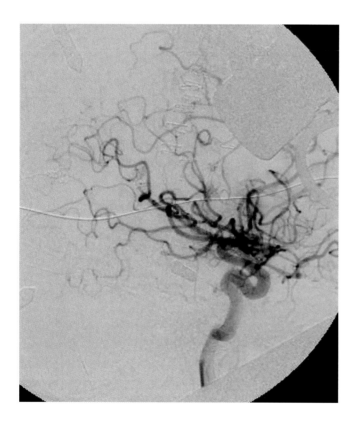

Figure 5.12. (x) Postoperative lateral internal carotid artery angiogram demonstrates complete removal of the arteriovenous malformation.

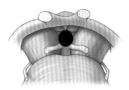

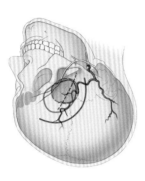

Case 5.13

- Diagnosis: Midbrain cavernous malformation (related anatomy: pp. **5, 6, 17, 18, 26, 27, 39, 42**)

- Preoperative examination: Intubated, right side flickering, and left side withdrawing

- Approach: Right orbitozygomatic (related approach: pp. **144–160**)

- Positioning: Supine

- Monitoring: Somatosensory evoked potentials and motor evoked potentials

- Outcome: Complete removal of lesion; the patient requires a tracheotomy but is able to follow commands on the left side and to flex the right side.

See Video 5.13 and Animations 5.2 and 5.3

Figure 5.13. A 59-year-old man presented with sudden-onset slurring of speech and right-sided hemiplegia.

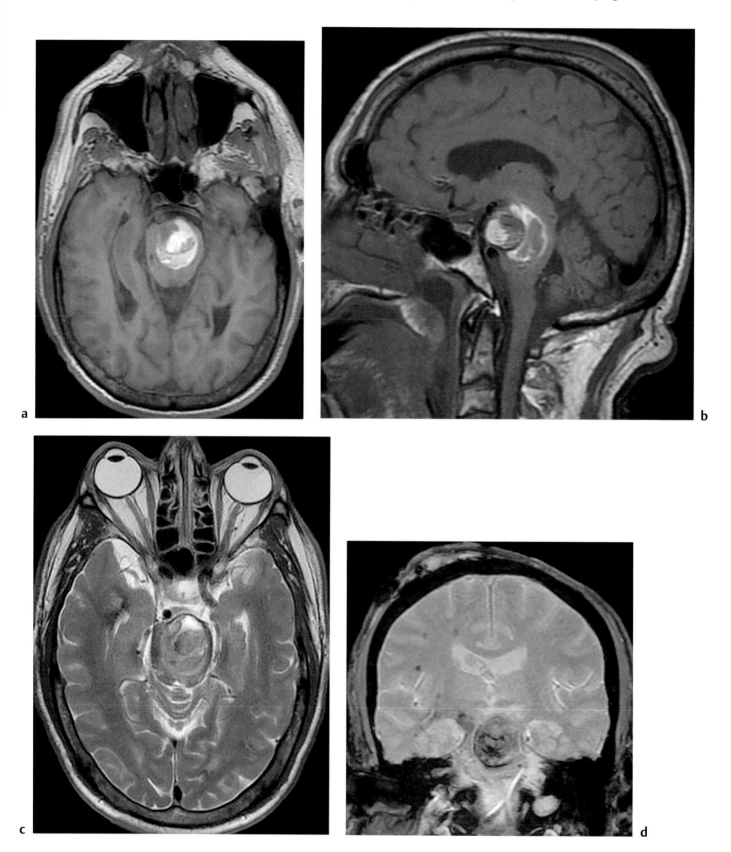

Figure 5.13. **(a)** Axial and **(b)** sagittal T1-weighted, **(c)** axial T2-weighted, and **(d)** coronal gradient-echo magnetic resonance images demonstrate a large mesencephalopontine hemorrhage caused by rupture of a cavernous malformation.

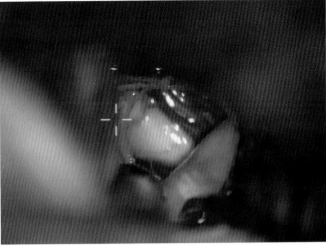

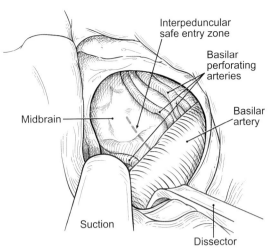

Figure 5.13. (e) The lesion was approached using a right orbitozygomatic craniotomy via the interpeduncular safe entry zone (*dashed line*). The exposure of the lesion is akin to that used for exposing aneurysms at the basilar apex. In general, several working corridors must be exposed. These include the carotid-oculomotor, carotid-optic, and supracarotid working corridors. It is common to visualize the lesion and brainstem using one viewing corridor, while using

a second corridor to perform the resection. In this case, the hemorrhage and the cavernous malformation extend into the centromedian midbrain. Thus, it is not possible to use the anterior mesencephalic safe entry zone, which is located more laterally, because the motor tracts are likely shifted laterally and might be injured. Therefore, the surgeon used the carotid-optic window to arrive at the interpeduncular fossa.

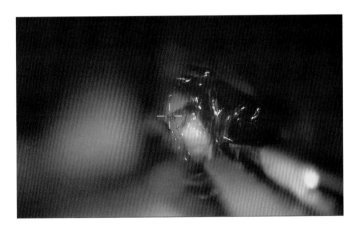

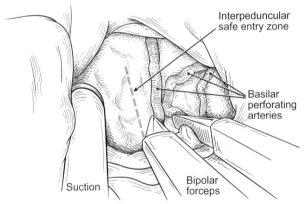

Figure 5.13. (f) The basilar artery is mobilized carefully to avoid injury to the basilar perforators. Basilar artery mobilization provides the surgeon with a small entry corridor in the midline, at a region called the interpeduncular fossa safe entry zone (*dashed line*), to remove lesions in the centromedian mesencephalon.

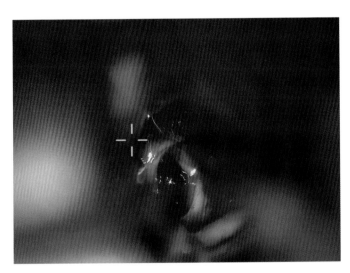

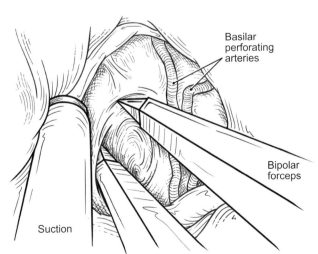

Figure 5.13. (g) The opening into the brainstem should run parallel to the ascending and descending fiber tracts, although they are sparse in the midline in this location, to minimize interrupting them.

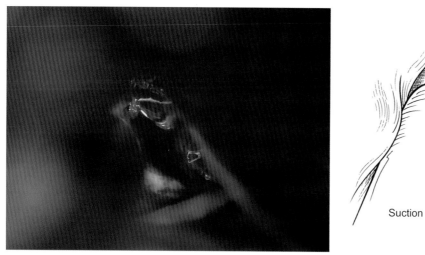
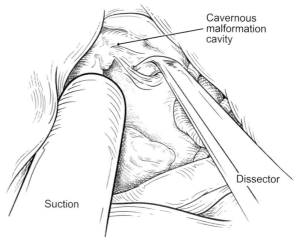

Figure 5.13. (h) The lesion is identified and suction is used to evacuate the blood to decompress the brainstem.

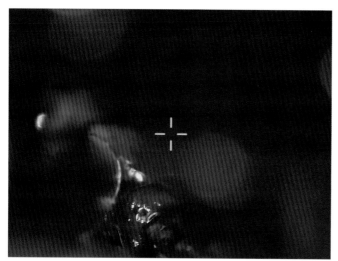
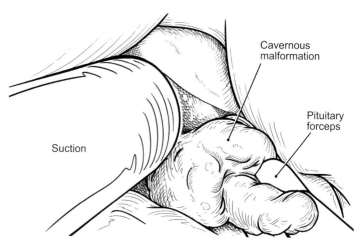

Figure 5.13. (i) The use of lighted bipolar forceps and suction cannulas can greatly facilitate the resection of lesions in deep surgical corridors. In this case, the lighted suction cannula provides illumination and countertraction as the cavernous malformation is mobilized.

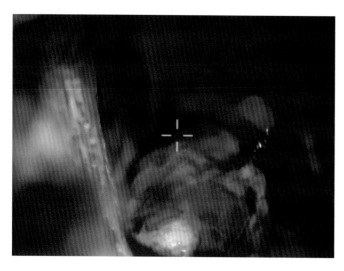
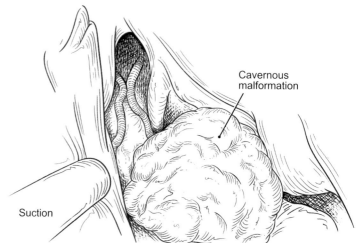

Figure 5.13. (j) The lesion is resected piecemeal and removed.

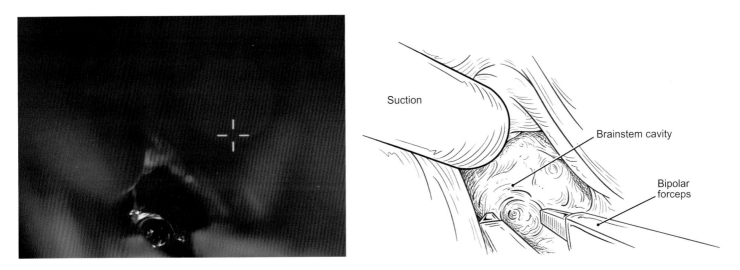

Figure 5.13. (k) The resection bed is inspected for remnants of cavernous malformation, which is facilitated by the increased illumination afforded by the lighted instruments, and hemostasis is obtained.

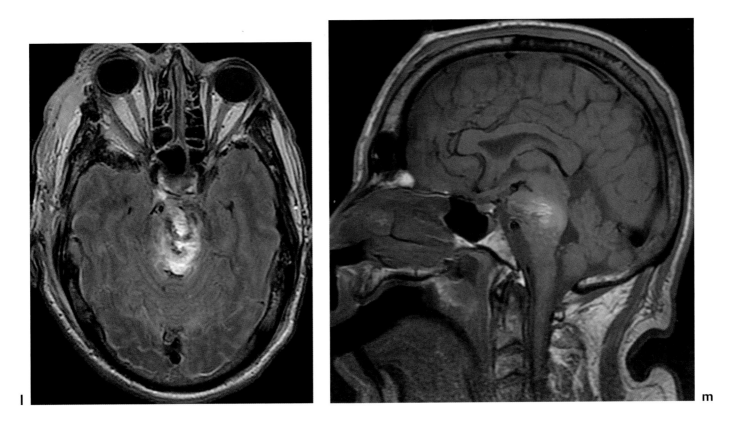

Figure 5.13. Postoperative **(l)** axial and **(m)** sagittal T1-weighted magnetic resonance images demonstrate complete removal of the lesion.

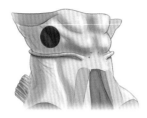

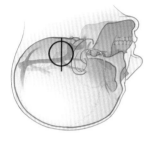

Case 5.14

- Diagnosis: Midbrain cavernous malformation (related anatomy: pp. **13, 38, 43**)
- Preoperative examination: Left arm 4/5; bilateral dysmetria
- Approach: Left supracerebellar infratentorial (related approach: pp. **238–246**)
- Positioning: Prone
- Monitoring: Somatosensory evoked potentials and motor evoked potentials
- Outcome: Complete removal of lesion; bilateral intranuclear ophthalmoplegia, Parinaud syndrome, right facial droop, proprioceptive deficit, and right hemiparesis (arm 2/5; leg 4–/5)

See Video 5.14 and Animations 5.2 and 5.4

Figure 5.14. A 56-year-old man presented with diplopia on right gaze.

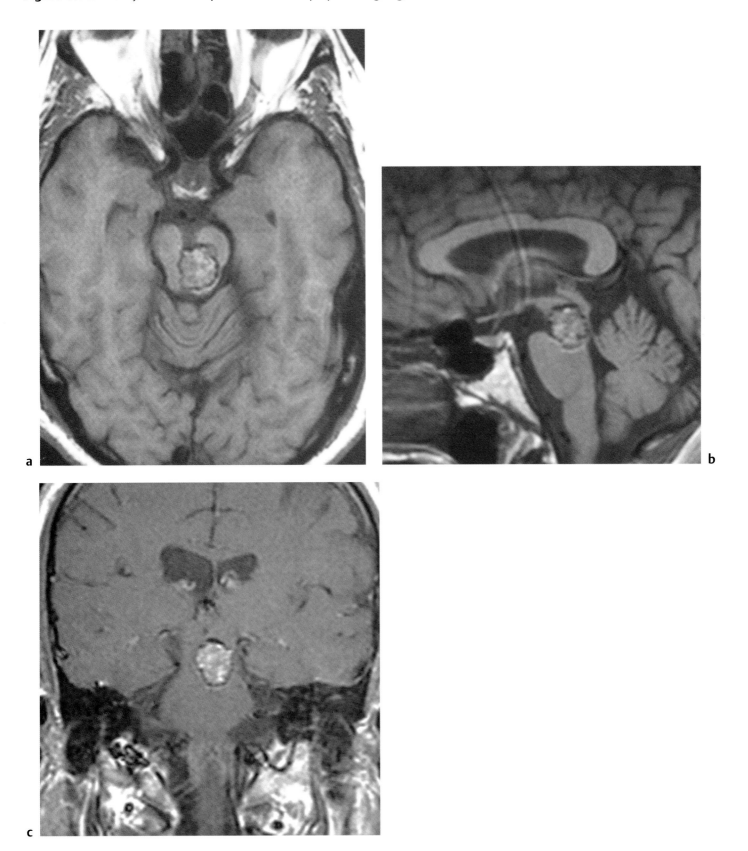

Figure 5.14. **(a)** Axial, **(b)** sagittal, and **(c)** coronal T1-weighted magnetic resonance images demonstrate a cavernous malformation in the midbrain of a patient with a history of three prior hemorrhages.

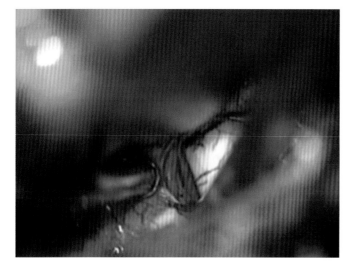

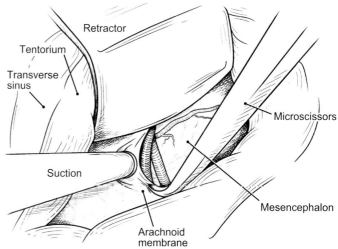

Figure 5.14. (d) The lesion is accessed using a left supracerebellar infratentorial approach via the lateral mesencephalic sulcus safe entry zone. The opening of the potential space between the cerebellum and the tentorium enables the surgeon to arrive at the mesencephalon posteriorly, effectively avoiding motor fibers. Dissection of the arachnoid membrane enables the mobilization of vessels from the brainstem surface, which facilitates the selection of an ideal point of entry into the brainstem. The optimal point of entry is often through the lesion when it abuts a pial or an ependymal surface, but when the lesion is deep, a safe entry zone provides the path least likely to cause morbidity.

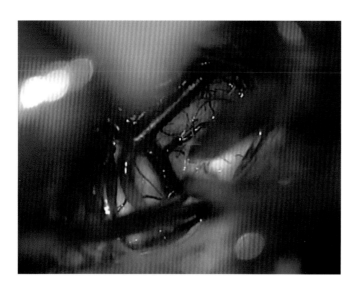

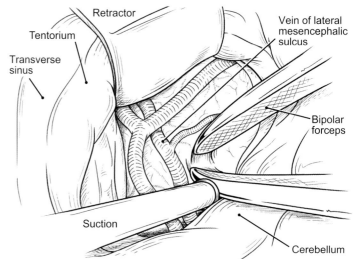

Figure 5.14. (e) Mobilization of the vein of the lateral mesencephalic sulcus enables the surgeon to use this safe entry zone to approach deep-seated lesions in the dorsolateral midbrain. In this case, the surface of the brainstem has hemosiderin discoloration from prior hemorrhages.

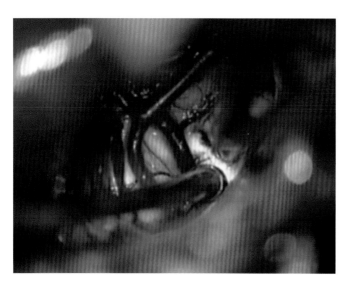

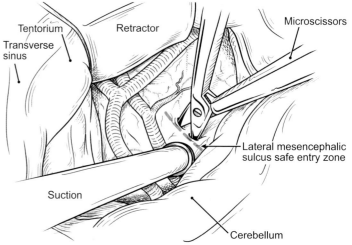

Figure 5.14. (f) A sharp opening is made into the brainstem at the lateral mesencephalic sulcus safe entry zone (*dashed line*) and is expanded using microscissors. The opening may also be expanded with microforceps, using a spreading maneuver to increase working room.

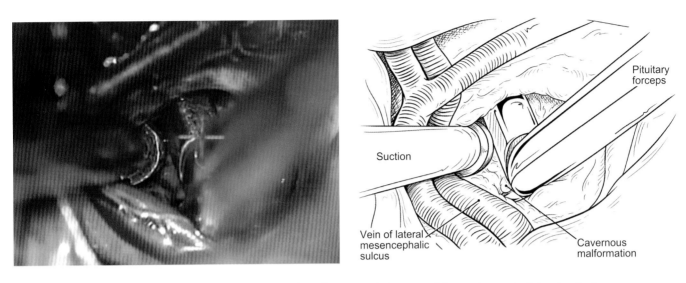

Figure 5.14. (g) The lesion is debulked, mobilized, and resected piecemeal from the underlying brainstem.

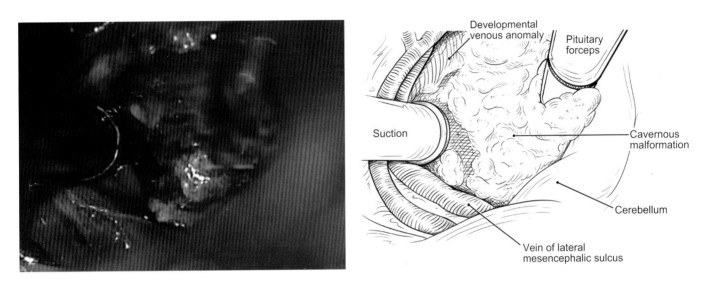

Figure 5.14. (h) Cavernous malformations are often associated with developmental venous anomalies. In this case, a developmental venous anomaly could be visualized deep within the resection cavity. These structures should be preserved to achieve the optimal outcome after resection of the cavernous malformation.

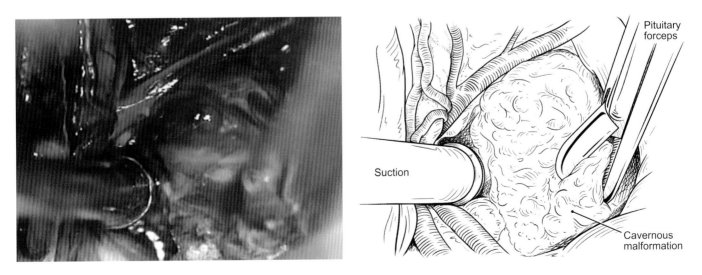

Figure 5.14. (i) The cavernous malformation is peeled from the brainstem using suction to provide countertraction as the pituitary forceps mobilize the lesion.

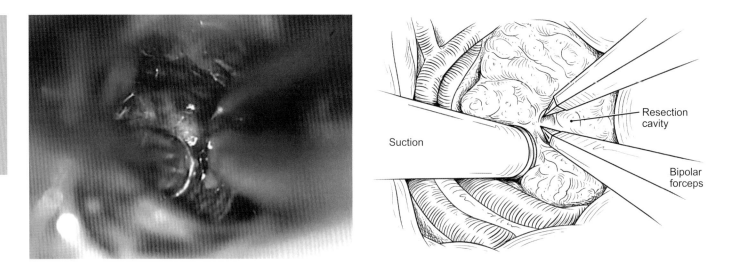

Figure 5.14. **(j)** The resection cavity is inspected for cavernous malformation remnants, and bipolar cautery on a low setting is used to obtain hemostasis.

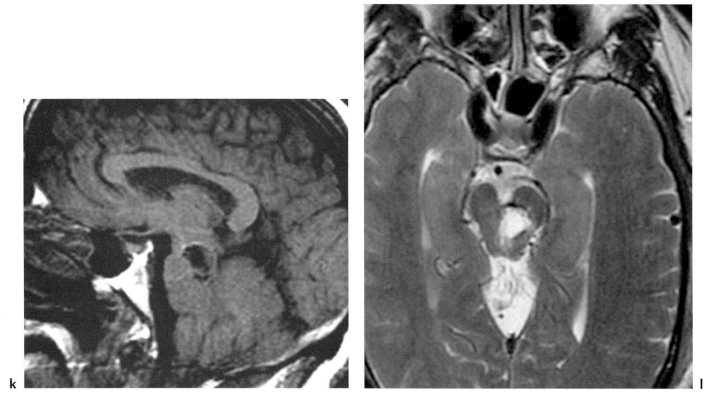

Figure 5.14. Postoperative **(k)** sagittal T1-weighted and **(l)** axial T2-weighted magnetic resonance images demonstrate complete removal of the lesion.

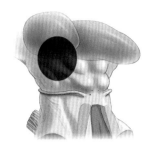

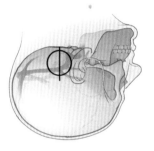

Case 5.15

- Diagnosis: Thalamic/midbrain cavernous malformation (related anatomy: pp. **18, 38, 43**)

- Preoperative examination: Gait instability, bilateral abducens nerve (CN VI) palsy, and partial bilateral oculomotor nerve (CN III) palsy

- Approach: Left lateral supracerebellar infratentorial and transtentorial (related approach: pp. **238–246**)

- Positioning: Prone

- Monitoring: Somatosensory evoked potentials and motor evoked potentials

- Outcome: Complete removal of lesion; postoperatively, the patient is unable to mobilize but by 4.5-month follow-up, he is able to ambulate without assistance; preoperative cranial nerve deficits persist but are stable.

See Video 5.15 and Animations 5.2 and 5.4

Figure 5.15. A 67-year-old man with a midbrain cavernous malformation presented after a prior unsuccessful resection attempt via a subtemporal approach at an outside institution.

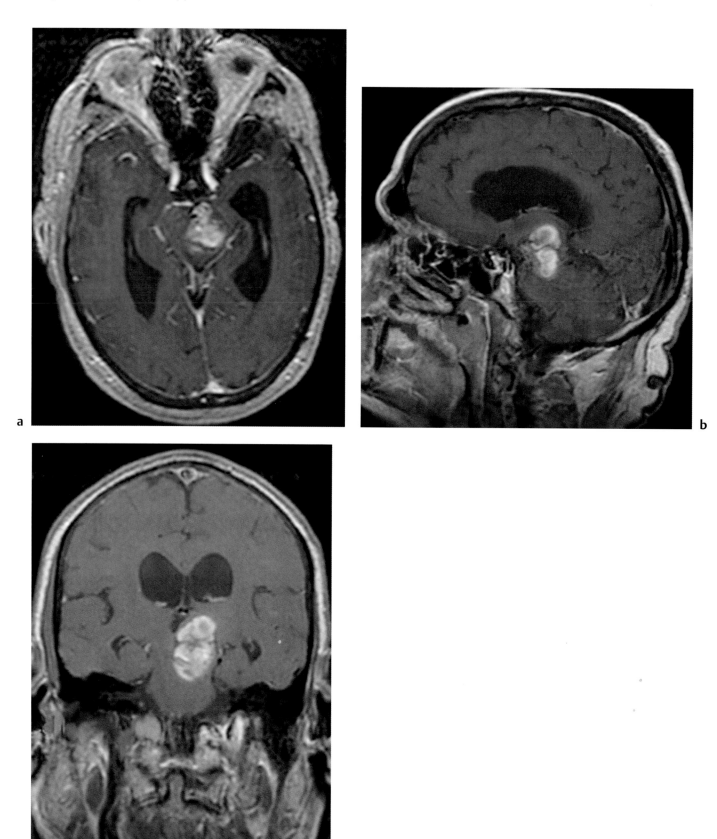

Figure 5.15. **(a)** Axial, **(b)** sagittal, and **(c)** coronal T1-weighted magnetic resonance images demonstrate a midbrain cavernous malformation with evidence of hemorrhage.

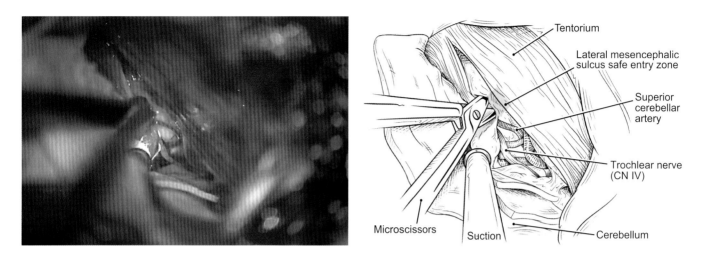

Figure 5.15. (d) The lesion is accessed using a left supracerebellar infratentorial approach, enabling the surgeon to arrive at the midbrain from a posterior or posterolateral direction. Release of cerebrospinal fluid and dissection of the arachnoid membrane result in visualization of the trochlear nerve (CN IV) and branches of the superior cerebellar artery, which are key landmarks to identify the lateral mesencephalic sulcus safe entry zone (*blue area*).

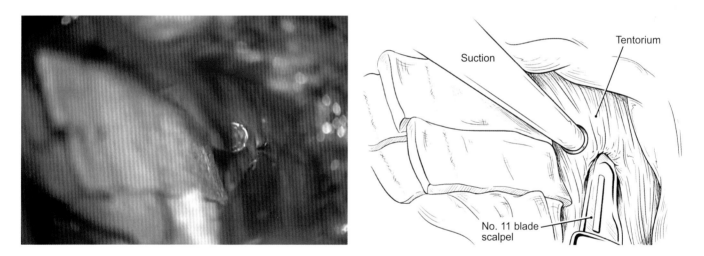

Figure 5.15. (e) In cases that require supratentorial visualization, the tentorium can be cut to obtain a superior view. This transtentorial approach can also be used to expose the posterior mesial temporal region and the thalamus.

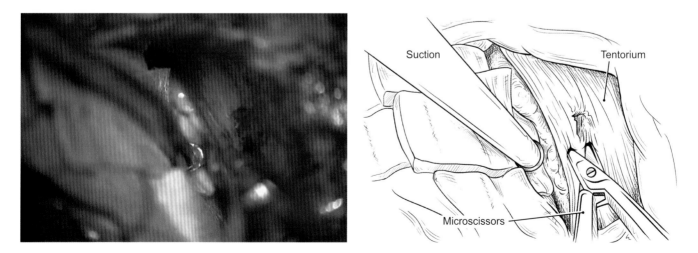

Figure 5.15. (f) The tentorium is cut with microscissors after being coagulated using bipolar cautery. Because the tentorium may contain venous lakes, care should be taken when coagulating and cutting it.

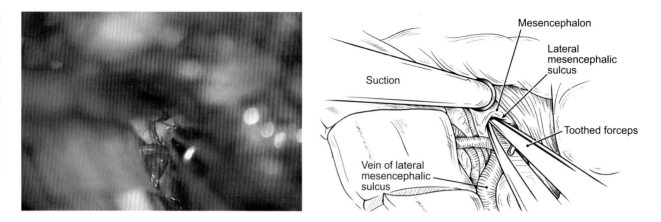

Figure 5.15. (g) Cutting the tentorium provides better visualization of the top of the midbrain and the thalamus. Neuronavigation is then used to select an ideal point of entry into the brainstem to resect the lesion.

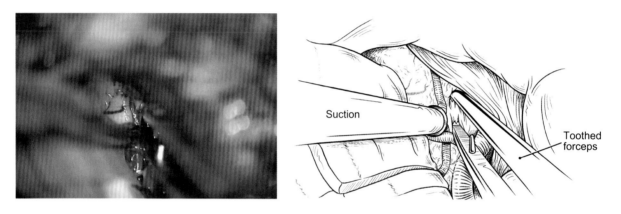

Figure 5.15. (h) The opening is expanded parallel to the ascending and descending fibers.

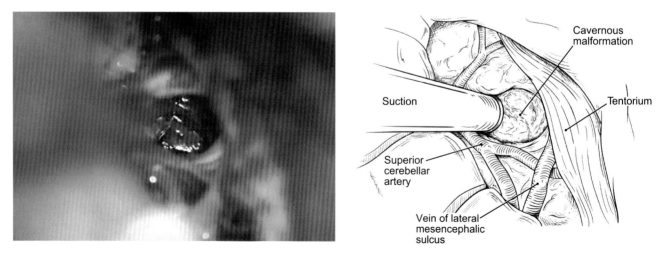

Figure 5.15. (i) The lesion is visualized and debulked.

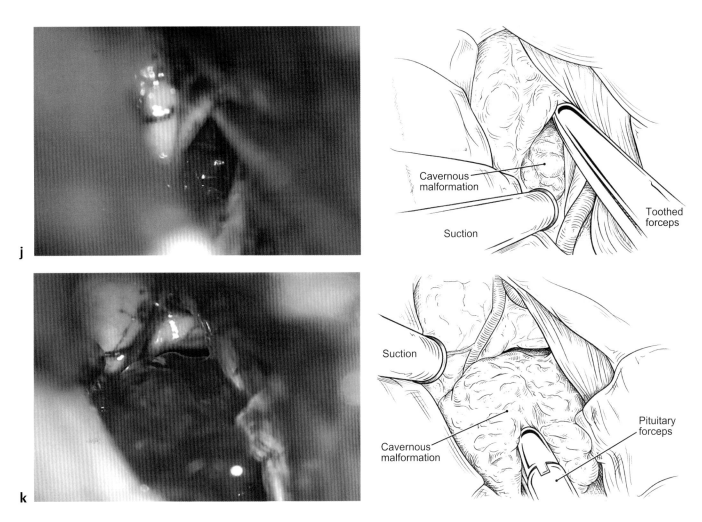

Figure 5.15. (j,k) Once fully mobilized, the cavernous malformation is removed piecemeal.

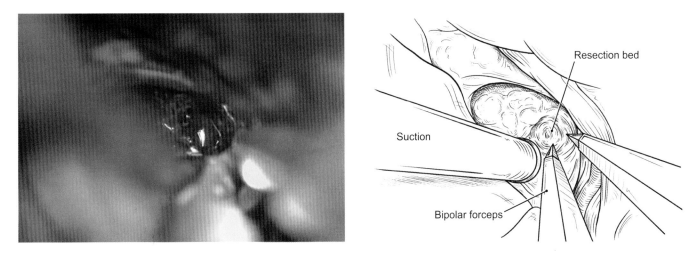

Figure 5.15. (l) The resection bed is inspected, and hemostasis is obtained.

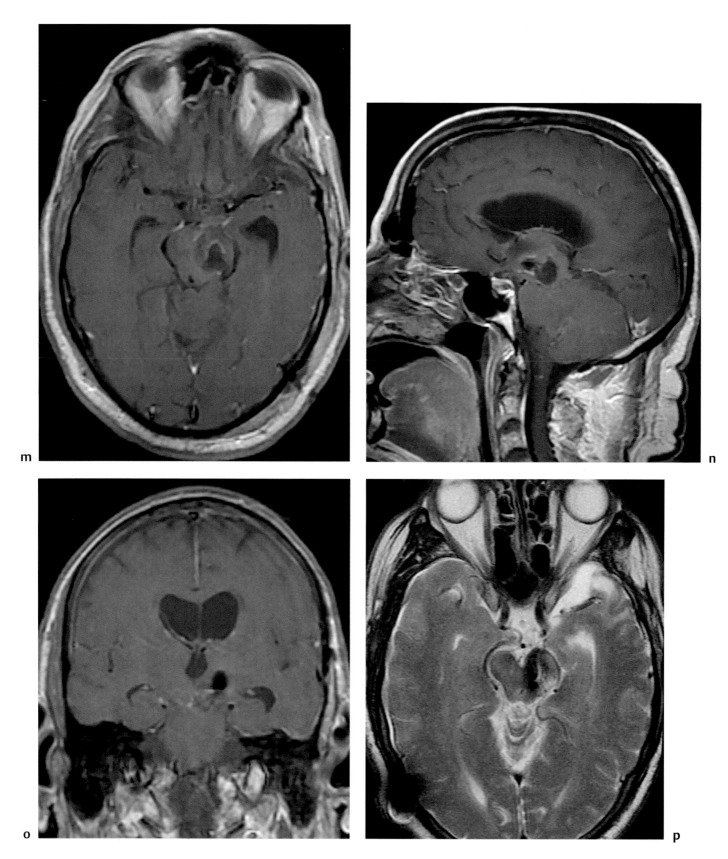

Figure 5.15. Postoperative **(m)** axial, **(n)** sagittal, and **(o)** coronal T1-weighted and **(p)** axial T2-weighted magnetic resonance images confirm complete removal of the lesion.

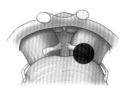

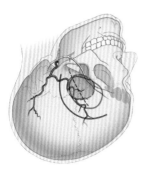

Case 5.16

- Diagnosis: Pontine cavernous malformation (related anatomy: pp. **5, 6, 17, 18, 26, 27, 39, 42**)

- Preoperative examination: Difficulty with tandem walk and right arm pronator drift

- Approach: Left orbitozygomatic craniotomy (related approach: pp. **144–160**)

- Positioning: Supine

- Monitoring: Somatosensory evoked potentials and motor evoked potentials

- Outcome: Complete removal of lesion; transient worsening of right arm weakness; otherwise, neurologic status is unchanged.

See Video 5.16 and Animations 5.2 and 5.3

Figure 5.16. A 26-year-old woman presented with difficulty with tandem gait and right arm pronator drift.

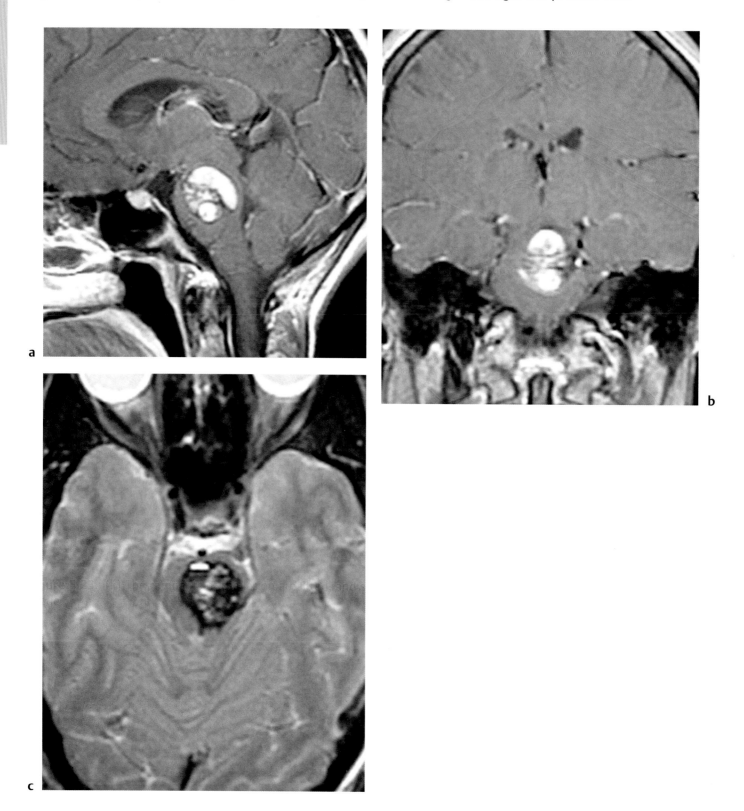

Figure 5.16. (a) Sagittal and **(b)** coronal T1-weighted and **(c)** axial T2-weighted magnetic resonance images demonstrate a large pontine cavernous malformation with evidence of hemorrhage.

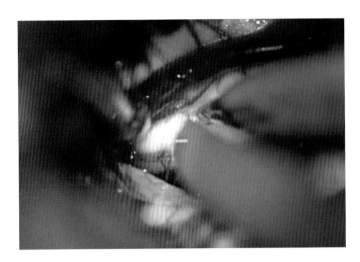

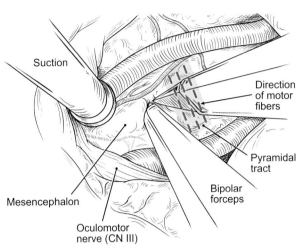

Figure 5.16. (d) The lesion is exposed using a left orbitozygomatic craniotomy. The cavernous malformation is approached lateral to and slightly below the oculomotor nerve (CN III). Neuronavigation can be used to optimize the point of entry into the brainstem. The point of entry should minimally transgress the brainstem and avoid the critical motor fibers (*dashed lines*) found anteriorly in the medial three-fifths of the cerebral peduncle. In many cases, the hemorrhage and cavernous malformation displace critical tracts (*green area*) and provide a path for resection of even the largest lesions. For ventral midbrain lesions, the anterior mesencephalic safe entry zone zone, which is bound superiorly by the posterior cerebral artery, inferiorly by the superior cerebellar artery, and medially by the oculomotor nerve, can be used.

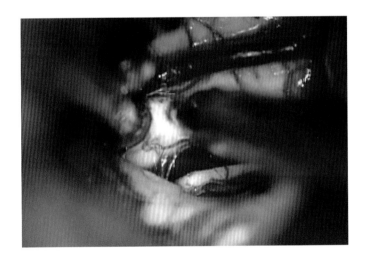

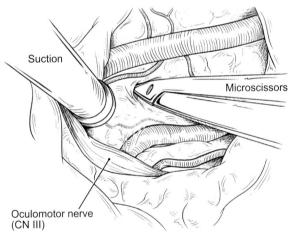

Figure 5.16. (e) Sharp dissection is used to make a small opening into the brainstem.

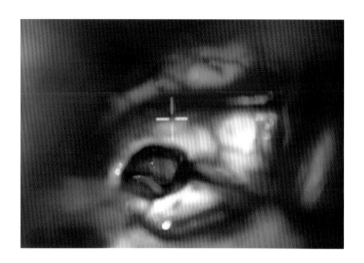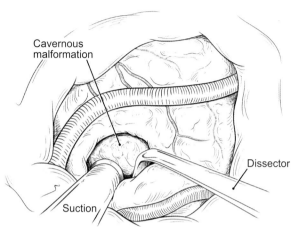

Figure 5.16. (f) The opening into the brainstem is expanded by spreading the fibers enough to place a small suction cannula and microdissector into the cavity to mobilize the lesion.

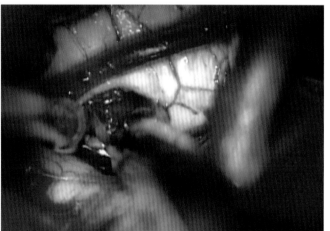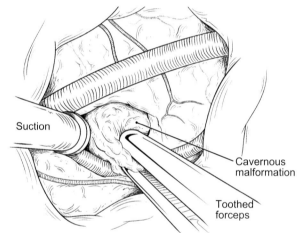

Figure 5.16. (g) The lesion is mobilized, dissected, and removed piecemeal.

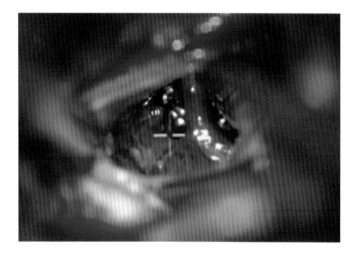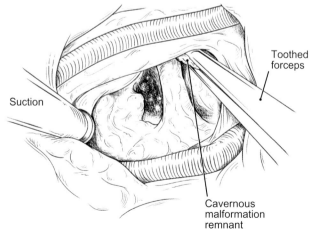

Figure 5.16. (h) Remnants of the cavernous malformation are removed using toothed forceps.

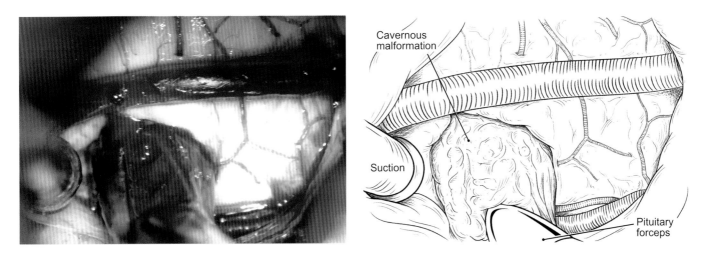

Figure 5.16. **(i)** As the cavernous malformation is removed, traction on the brainstem is minimized.

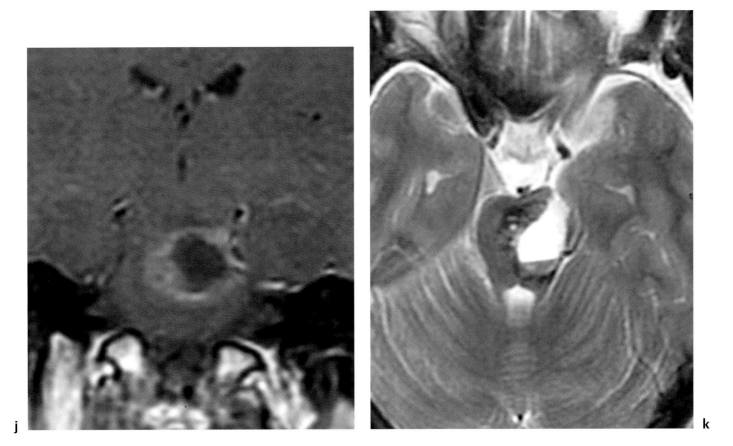

Figure 5.16. Postoperative **(j)** coronal T1-weighted and **(k)** axial T2-weighted magnetic resonance images demonstrate complete resection of the lesion, with some fluid in the resection cavity. The T2-weighted magnetic resonance image also shows the pathway into the brainstem to remove the lesion.

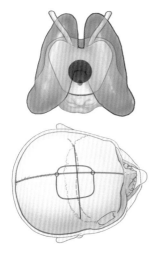

Case 5.17

- Diagnosis: Midbrain cavernous malformation (related anatomy: pp. **3–12, 14–16**)
- Preoperative examination: Neurologically intact
- Approach: Right posterior interhemispheric transcallosal interforniceal
- Positioning: Semi-sitting
- Monitoring: Somatosensory evoked potentials and motor evoked potentials
- Outcome: Complete removal of lesion; no new deficit; memory is stable.

See Video 5.17 and Animation 5.2

Figure 5.17. An 18-year-old man presented with progressive memory loss.

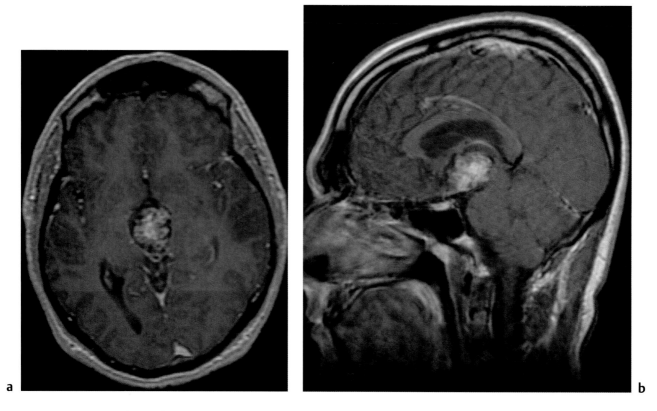

a   b

Figure 5.17. (a) Axial and **(b)** sagittal T1-weighted magnetic resonance images demonstrate a midbrain cavernous malformation with evidence of hemorrhage.

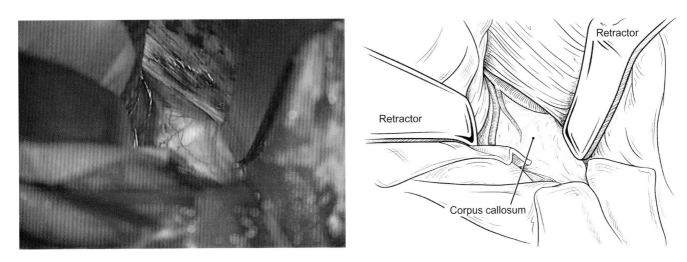

Figure 5.17. (c) The lesion was accessed using a posterior interhemispheric transcallosal approach. Although retractors are rarely used to expand the operative field, retractors are gently placed on the parieto-occipital lobes to expand the interhemispheric exposure in this case.

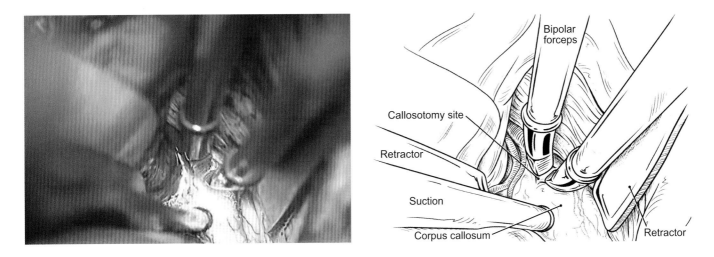

Figure 5.17. (d) Neuronavigation imaging is used to select the optimal site for the callosotomy.

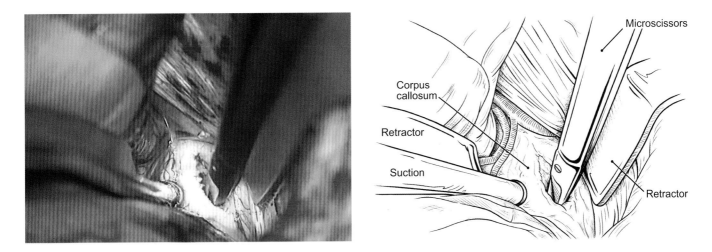

Figure 5.17. (e) Sharp dissection is used to expand the opening in the corpus callosum.

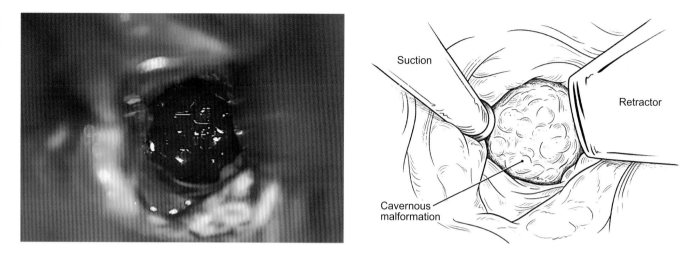

Figure 5.17. (f) The lesion is visualized at the depth of the cavity after the opening is further expanded.

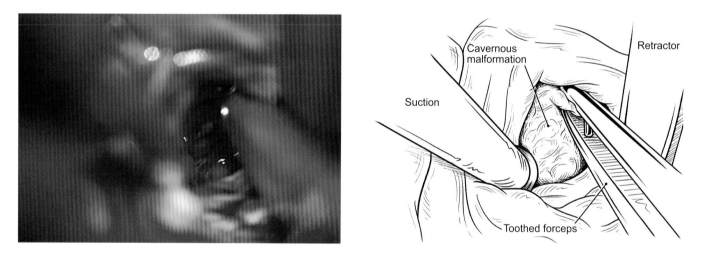

Figure 5.17. (g) A combination of microdissectors and toothed forceps is used to mobilize the lesion from the adjacent brainstem.

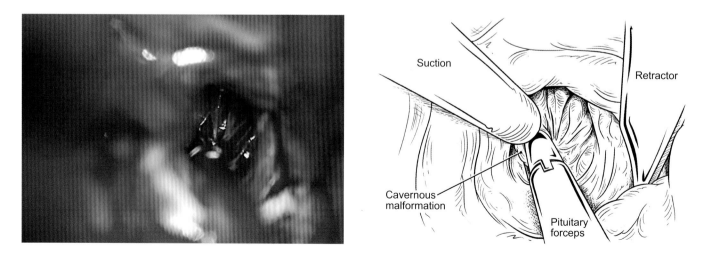

Figure 5.17. (h) Remnants of the cavernous malformation are peeled from the brainstem using pituitary forceps and suction.

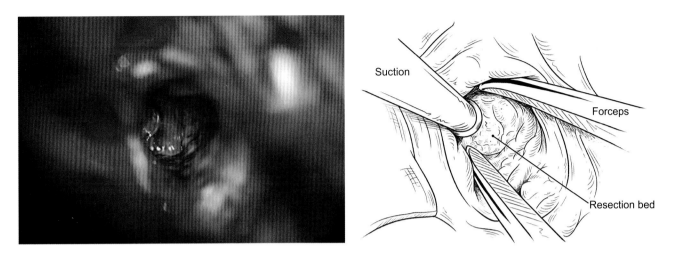

Figure 5.17. (i) The resection bed is inspected to ensure that no remnant is left behind and to confirm that hemostasis is obtained.

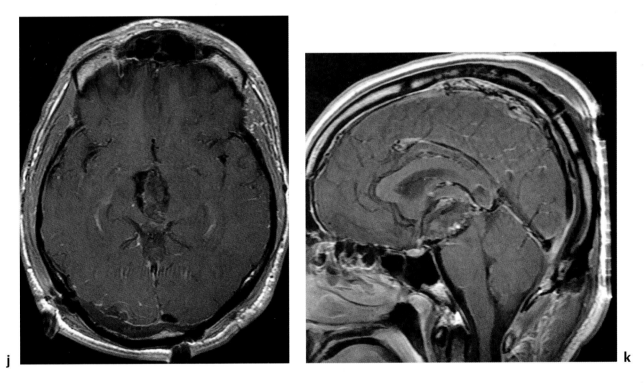

j

k

Figure 5.17. Postoperative **(j)** axial and **(k)** sagittal T1-weighted magnetic resonance images demonstrate complete removal of the lesion and show the location of the craniotomy used for the posterior interhemispheric approach.

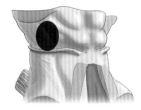

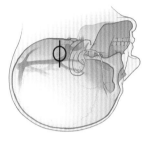

Case 5.18

- Diagnosis: Midbrain cavernous malformation (related anatomy: pp. **18, 38, 43**)
- Preoperative examination: Neurologically intact
- Approach: Left lateral supracerebellar infratentorial (related approach: pp. **238–246**)
- Positioning: Supine
- Monitoring: Somatosensory evoked potentials and motor evoked potentials
- Outcome: Complete removal of lesion; diminished sensation on right side of body; otherwise, the patient is neurologically intact.

See Video 5.18 and Animations 5.2 and 5.4

Figure 5.18. A 45-year-old woman presented after an episode of right arm and leg numbness.

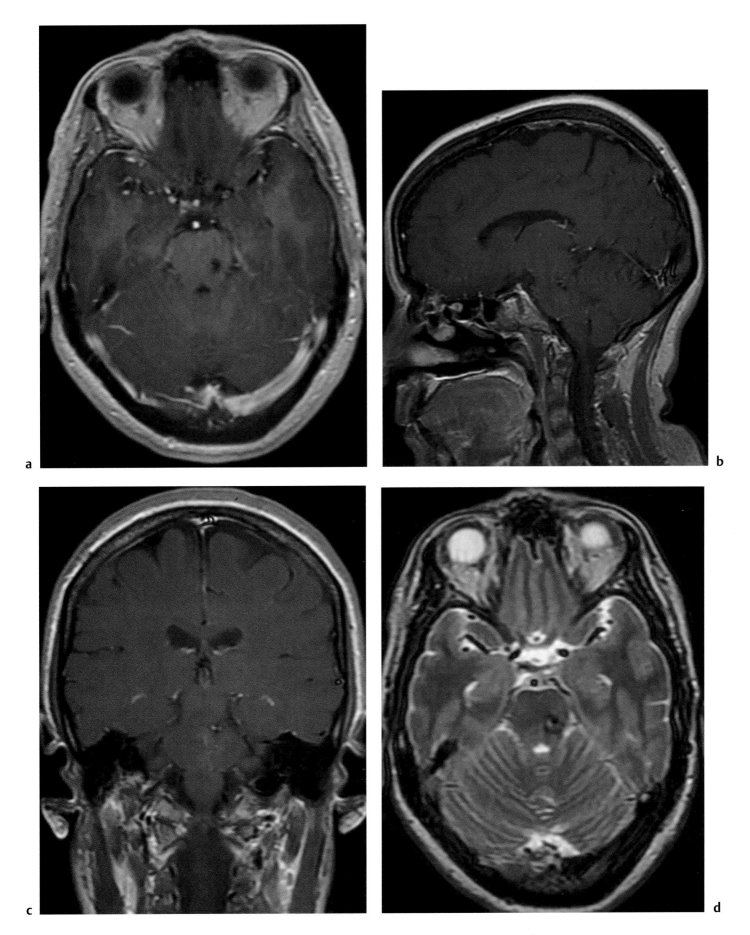

Figure 5.18. (a) Axial, **(b)** sagittal, and **(c)** coronal T1-weighted and **(d)** axial T2-weighted magnetic resonance images demonstrate a left lateral mesencephalic cavernous malformation.

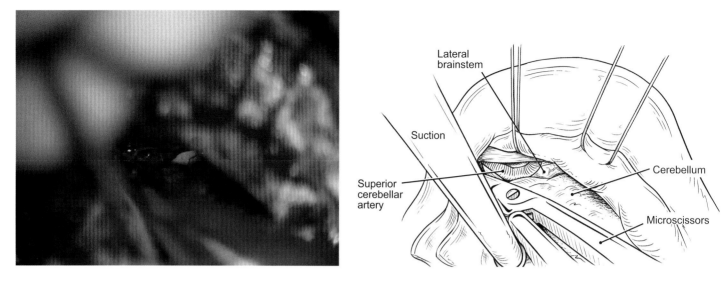

Figure 5.18. (e) The lesion is approached using a left lateral supracerebellar infratentorial craniotomy. The release of cerebrospinal fluid from the cerebellopontine angle enables the surgeon to visualize the lateral brainstem and obtain the cerebellar relaxation necessary for the supracerebellar infratentorial approach.

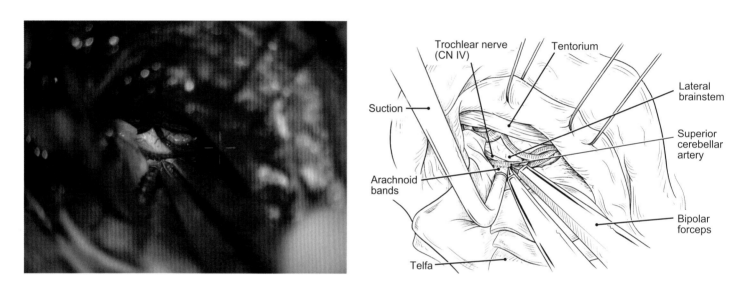

Figure 5.18. (f) Disconnection of arachnoid bands tethering the cerebellum to the tentorium aids visualization of the lateral brainstem. The trochlear nerve (CN IV) and the superior cerebellar artery are visualized.

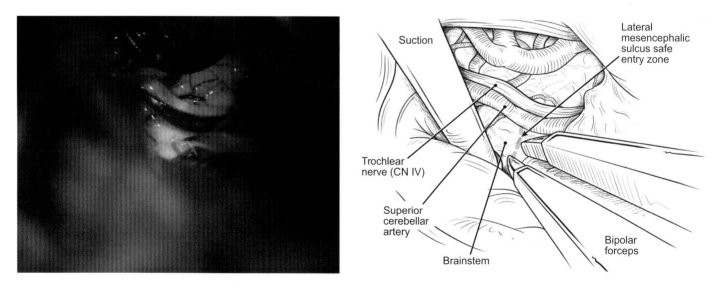

Figure 5.18. (g) The use of intraoperative neuronavigation enables selection of an ideal point of entry into the brainstem, the lateral mesencephalic sulcus safe entry zone (*dashed line*), which minimally traverses the normal anatomy. The courses of the trochlear nerve and the superior cerebellar artery as they traverse the vein of the lateral mesencephalic sulcus are reliable landmarks for identifying the lateral mesencephalic sulcus safe entry zone.

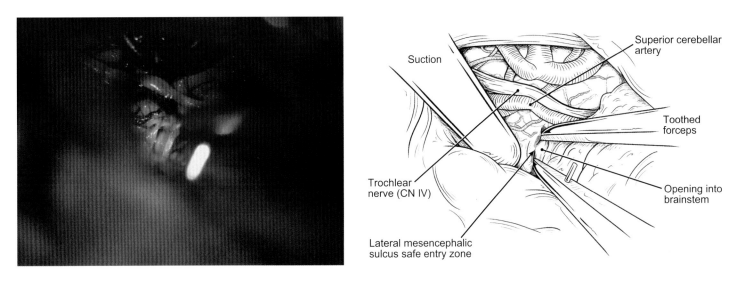

Figure 5.18. (h) The opening into the brainstem using the lateral mesencephalic sulcus safe entry zone (*dashed line*) is made sharply using microscissors or toothed forceps and is minimally expanded to limit interruption of the ascending and descending tracts.

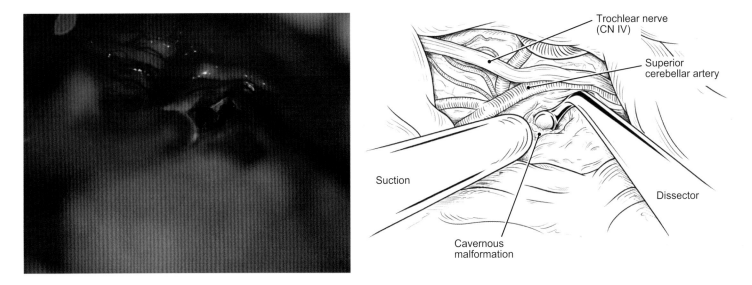

Figure 5.18. (i) After the cavernous malformation is entered, a microdissector is used to mobilize it from the brainstem. Lighted instruments, such as a suction cannula, greatly facilitate visualization at the depth of the cavity.

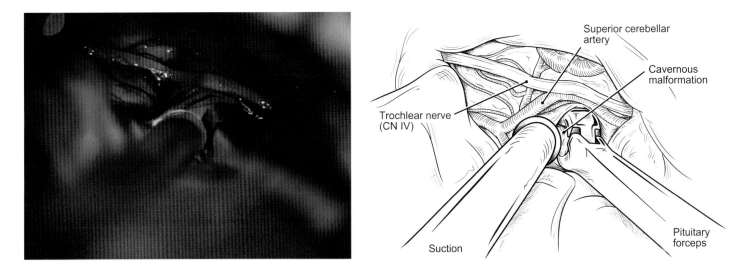

Figure 5.18. (j) Microinstruments, such as pituitary forceps and suction cannulas, are used to remove the lesion piecemeal.

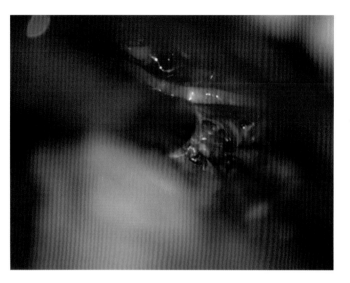
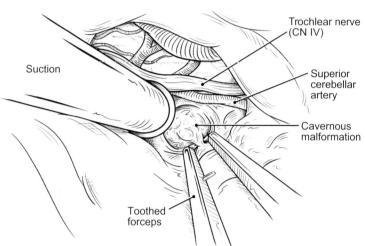

Figure 5.18. (k) Toothed forceps are essential for peeling the cavernous malformation remnants from the adjacent brainstem.

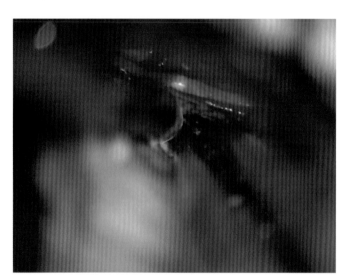
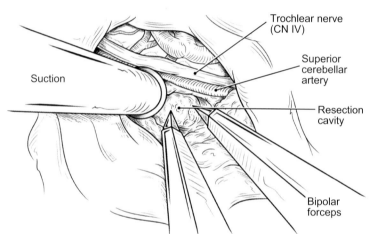

Figure 5.18. (l) Selective use of bipolar forceps to cauterize bleeders prevents injury to critical structures in the brainstem. When venous bleeding from the resection cavity occurs, the patient's head should be elevated, carbon dioxide levels should be optimized, and hemostatic agents should be used to control the bleeding. The use of bipolar forceps in the brainstem should be minimized, and any developmental venous anomalies should be preserved.

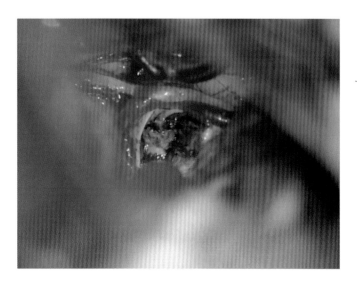
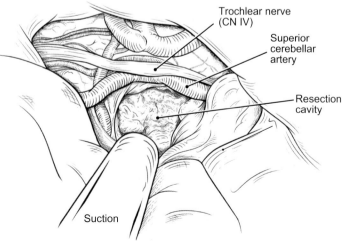

Figure 5.18. (m) Final inspection of the resection cavity shows complete removal of the lesion.

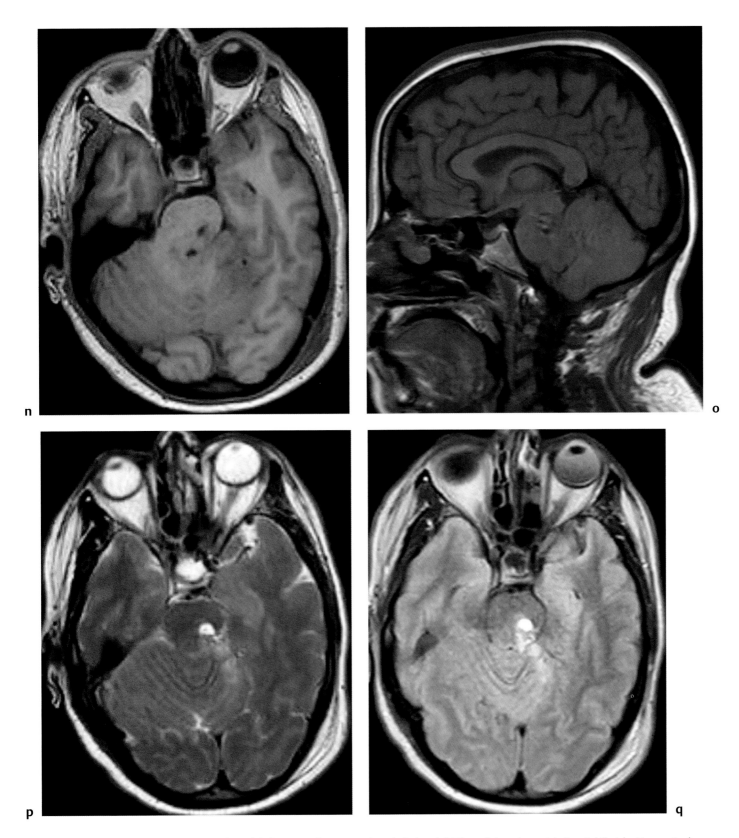

Figure 5.18. Postoperative **(n)** axial and **(o)** sagittal T1-weighted, **(p)** axial T2-weighted, and **(q)** axial fluid-attenuated inversion recovery (FLAIR) magnetic resonance images confirm complete removal of the lesion.

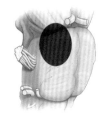

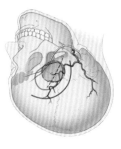

Case 5.19

- Diagnosis: Pontomesencephalic cavernous malformation (related anatomy: pp. **5, 6, 17, 18, 26, 27, 39, 42**)

- Preoperative examination: Motor discoordination with fine movement in left hand

- Approach: Right orbitozygomatic (related approach: pp. **144–160**)

- Positioning: Supine, with head rotated to contralateral side and neck extended

- Monitoring: Somatosensory evoked potentials and motor evoked potentials

- Outcome: Complete removal of lesion; neurologic status is unchanged.

See Video 5.19 and Animations 5.2 and 5.3

Figure 5.19. A 21-year-old man presented with subtle left hand motor discoordination and a history of sudden-onset headache, diplopia, and left hemiparesis 6 months earlier.

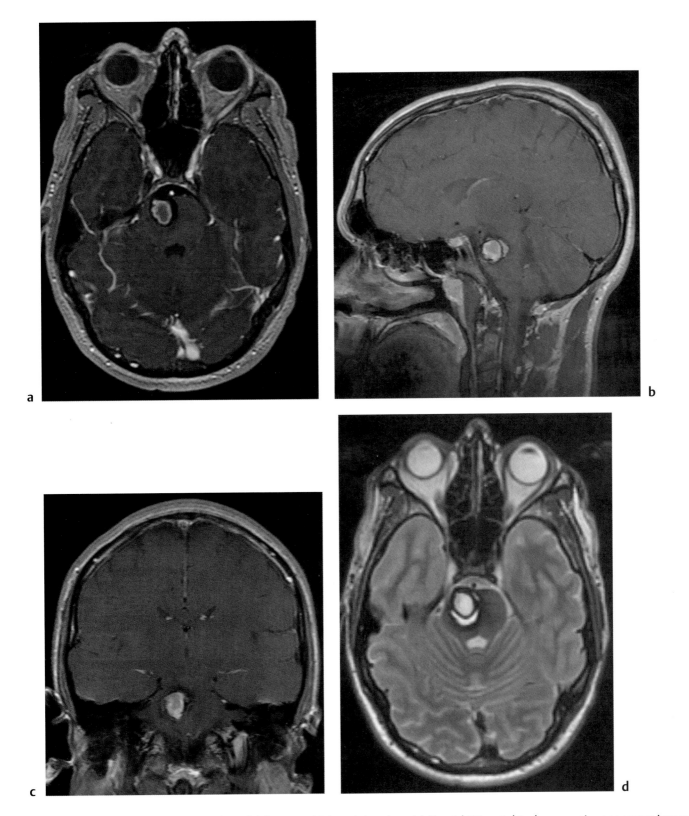

Figure 5.19. **(a)** Axial, **(b)** sagittal, and **(c)** coronal T1-weighted and **(d)** axial T2-weighted magnetic resonance images demonstrate a cavernous malformation in the right pontomesencephalic junction.

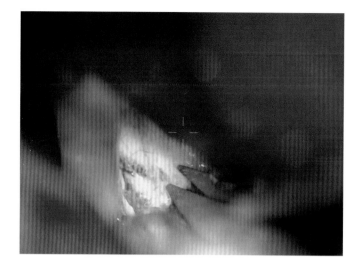
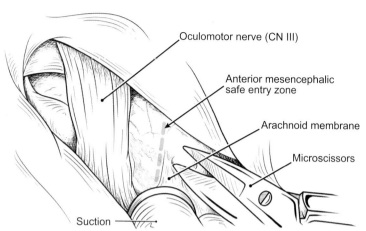

Figure 5.19. (e) The lesion was approached using a right orbitozygomatic craniotomy via the anterior mesencephalic safe entry zone (*dashed line*). The key to this operation is to position the patient with the head rotated to the contralateral side and the neck extended to enable the frontal and temporal lobes to fall away once the sylvian fissure is widely split. In this case, the lesion had displaced the motor tracts, which are ventrally and laterally located in the middle three-fifths of the cerebral peduncle. The anterior mesencephalic safe entry zone is reached by disconnecting the arachnoid membrane lateral to the oculomotor nerve (CN III), which enables the temporal lobe to fall away while the oculomotor nerve remains medially displaced. In the space between the posterior cerebral artery and the superior cerebellar artery just lateral to the oculomotor nerve, the brainstem can be entered to resect intrinsic lesions.

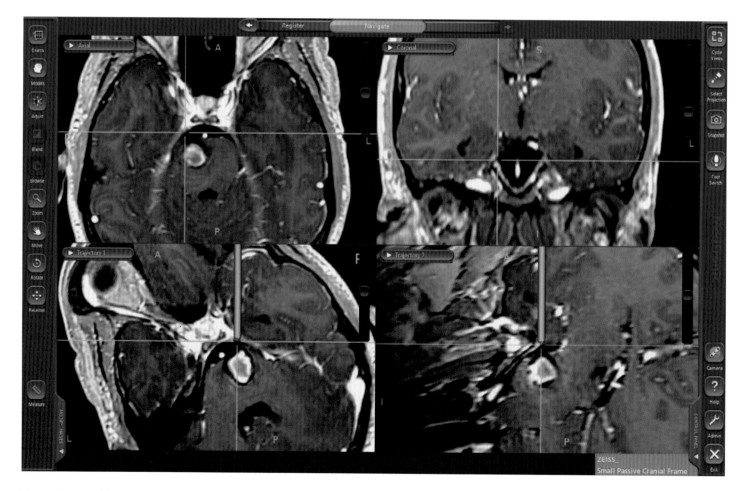

Figure 5.19. (f) Intraoperative neuronavigation images assist with the selection of entry points into the brainstem when the lesion does not abut a pial or an ependymal surface or when there is no obvious hemosiderin staining of the surface of the brainstem to assist with the selection of a point of entry.

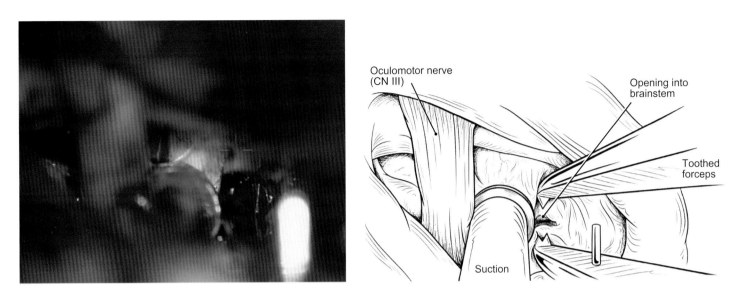

Figure 5.19. (g) Toothed forceps are used to make a small opening in the brainstem just lateral to the oculomotor nerve. The brainstem fibers are split to minimize the surgical footprint.

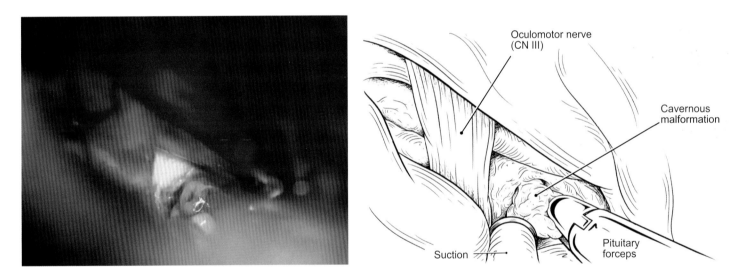

Figure 5.19. (h) Pituitary forceps are used to remove the lesion piecemeal.

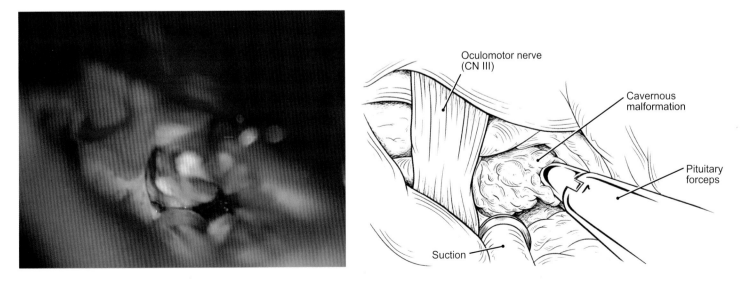

Figure 5.19. (i) The suction cannula provides countertraction and dynamic retraction as the lesion is mobilized.

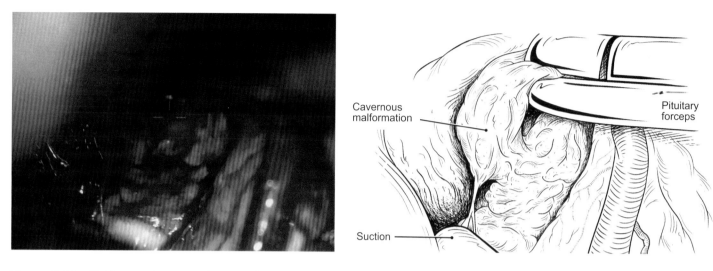

Figure 5.19. (j) The suction cannula is used as a microdissector to disconnect the cavernous malformation from the brainstem while the pituitary forceps provide traction on the lesion.

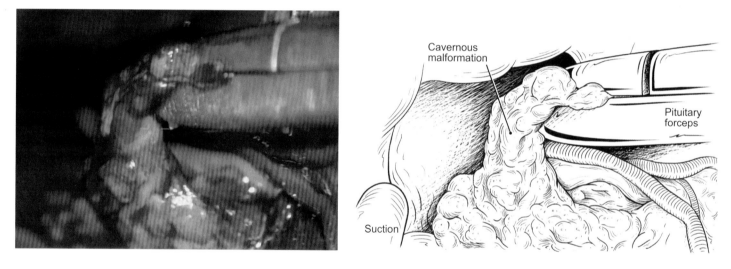

Figure 5.19. (k) Pituitary forceps are used to remove the remnants of the cavernous malformation from the resection cavity.

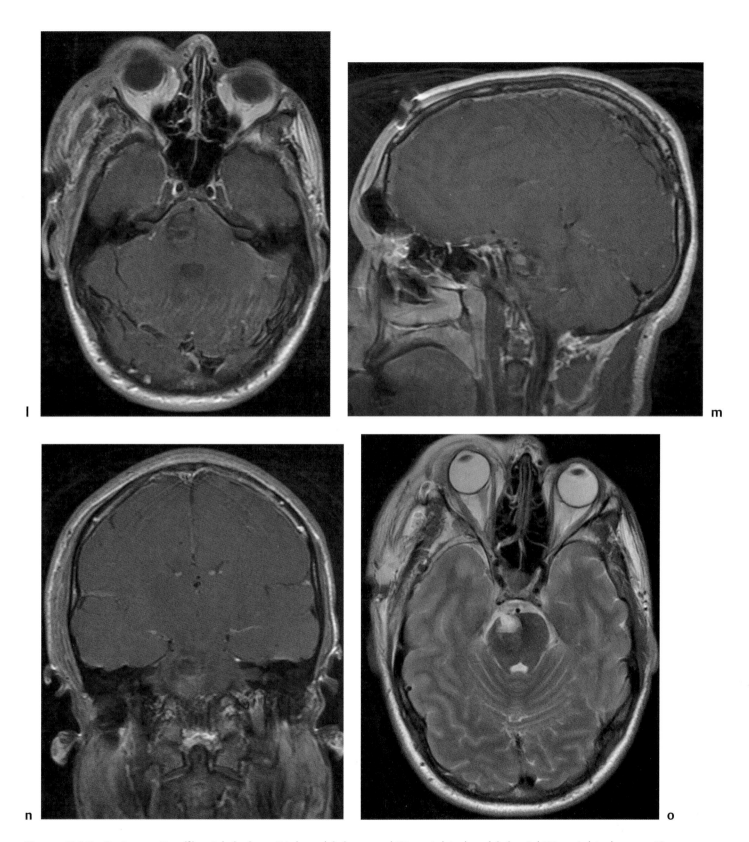

Figure 5.19. Postoperative **(l)** axial, **(m)** sagittal, and **(n)** coronal T1-weighted and **(o)** axial T2-weighted magnetic resonance images confirm complete removal of the cavernous malformation.

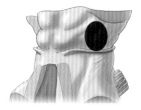

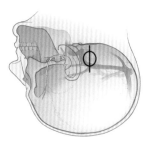

Case 5.20

- Diagnosis: Midbrain pilocytic astrocytoma (related anatomy: pp. **18, 38, 43**)

- Preoperative examination: Impaired upgaze; disconjugate gaze (worse on right gaze); mild left facial weakness; and mild left arm and leg weakness

- Approach: Right lateral supracerebellar infratentorial and transtentorial (related approach: pp. **238–246**)

- Positioning: Supine

- Monitoring: Somatosensory evoked potentials and motor evoked potentials

- Outcome: Subtotal resection of lesion; neurologic status is unchanged.

See Video 5.20

Figure 5.20. A 52-year-old man previously diagnosed with a midbrain pilocytic astrocytoma presented after multiple prior biopsies and radiotherapy.

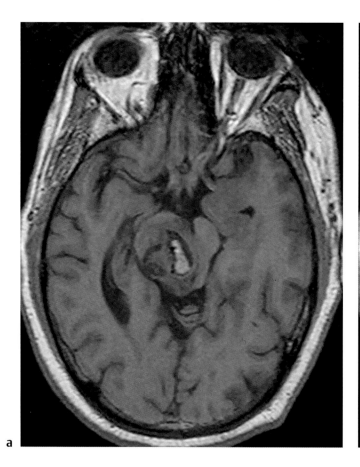

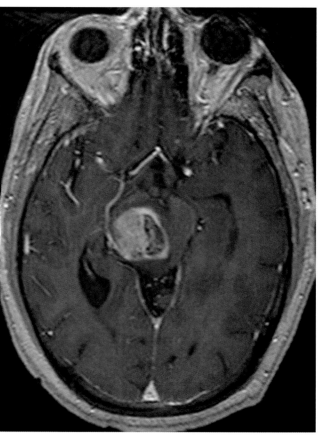

a

b

Figure 5.20. (a) Axial T1-weighted without contrast and **(b)** axial T1-weighted with contrast magnetic resonance images demonstrate a large, highly contrast-enhancing lesion in the midbrain. The lesion was accessed using a right lateral supracerebellar infratentorial and transtentorial approach.

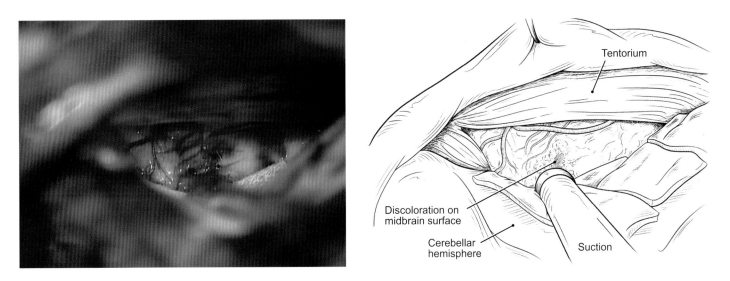

Figure 5.20. (c) Discoloration on the surface of the brainstem signifies the site of the lesion, and a biopsy specimen is obtained. The biopsy results indicate that the lesion is a juvenile pilocytic astrocytoma, which requires complete removal, if possible.

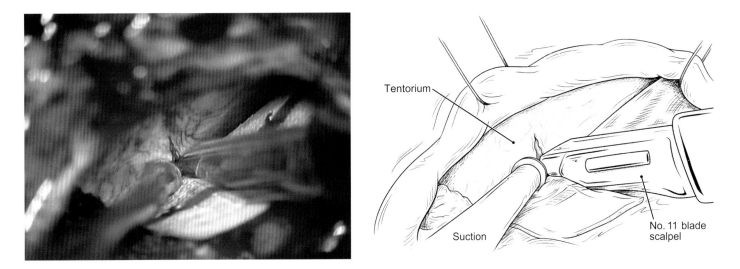

Figure 5.20. (d) The superior extension of the tumor is exposed by coagulating and cutting the tentorium to better visualize the lesion.

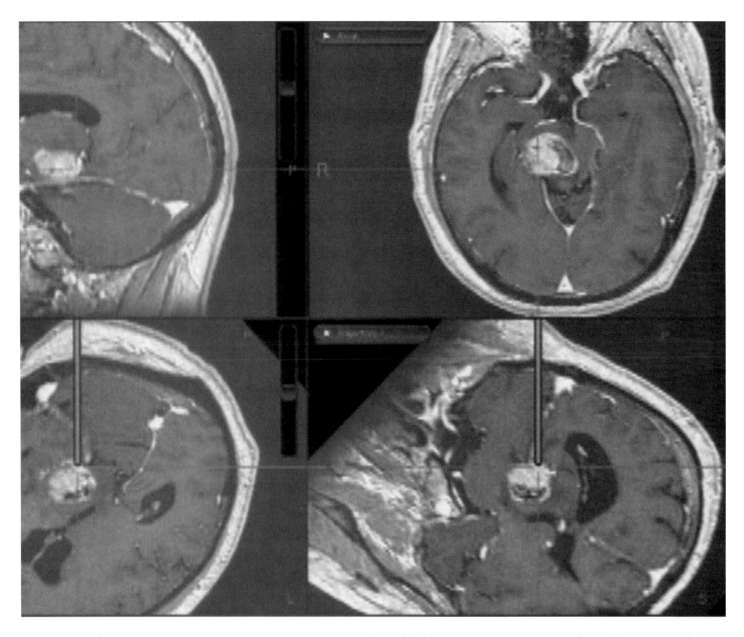

Figure 5.20. (e) Intraoperative neuronavigation images show the added exposure and trajectory afforded by incising the tentorium.

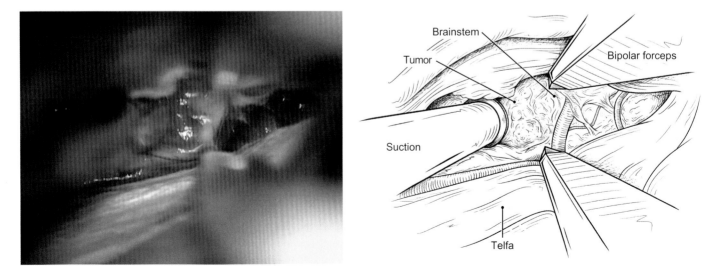

Figure 5.20. (f) The tumor is debulked internally and resected piecemeal. The gelatinous nature of the tumor enables it to be readily distinguished from adjacent normal brain tissue, but this distinction is not always possible.

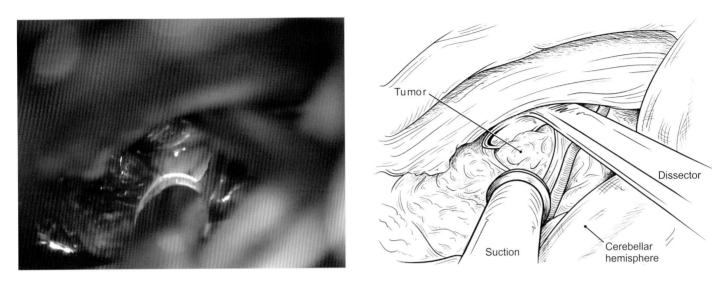

Figure 5.20. (g) Tumor removal continues until the boundary with the normal brain tissue is reached. Neuronavigation can help identify this interface, but other factors, such as tumor consistency and response to suction and cautery, can also help identify it.

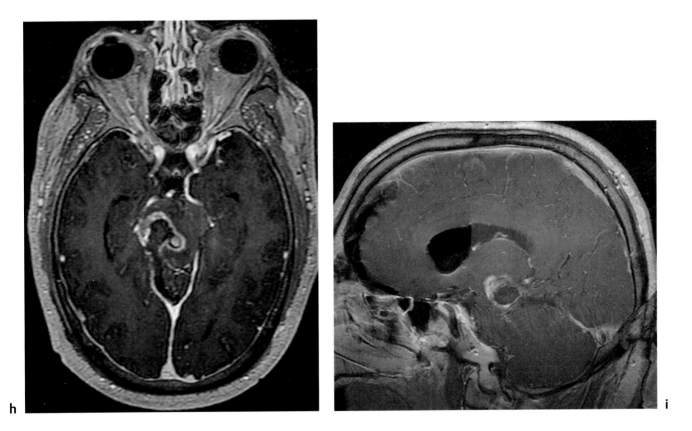

Figure 5.20. Postoperative **(h)** axial T1-weighted and **(i)** sagittal T1-weighted with contrast magnetic resonance images confirm subtotal removal of the lesion.

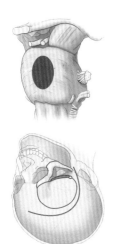

Case 5.21

• Diagnosis: Complex basilar artery aneurysm (related anatomy: pp. **27–29**)
• Preoperative examination: Neurologically intact
• Approach: Right orbitozygomatic (related approach: pp. **144–160**)
• Positioning: Supine
• Monitoring: Somatosensory evoked potentials and motor evoked potentials
• Outcome: Aneurysm occluded; bypass patent; patient is neurologically intact.

See Video 5.21

Figure 5.21. A 50-year-old man presented with headaches. Angiograms showed a dissecting basilar artery aneurysm.

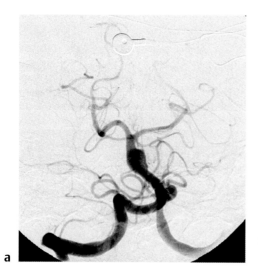
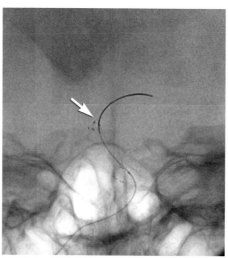

a
b

Figure 5.21. (a) Transfacial vertebral artery angiogram shows a dissecting basilar artery aneurysm in a 50-year-old patient with headaches who had endovascular treatment of the lesion. **(b)** An unsubtracted transfacial angiogram shows the stent (*arrow*) placed in the aneurysm to enable the injured vessel wall to heal.

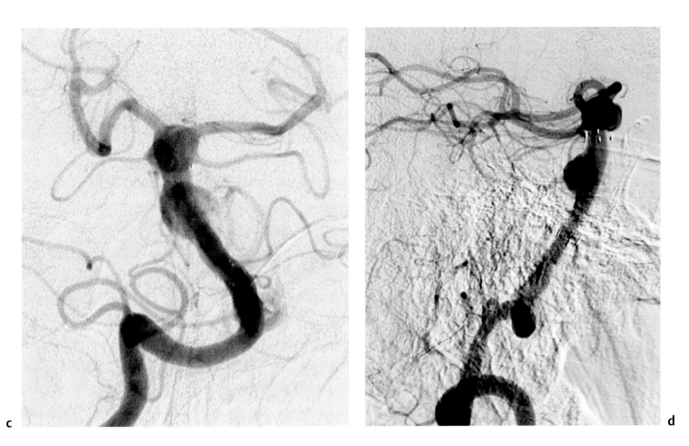

c   d

Figure 5.21. (c) Thirteen months after stent placement, further enlargement of the aneurysm is observed on a transfacial vertebral artery angiogram. **(d)** Lateral vertebral artery angiogram demonstrates progressive enlargement of the original aneurysm through the stent and disease progression distal to the stent. The patient underwent an Allcock test.

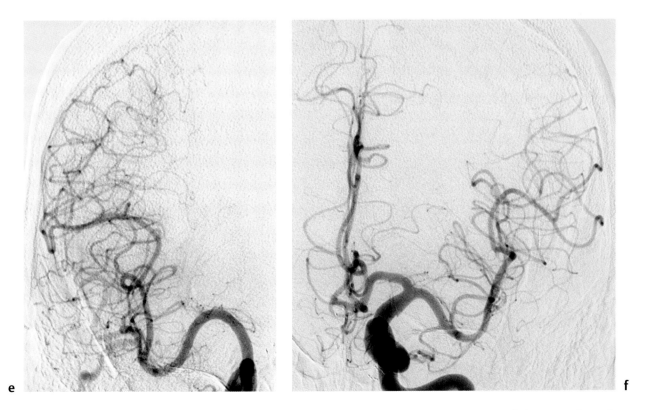

e   f

Figure 5.21. (e,f) Anteroposterior internal carotid artery angiograms with compression of the contralateral internal carotid artery show no significant posterior communicating artery contribution as a collateral. The decision is made to disconnect the anterior and posterior circulations by occluding the basilar artery below the superior cerebellar arteries and to revascularize the basilar apex using a superficial temporal artery-to-superior cerebellar artery bypass.

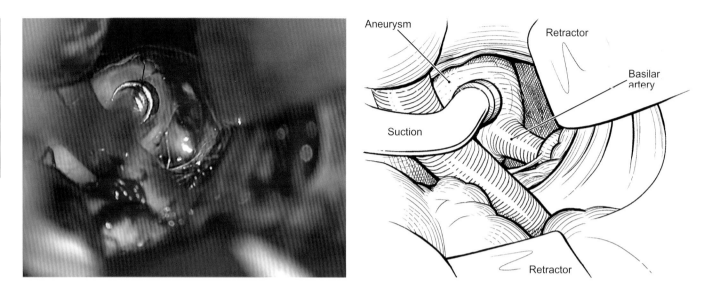

Figure 5.21. (g) Through a right orbitozygomatic approach, the distal basilar artery aneurysm is visible.

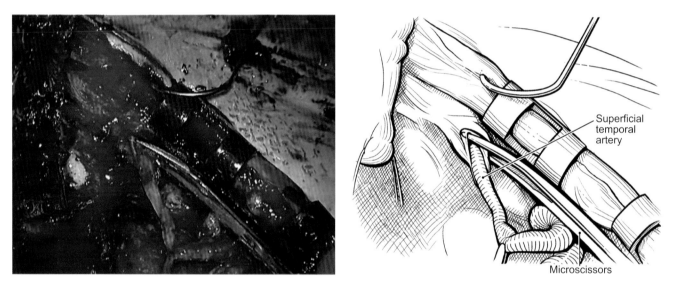

Figure 5.21. (h) The superficial temporal artery is freed and prepared for anastomosis.

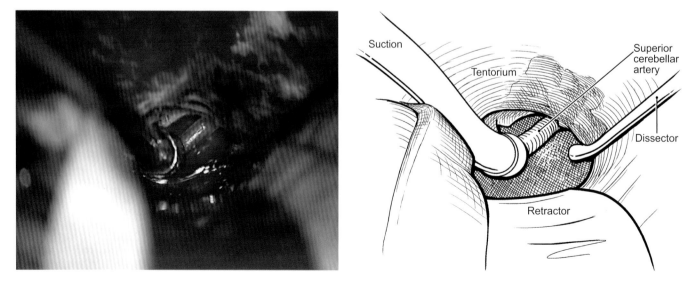

Figure 5.21. (i) The superior cerebellar artery is exposed through an incision in the tentorium.

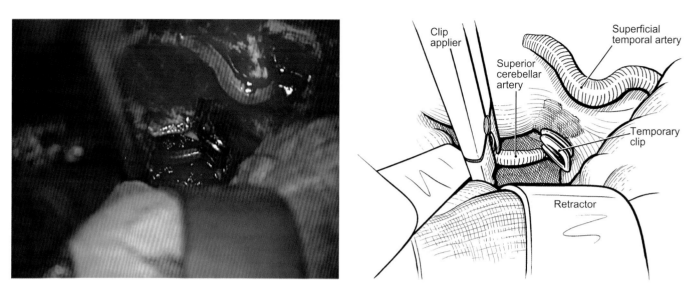

Figure 5.21. **(j)** Temporary clips are placed on the superior cerebellar artery.

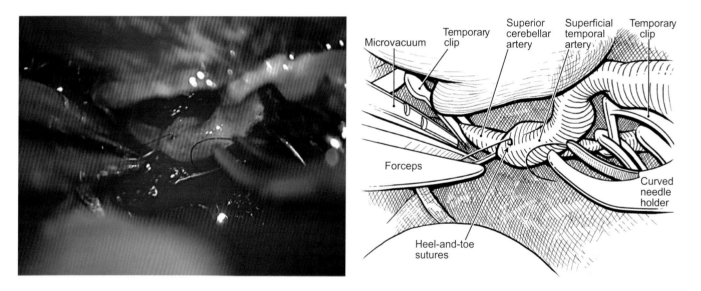

Figure 5.21. **(k)** After the superior cerebellar artery arteriotomy is made, the cut end of the superficial temporal artery is tacked to the superior cerebellar artery with heel-and-toe sutures.

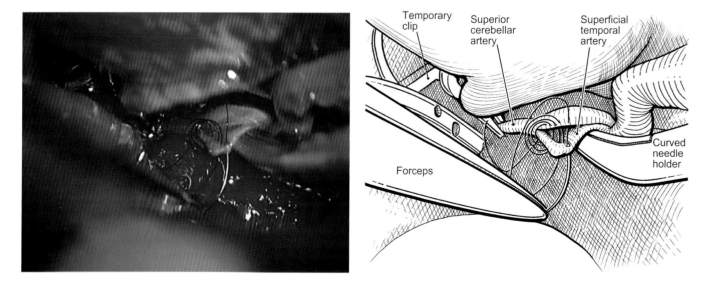

Figure 5.21. **(l)** Continuous running sutures are placed loosely in the back wall of the anastomosis.

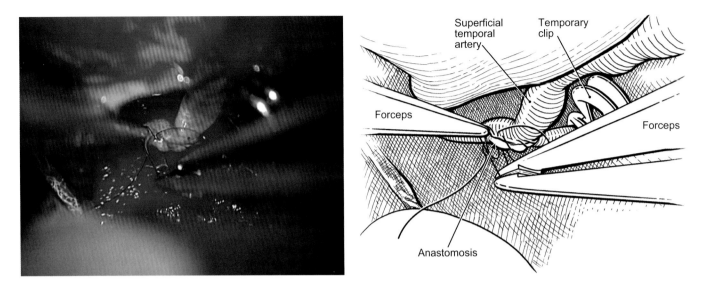

Figure 5.21. (m) The sutures are tightened.

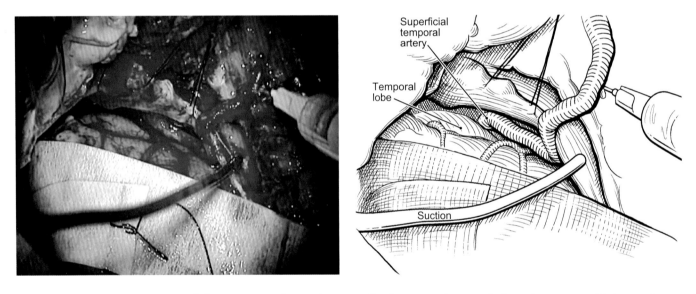

Figure 5.21. (n) An overview of the exposure shows the superficial temporal artery below the temporal lobe on its way to the site of the anastomosis.

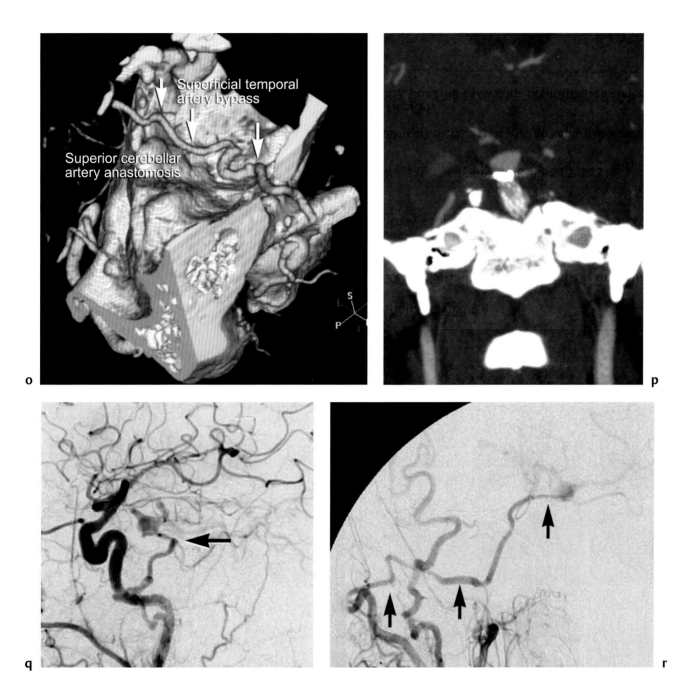

Figure 5.21. **(o)** Three-dimensional reconstruction shows the superficial temporal artery-to-superior cerebellar artery bypass (*arrows*). **(p)** Computed tomography angiogram shows the clips above the stent (placed during a prior hospitalization) and below the superior cerebellar artery.

(q) Lateral right common carotid artery angiogram demonstrates the superficial temporal artery-to-superior cerebellar artery bypass (*arrow*). **(r)** Close-up anteroposterior angiographic view shows the superficial temporal artery-to-superior cerebellar artery bypass (*arrows*).

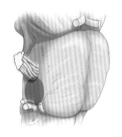

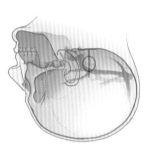

Case 5.22

- Diagnosis: Cerebellopontine angle arteriovenous malformation (related anatomy: pp. **51, 56, 62, 118–124**)

- Preoperative examination: Mild right-sided hearing loss

- Approach: Right retrosigmoid craniotomy (related approach: pp. **212–222**)

- Positioning: Supine

- Monitoring: Somatosensory evoked potentials and motor evoked potentials; trigeminal nerve (CN V), facial nerve (CN VII), and vestibulocochlear nerve (CN VIII)

- Outcome: Complete removal of lesion; neurologic status is unchanged.

See Video 5.22

Figure 5.22. A 57-year-old man presented with mild right-sided hearing loss.

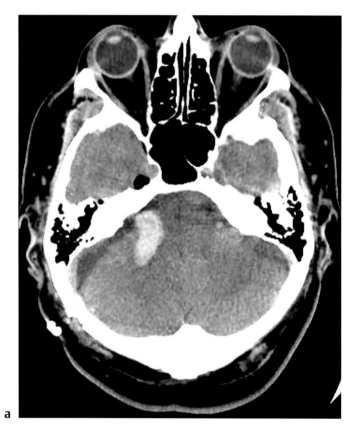

a

Figure 5.22. (a) Axial computed tomogram of a 57-year-old man with a decrease in hearing on the right demonstrates a hemorrhage in the cerebellopontine angle and mild displacement of the pons.

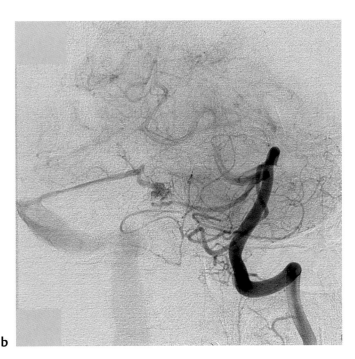

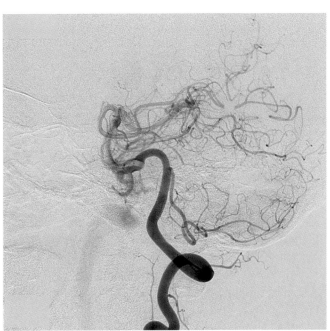

b   c

Figure 5.22. **(b)** Left transfacial and **(c)** lateral vertebral artery angiograms demonstrate a small brainstem arteriovenous malformation fed by branches of the anterior inferior cerebellar artery and draining into the deep venous circulation.

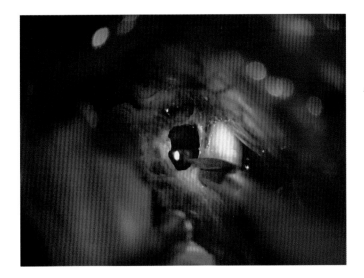

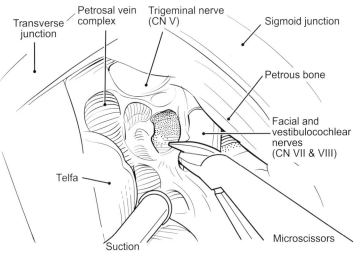

Figure 5.22. **(d)** The lesion is approached using a right retrosigmoid craniotomy.

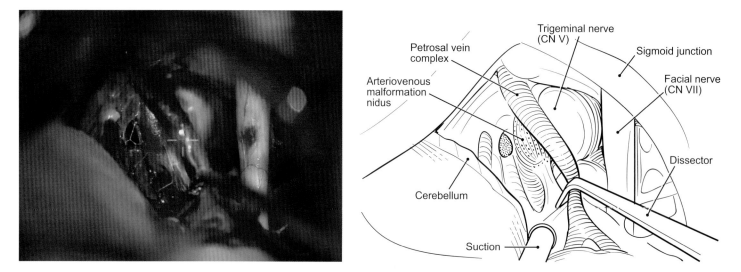

Figure 5.22. (e) Sharp dissection of the arachnoid membrane overlying the facial (CN VII) and vestibulocochlear nerve (CN VIII) complex and the petrosal vein complex aids visualization of the arteriovenous malformation nidus and facilitates understanding its angioarchitecture.

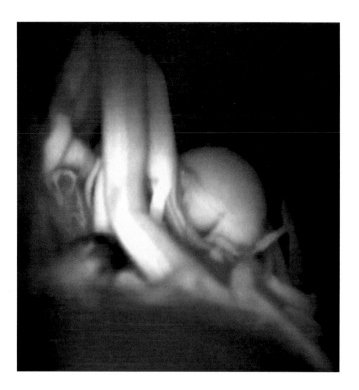

Figure 5.22. (f) Indocyanine green angiography helps delineate the arterial input and venous drainage of superficial arteriovenous malformations.

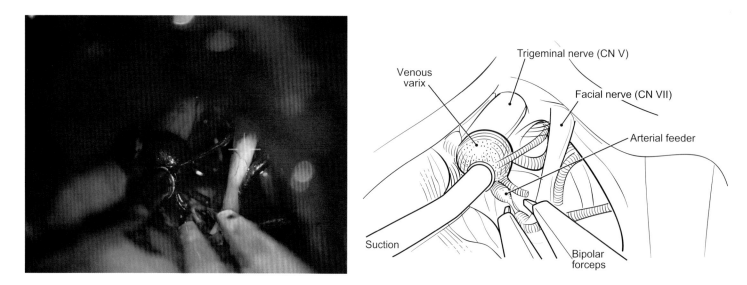

Figure 5.22. (g) Once the arteriovenous malformation is visualized, its arterial feeders can be coagulated sequentially and sharply disconnected.

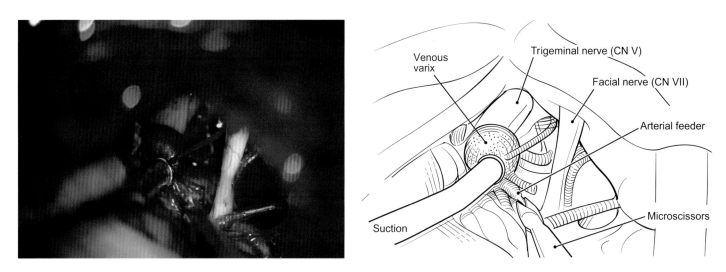

Figure 5.22. **(h)** Arterial feeders on the surface are carefully pruned after being coagulated, and the arteriovenous malformation is mobilized circumferentially before entering the brainstem parenchyma, where untoward damage to critical nuclei could occur.

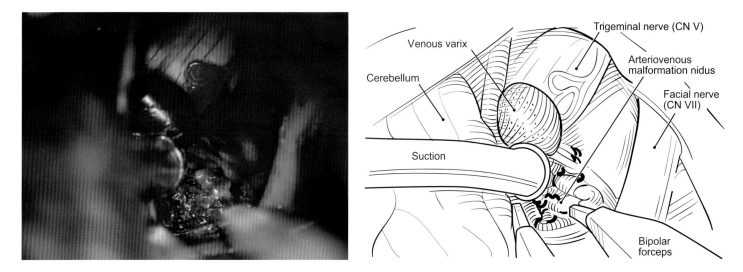

Figure 5.22. **(i)** When arterial feeders enter the brainstem parenchyma, the lesion can be coagulated and left in situ. This maneuver, which is akin to the technique used for resection of glomus-type arteriovenous malformations in the spinal cord, minimizes injury to the blood supply of the normal brainstem.

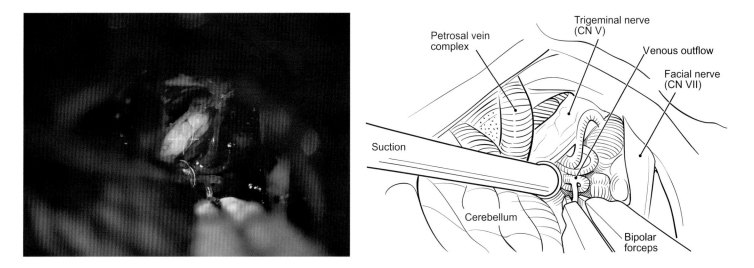

Figure 5.22. **(j)** Final devascularization of the arteriovenous malformation enables the surgeon to prune its venous outflow.

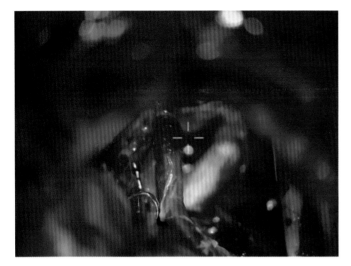
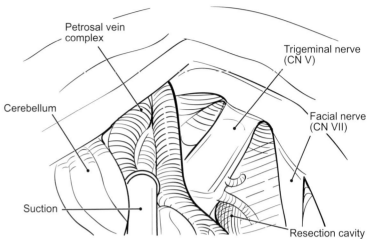

Figure 5.22. (k) The resection cavity is visualized.

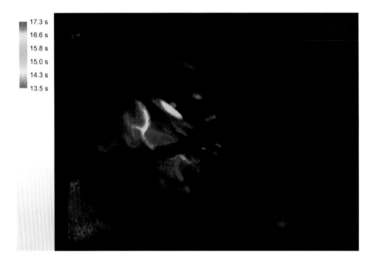

Figure 5.22. (l) After removal of the arteriovenous malformation, indocyanine green angiography indicates no further abnormal shunting.

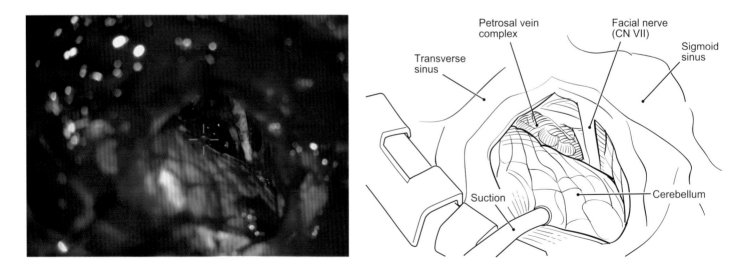

Figure 5.22. (m) A low-magnification view of the approach demonstrates the intact cerebellar surface and preservation of the petrosal vein complex.

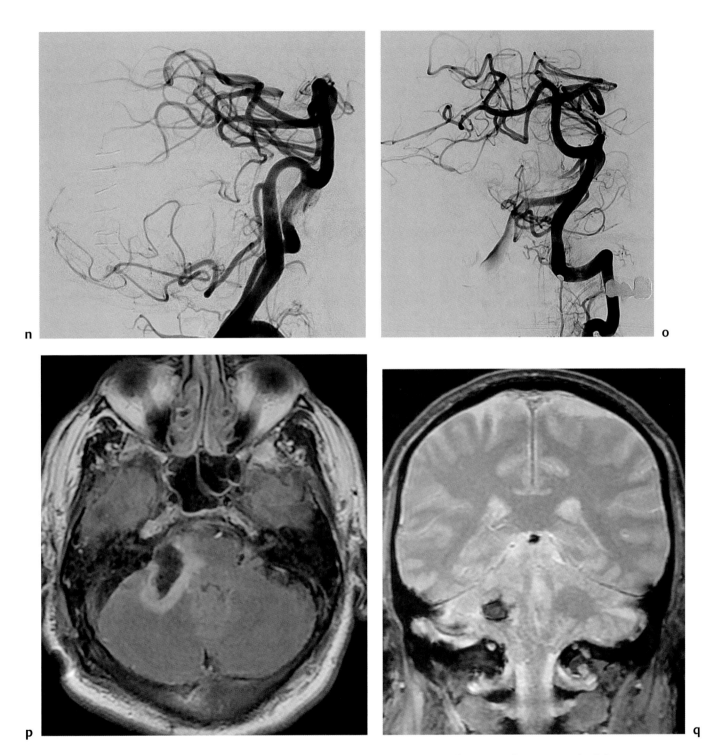

Figure 5.22. **(n)** Lateral and **(o)** transfacial vertebral artery angiograms confirm complete removal of the arteriovenous malformation. Postoperative **(p)** axial T1-weighted and **(q)** coronal gradient-echo magnetic resonance images demonstrate complete removal of the arteriovenous malformation.

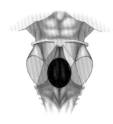

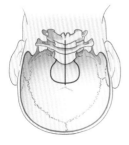

Case 5.23

- Diagnosis: Fourth ventricle cavernous malformation (related anatomy: pp. **25, 26, 29, 31, 57–59**)

- Preoperative examination: Progressive right-sided weakness (4/5), ataxia, and dysarthria of 5 months' duration

- Approach: Midline suboccipital craniotomy (related approach: pp. **200–211**)

- Positioning: Prone

- Monitoring: Somatosensory evoked potentials and motor evoked potentials

- Outcome: Complete removal of lesion; new bilateral abducens nerve (CN VI) palsy

See Video 5.23 and Animations 5.2 and 5.5

Figure 5.23. A 68-year-old man presented with progressive right-sided weakness, ataxia, and dysarthria of 5 months' duration.

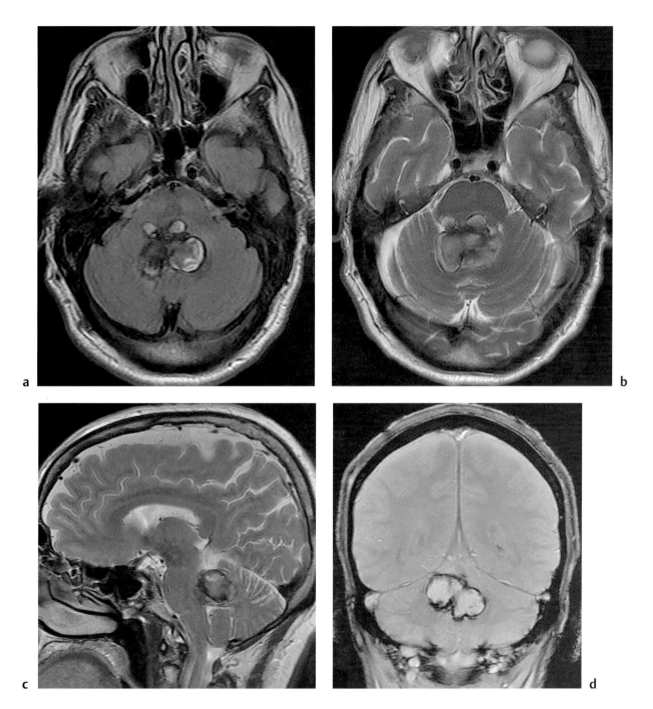

Figure 5.23. **(a)** Axial T1-weighted magnetic resonance image with contrast and **(b)** axial and **(c)** sagittal T2-weighted and **(d)** coronal gradient-echo magnetic resonance images demonstrate a cavernous malformation in the dorsal brainstem, exophytic from the fourth ventricle.

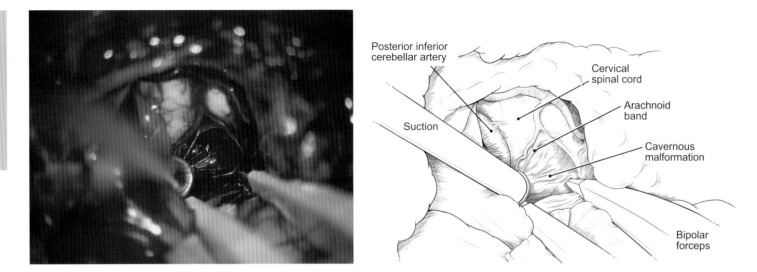

Figure 5.23. (e) The lesion is approached using a midline suboccipital craniotomy with the patient prone. The key to approaching this type of lesion is to maximally flex the neck. The skin incision should be made to at least the C2 vertebra to provide the uphill approach necessary to reach the lesion. The cerebellar hemispheres are mobilized by dissecting the arachnoid bands tethering them.

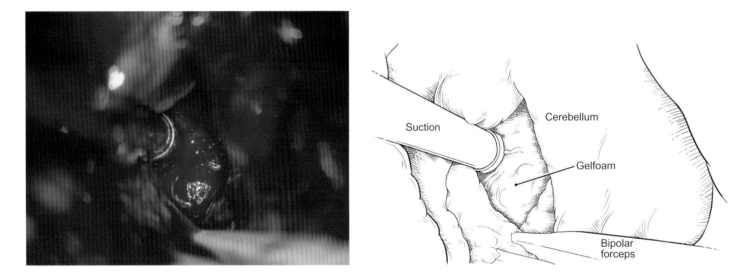

Figure 5.23. (f) After mobilization of the cerebellar hemispheres, a piece of Gelfoam is placed in the fourth ventricle to prevent blood from collecting in the ventricular system and obstructing it.

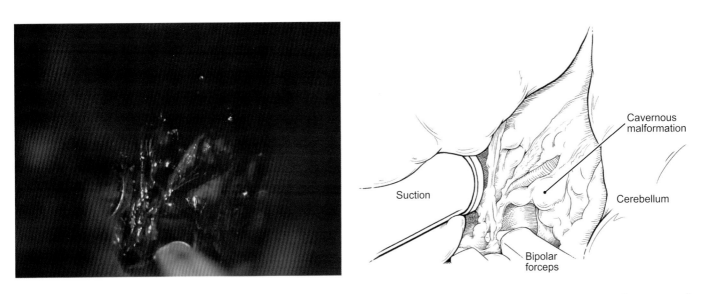

Figure 5.23. (g) The exophytic portion of the cavernous malformation is visualized and coagulated to debulk it internally.

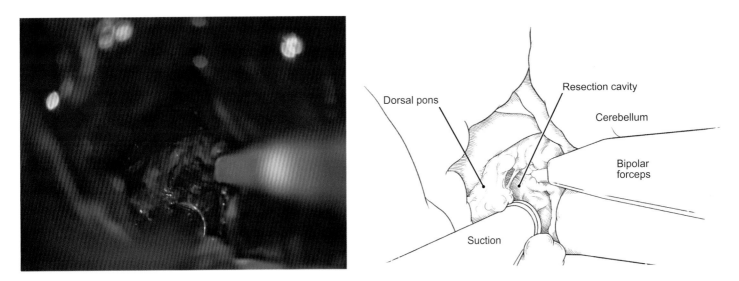

Figure 5.23. (h) Suction and cautery are used to evacuate blood products of various ages from the resection cavity.

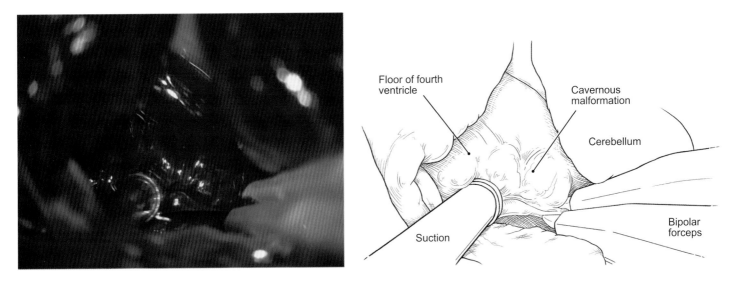

Figure 5.23. (i) The lesion is mobilized from the floor of the fourth ventricle (at the depth of the field of view).

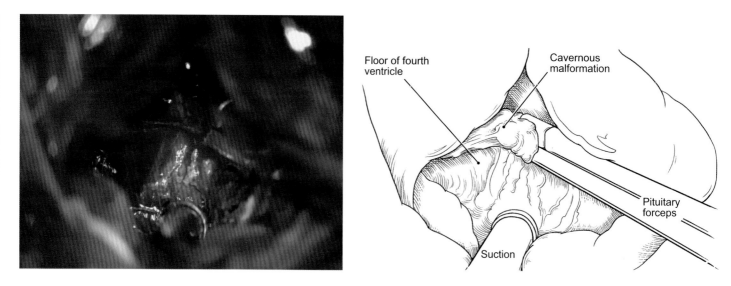

Figure 5.23. (j) Once mobilized, the cavernous malformation is removed using pituitary forceps and toothed forceps.

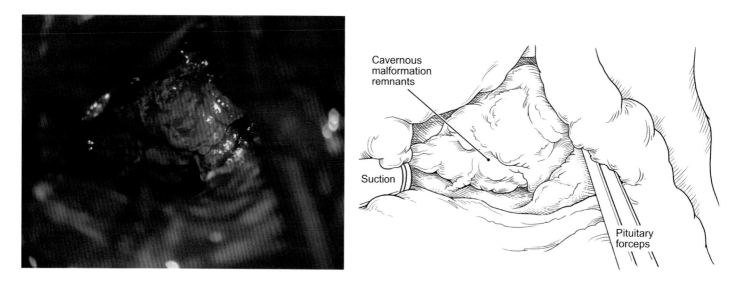

Figure 5.23. (k) The remnants of the lesion are lifted, and suction is used to disconnect them from the adjacent brainstem tissue.

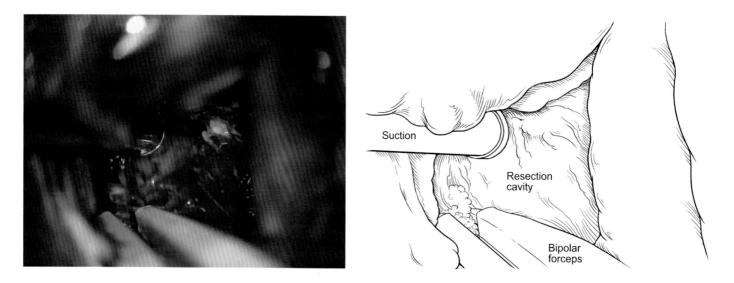

Figure 5.23. (l) After complete removal of the lesion, the resection cavity is inspected and hemostasis is obtained.

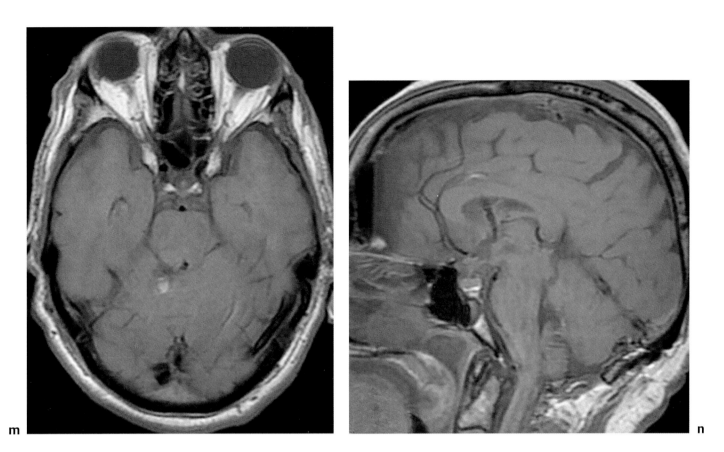

Figure 5.23. Postoperative **(m)** axial and **(n)** sagittal T1-weighted magnetic resonance images confirm complete removal of the lesion.

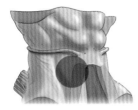

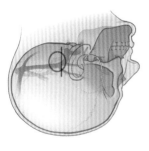

Case 5.24

- Diagnosis: Pontomesencephalic cavernous malformation (related anatomy: pp. **18, 38, 43**)

- Preoperative examination: Right facial nerve (CN VII) and hypoglossal nerve (CN XII) palsies from prior hemorrhages; new worsening of left oculomotor nerve (CN III) palsy

- Approach: Left lateral supracerebellar infratentorial (related approach: pp. **238–246**)

- Positioning: Supine

- Monitoring: Somatosensory evoked potentials and motor evoked potentials

- Outcome: Complete removal of lesion; neurologic status is unchanged.

See Video 5.24 and Animations 5.2 and 5.4

Figure 5.24. A 25-year-old woman presented with sudden-onset nausea, vomiting, dizziness, headaches, neck pain, visual disturbances, and diplopia.

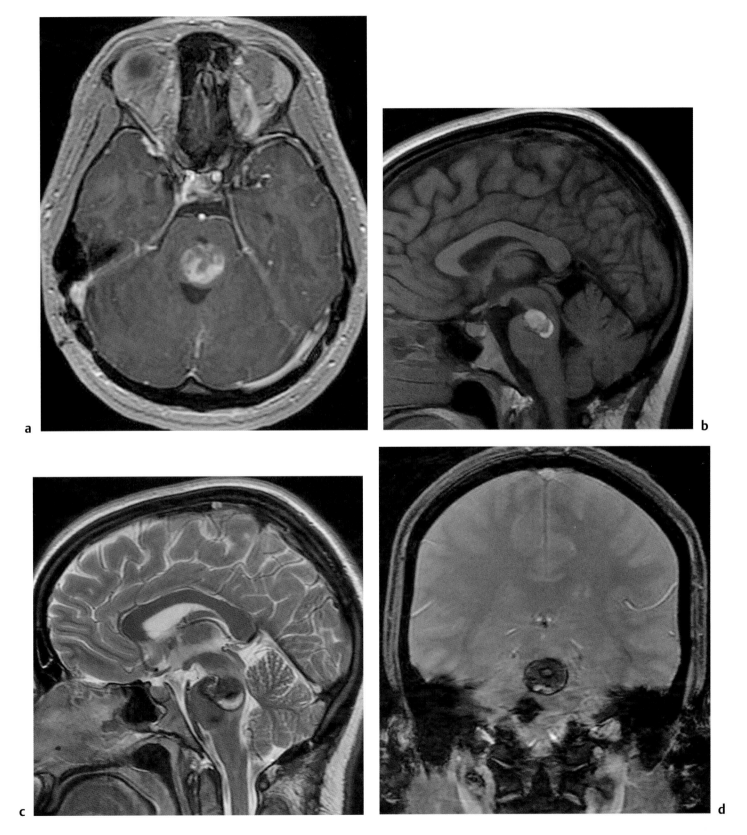

a

b

c

d

Figure 5.24. (a) Axial and **(b)** sagittal T1-weighted, **(c)** sagittal T2-weighted, and **(d)** coronal gradient-echo magnetic resonance images demonstrate a cavernous malformation with evidence of a recent hemorrhage.

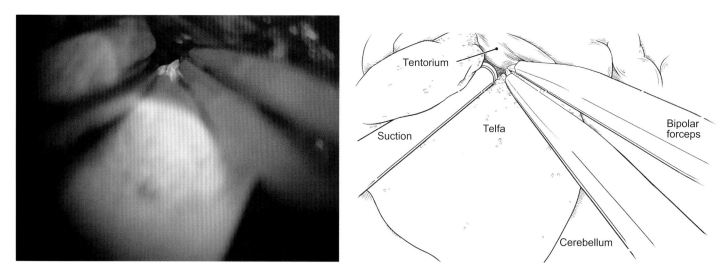

Figure 5.24. (e) The lesion is approached using a left lateral supracerebellar infratentorial craniotomy. Telfa is placed on the cerebellum to retract it and to develop the supracerebellar space used to arrive at the lateral brainstem surface for entry into the lesion.

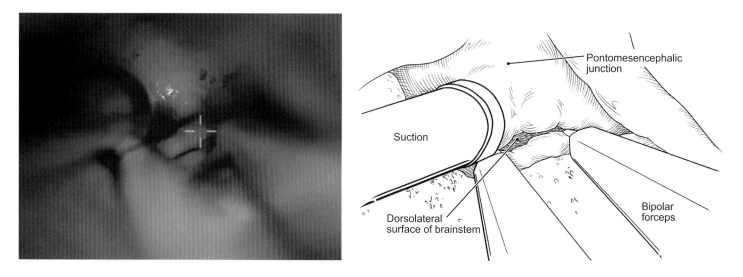

Figure 5.24. (f) The neuronavigation system is used to pinpoint the location for a small opening to be placed in the brainstem to access the lesion.

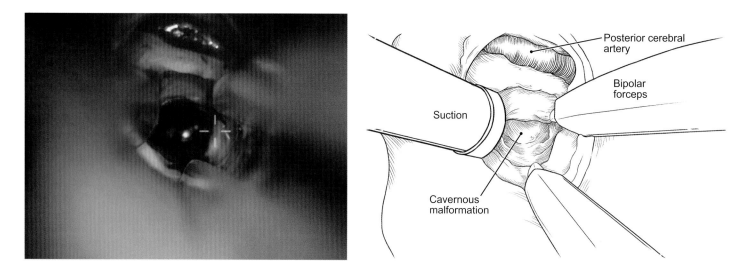

Figure 5.24. (g) Entry into the hemorrhage cavity of the cavernous malformation enables the release of blood products.

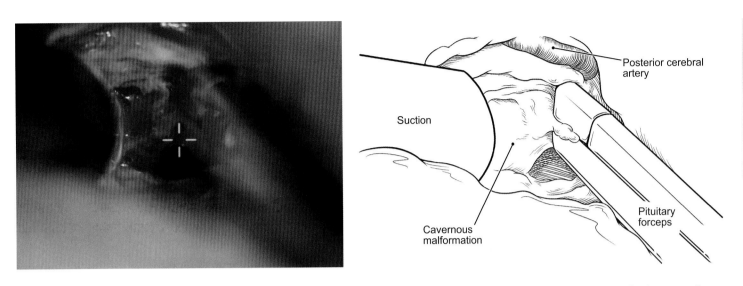

Figure 5.24. (h) The cavernous malformation is mobilized from the adjacent brainstem and bluntly dissected. The use of a lighted suction cannula provides illumination at the depth of the resection cavity.

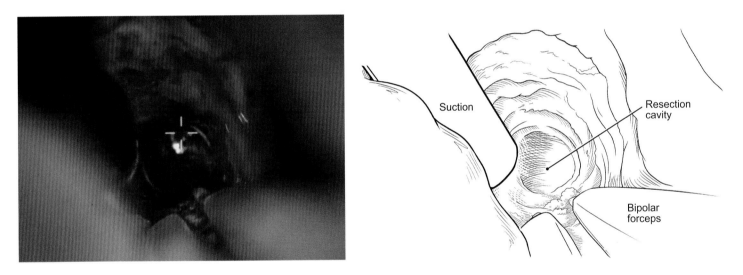

Figure 5.24. (i) Final inspection of the resection cavity ensures that no remnant of the cavernous malformation is left behind and that hemostasis is achieved.

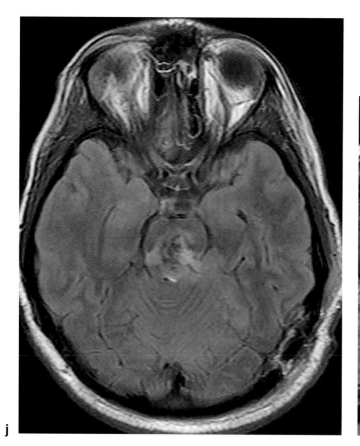
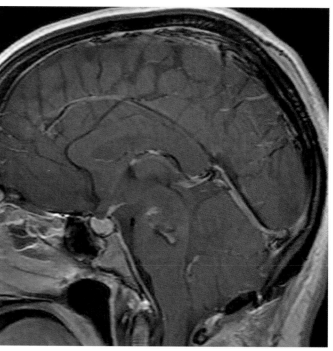

j

k

Figure 5.24. Postoperative **(j)** axial and **(k)** sagittal T1-weighted magnetic resonance images confirm complete removal of the lesion.

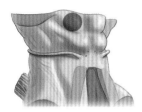

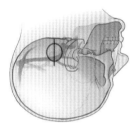

Case 5.25

- Diagnosis: Midbrain cavernous malformation (related anatomy: pp. **18, 38, 43**)
- Preoperative examination: Trochlear nerve (CN IV) palsy
- Approach: Left lateral supracerebellar infratentorial (related approach: pp. **238–246**)
- Positioning: Supine
- Monitoring: Somatosensory evoked potentials and motor evoked potentials
- Outcome: Complete removal of lesion; neurologic status is unchanged.

See Video 5.25 and Animations 5.2 and 5.4

Figure 5.25. A 30-year-old woman presented with diplopia.

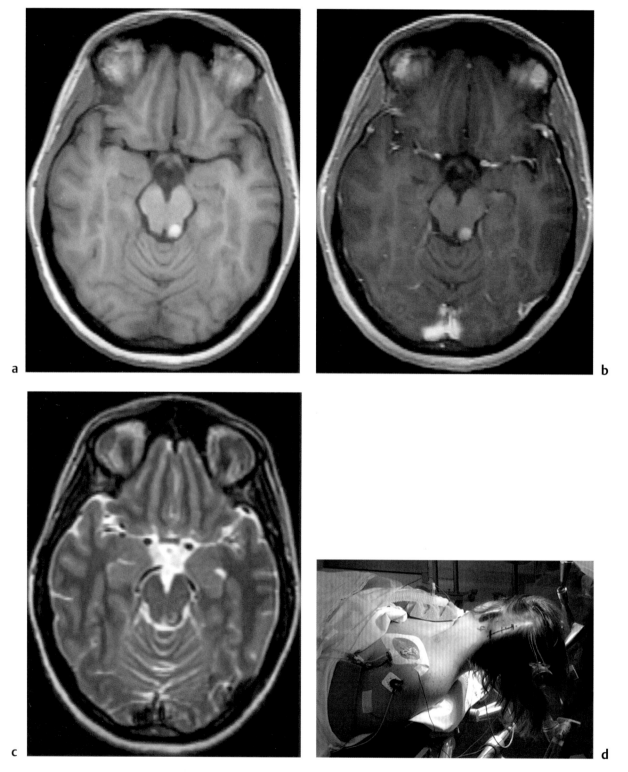

Figure 5.25 Axial T1-weighted magnetic resonance images **(a)** without and **(b)** with contrast and **(c)** axial T2-weighted magnetic resonance image demonstrate a cavernous malformation with evidence of recent hemorrhage. **(d)** The patient is positioned supine, with the head turned to the right, for a left lateral supracerebellar infratentorial approach to the dorsolateral brainstem.

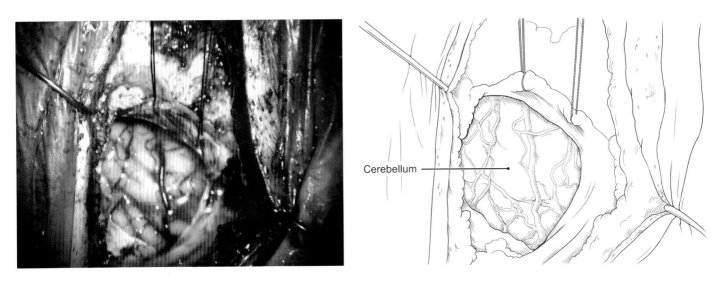

Figure 5.25. (e) The craniotomy should be placed to gain access to both the petrosal and the tentorial surfaces of the cerebellum. The petrosal surface of the cerebellum is important for gaining access to the cerebellopontine angle fissure to release cerebrospinal fluid. After adequate cerebellar relaxation is achieved, the tentorial surface of the cerebellum is dynamically retracted to arrive at the dorsolateral brainstem.

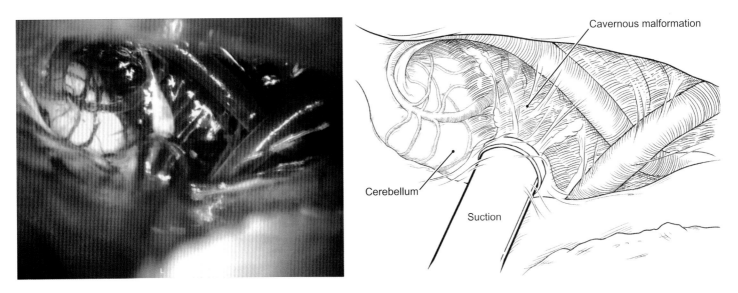

Figure 5.25. (f) Arachnoid bands that tether the cerebellum to the tentorium are dissected and evacuated, enabling the cerebellum to relax and demonstrating the cavernous malformation.

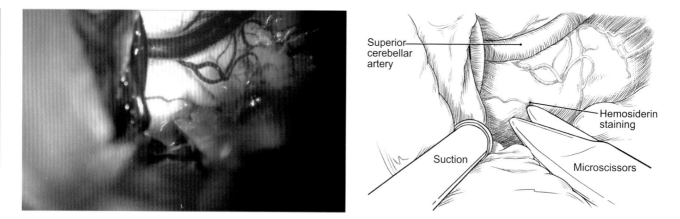

Figure 5.25. (g) The neuronavigation system is used to pinpoint the location for a small opening overlying the cavernous malformation. In this case, the lesion abuts a pial surface, so the lesion is approached directly rather than through the lateral mesencephalic sulcus proximal to the lesion. Alternatively, the lateral mesencephalic sulcus safe entry zone can be used to approach lesions in the mesencephalon that may be deep or that may not abut a pial surface directly.

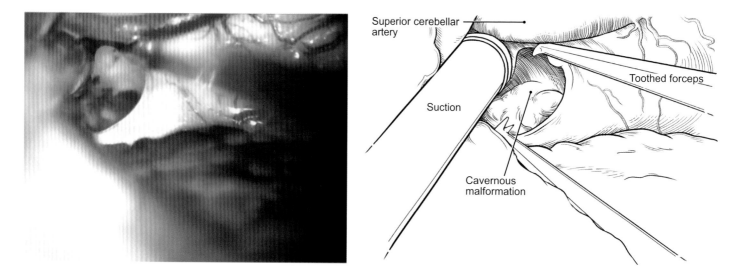

Figure 5.25. (h) Entry into the brainstem is expanded by using bipolar forceps or toothed forceps to spread the opening.

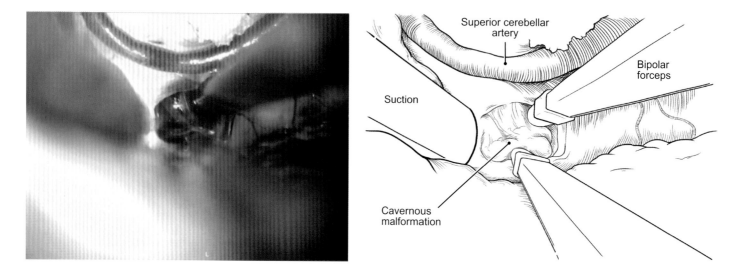

Figure 5.25. (i) The cavernous malformation is identified and peeled from the adjacent brainstem tissue.

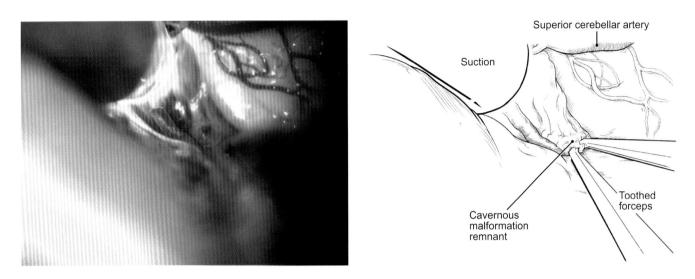

Figure 5.25. (j) The use of lighted microinstruments, such as a lighted suction cannula, provides better illumination at the depth of the cavity. Superficial and deep draining veins of the brainstem should not be disturbed.

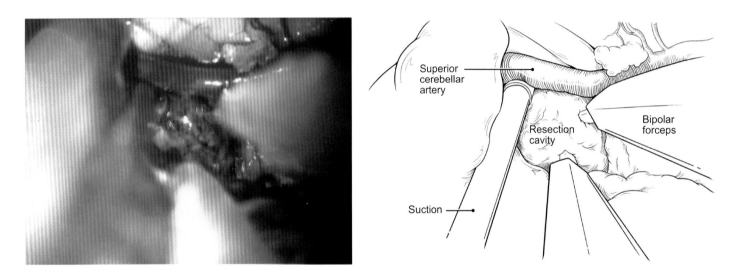

Figure 5.25. (k) Upon completion of the resection, the cavity is inspected and hemostasis is obtained. Care is taken to avoid interrupting the developmental venous anomaly associated with the lesion.

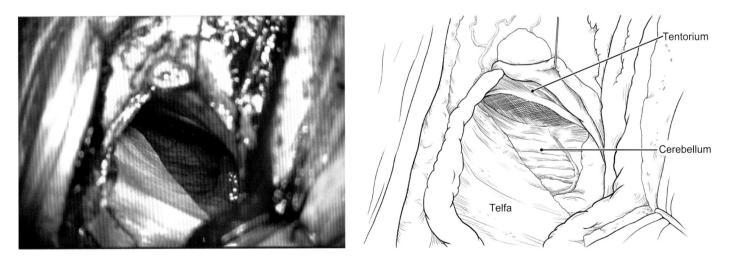

Figure 5.25. (l) Intraoperative photograph and illustration show the corridor made possible using the supracerebellar infratentorial approach.

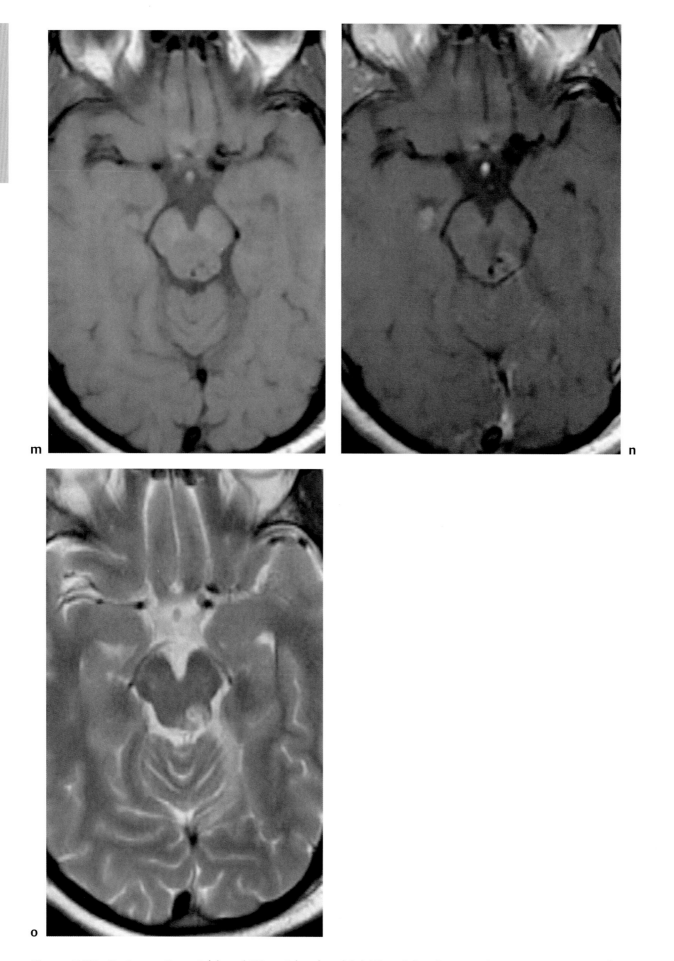

Figure 5.25. Postoperative axial **(m,n)** T1-weighted and **(o)** T2-weighted magnetic resonance images demonstrate complete removal of the lesion.

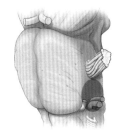

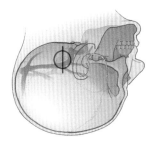

Case 5.26

- Diagnosis: Pontomedullary junction cavernous malformation (related anatomy: pp. **51, 56, 62, 81–84, 118–124**)

- Preoperative examination: Left facial nerve (CN VII) and hypoglossal nerve (CN XII) palsies

- Approach: Left retrosigmoid (related approach: pp. **212–222**)

- Positioning: Supine

- Monitoring: Somatosensory evoked potentials and motor evoked potentials; trigeminal (CN V), vestibulocochlear (CN VIII), glossopharyngeal (CN IX), vagus (CN X), and accessory (CN XI) nerves

- Outcome: Complete removal of lesion; neurologic status is unchanged.

See Video 5.26 and Animations 5.2 and 5.6

Figure 5.26. A 37-year-old man presented to an outside hospital with nausea, vertigo, and right-sided numbness.

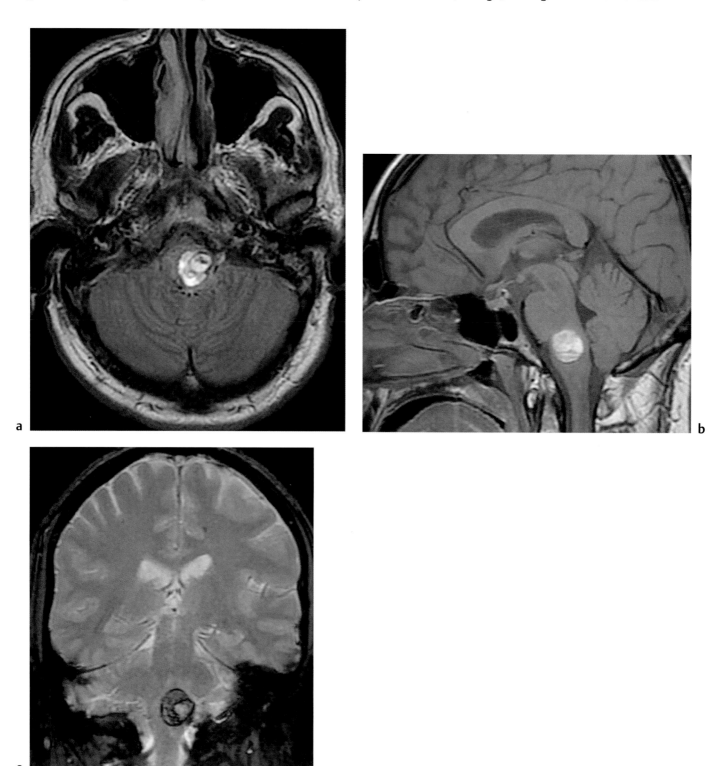

Figure 5.26. (a) Axial and (b) sagittal T1-weighted and (c) coronal gradient-echo magnetic resonance images demonstrate a cavernous malformation in the left pontomedullary junction with evidence of hemorrhage.

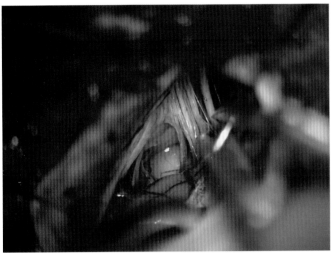

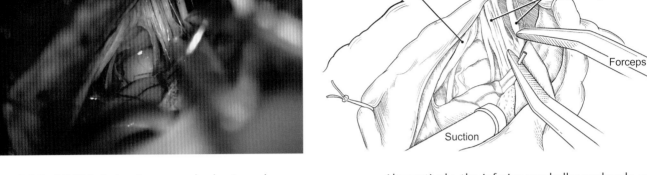

Figure 5.26. (d) This lesion is approached using a low retrosigmoid craniotomy where the lesion closely abuts a pial plane. This area can be approached by performing a low retrosigmoid craniotomy (alternatively, a far-lateral approach may be used) and by dissecting between the lower cranial nerves. Alternatively, the inferior cerebellar peduncle safe entry zone can be accessed between the lower cranial nerves and the facial–vestibulocochlear nerve (CN VII-VIII) complex. The arachnoid membrane over the lower cranial nerves is dissected to enable mobilization of these nerves.

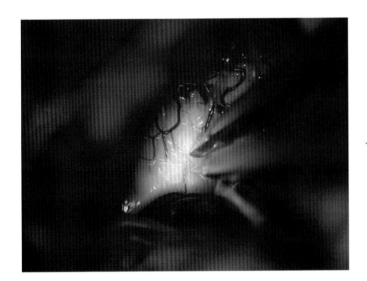

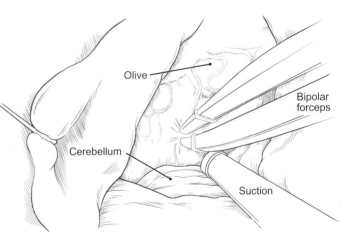

Figure 5.26. (e) The neuronavigation system is used to select the optimal point of entry into the brainstem, and a small opening is made adjacent to the takeoff of the vagus nerve (CN X). The pia is coagulated using bipolar cautery, and microscissors are then used to complete the opening.

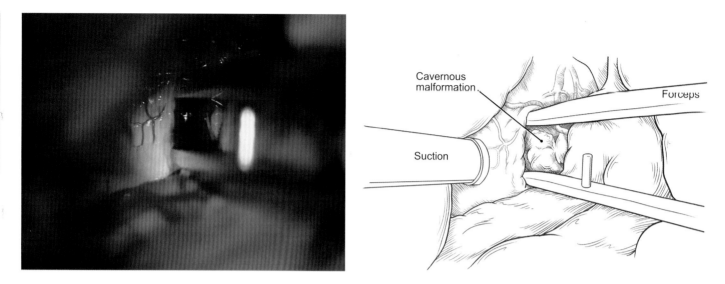

Figure 5.26. (f) Microforceps are used to spread the fibers, increasing the size of the opening into the brainstem.

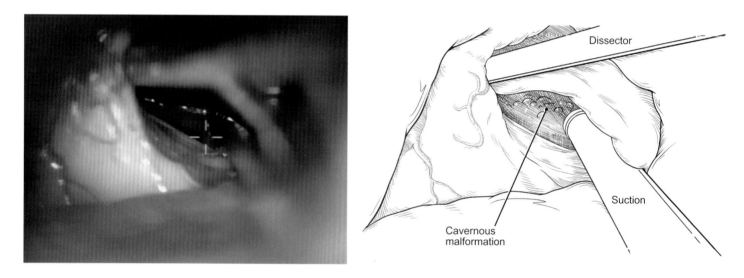

Figure 5.26. (g) The cavity of the cavernous malformation is entered, and the lesion is visualized.

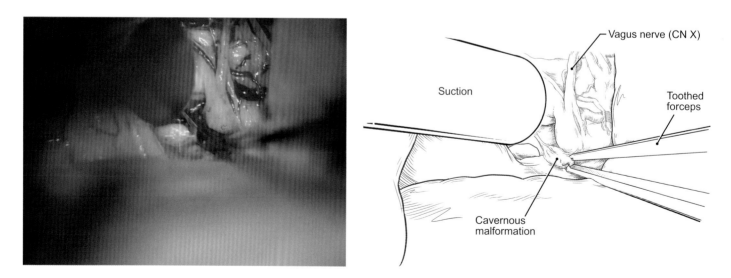

Figure 5.26. (h) The lesion is mobilized and bluntly dissected from adjacent tissue using toothed forceps, while lighted suction also provides illumination and countertraction.

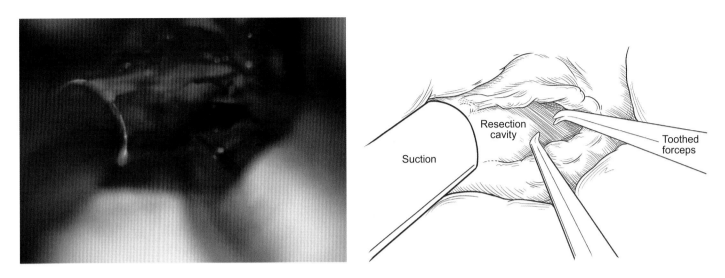

Figure 5.26. (i) A final inspection of the resection cavity demonstrates excellent hemostasis and no remnants of the cavernous malformation.

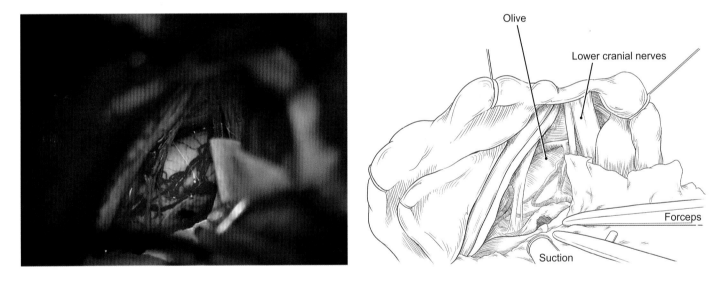

Figure 5.26. (j) A final view of the size of opening in the brainstem necessary to resect this lesion.

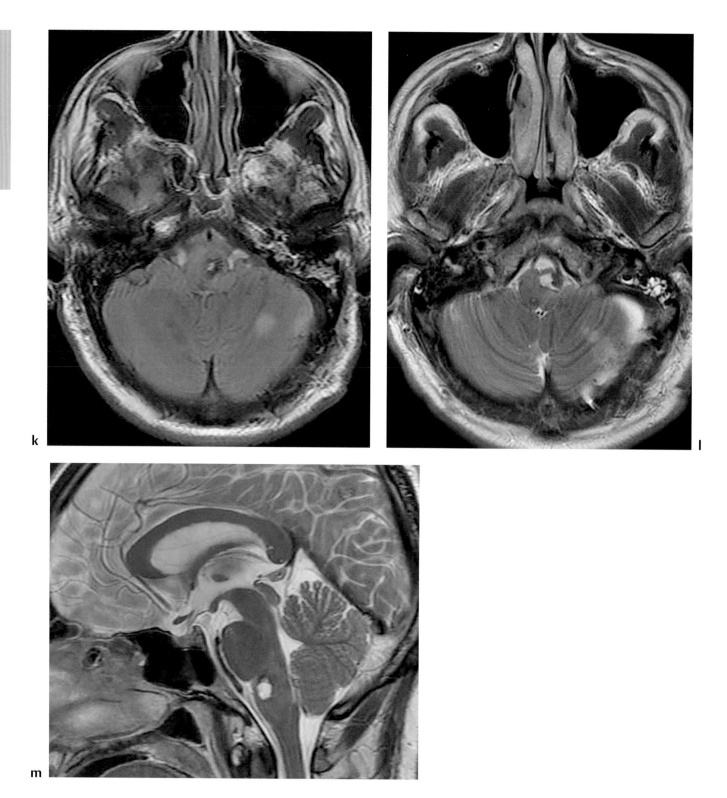

Figure 5.26. Postoperative **(k)** axial T1-weighted and **(l)** axial and **(m)** sagittal T2-weighted magnetic resonance images confirm complete removal of the lesion.

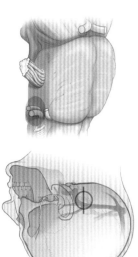

Case 5.27

- Diagnosis: Pontomedullary junction cavernous malformation (related anatomy: pp. **51, 56, 62, 118–124**)

- Preoperative examination: Right oculomotor nerve (CN III) palsy

- Approach: Right retrosigmoid (related approach: pp. **212–222**)

- Positioning: Supine

- Monitoring: Somatosensory evoked potentials and motor evoked potentials; trigeminal (CN V), facial (CN VII), and vestibulocochlear (CN VIII) nerves

- Outcome: Complete removal of lesion; neurologic status is unchanged.

See Video 5.27 and Animations 5.2 and 5.6

Figure 5.27. A 23-year-old woman presented with diplopia.

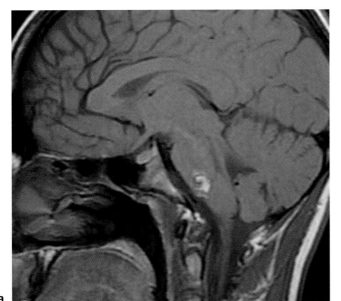

a

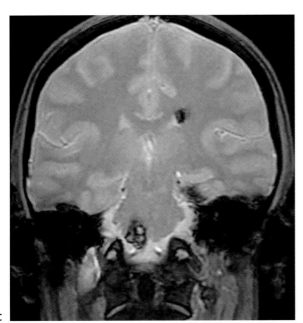

c

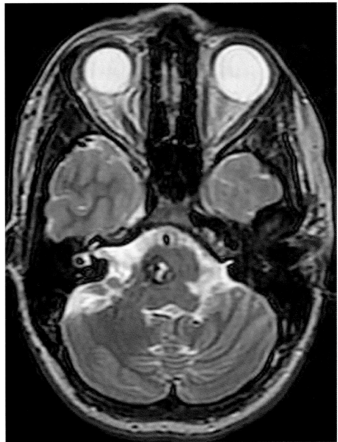

b

Figure 5.27. **(a)** Sagittal T1-weighted, **(b)** axial T2-weighted, and **(c)** coronal gradient-echo magnetic resonance images demonstrate a cavernous malformation in the pontomedullary junction. Note that the patient has another cavernous malformation.

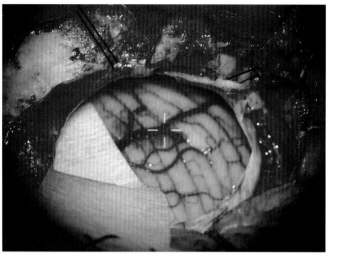
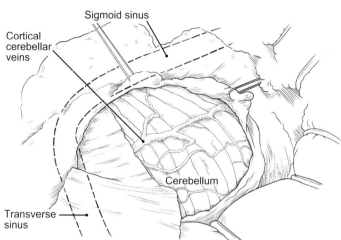

Figure 5.27. (d) The lesion is approached using a retrosigmoid craniotomy.

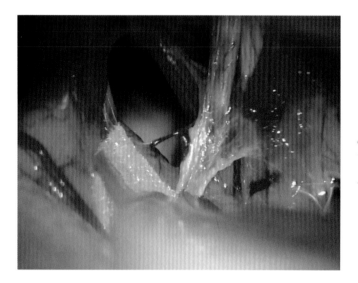
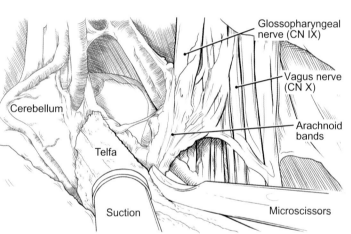

Figure 5.27. (e) Dissection of the arachnoid membrane enables the cerebellum to be dynamically retracted, exposing several safe entry zones on the lateral brainstem surface. Microscissors are used to sharply disconnect the arachnoid membrane from the lower cranial nerves.

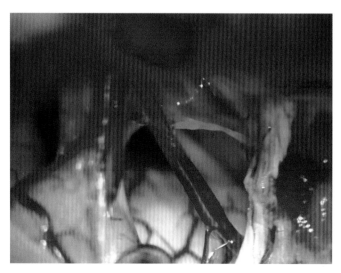
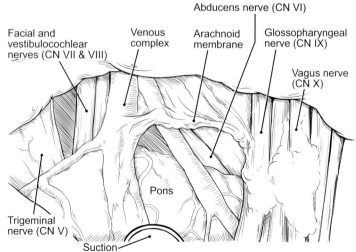

Figure 5.27. (f) Because of the location of this lesion, the inferior cerebellar peduncle is used to gain access to the lesion to resect it. The inferior cerebellar peduncle is accessed between the facial–vestibulocochlear nerve (CN VII-VIII) complex and the lower cranial nerves.

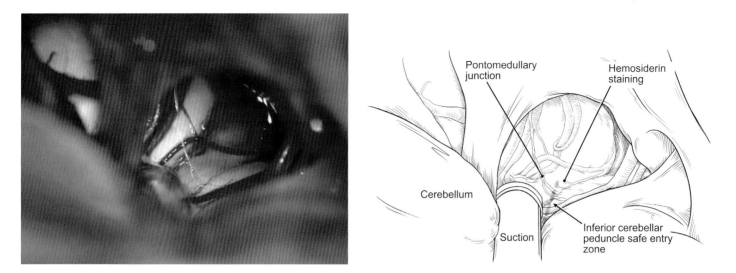

Figure 5.27. (g) A small area of hemosiderin discoloration on the surface of the brainstem corresponds to the neuronavigation site of optimal entry for access to the cavernous malformation. The blue dashed line demarcates the direction of the fibers in the inferior cerebellar peduncle.

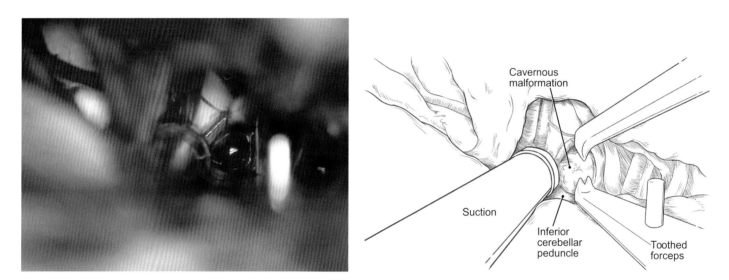

Figure 5.27. (h) Microforceps are used to make an opening into the pons. A spreading movement is used to expand the opening with minimal trauma.

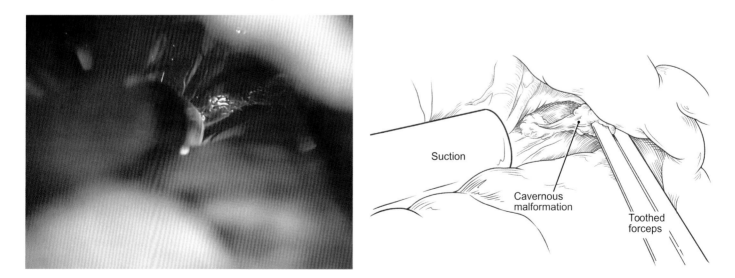

Figure 5.27. (i) The cavernous malformation is mobilized and resected piecemeal with the aid of a lighted suction cannula and toothed microforceps.

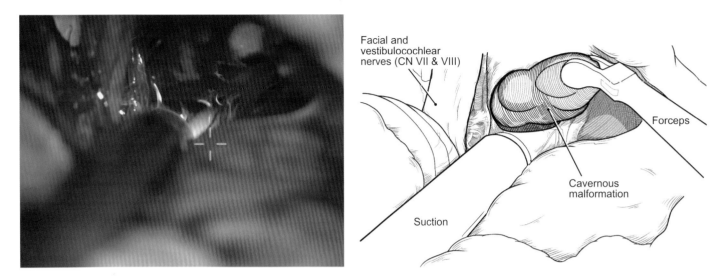

Figure 5.27. (j) Pituitary forceps are used to bluntly disconnect the lesion from the adjacent brainstem surface. Care is taken to avoid injury to the veins on the surface of the brainstem and to any developmental venous anomalies found in association with the cavernous malformation.

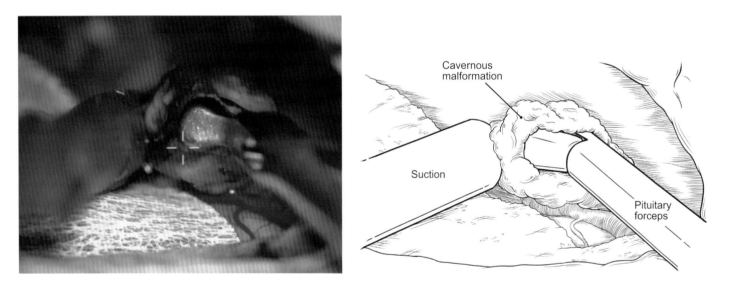

Figure 5.27. (k) The cavernous malformation is removed from the cavity.

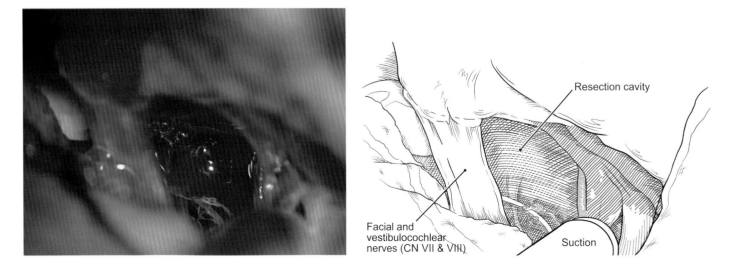

Figure 5.27. (l) A final inspection of the resection cavity is performed to ensure that hemostasis is achieved and that no remnant of the cavernous malformation is left behind.

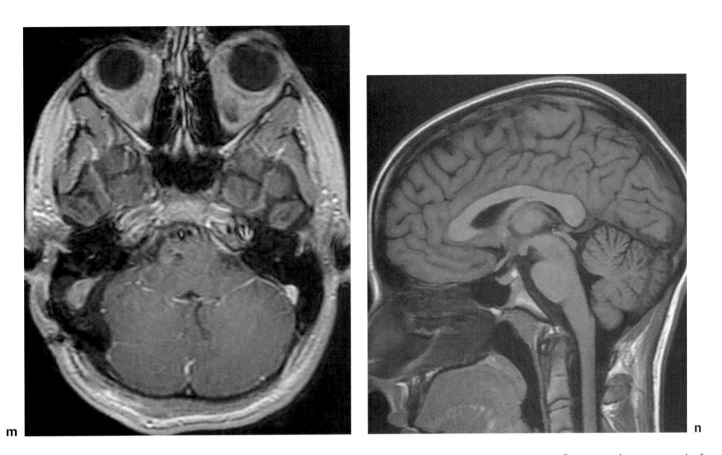

m

n

Figure 5.27. Postoperative **(m)** axial and **(n)** sagittal T1-weighted magnetic resonance images confirm complete removal of the lesion.

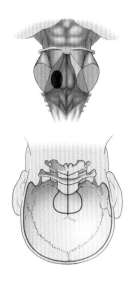

Case 5.28

- Diagnosis: Pontine cavernous malformation (related anatomy: pp. **25, 57–59**)
- Preoperative examination: Left intranuclear ophthalmoplegia
- Approach: Midline suboccipital telovelar (related approach: pp. **200–211**)
- Positioning: Prone
- Monitoring: Somatosensory evoked potentials and motor evoked potentials; facial nerve (CN VII)
- Outcome: Complete removal of lesion; neurologic status is unchanged.

See Video 5.28 and Animations 5.2 and 5.5

Figure 5.28. A 32-year-old woman presented with diplopia and a history of two prior hemorrhages.

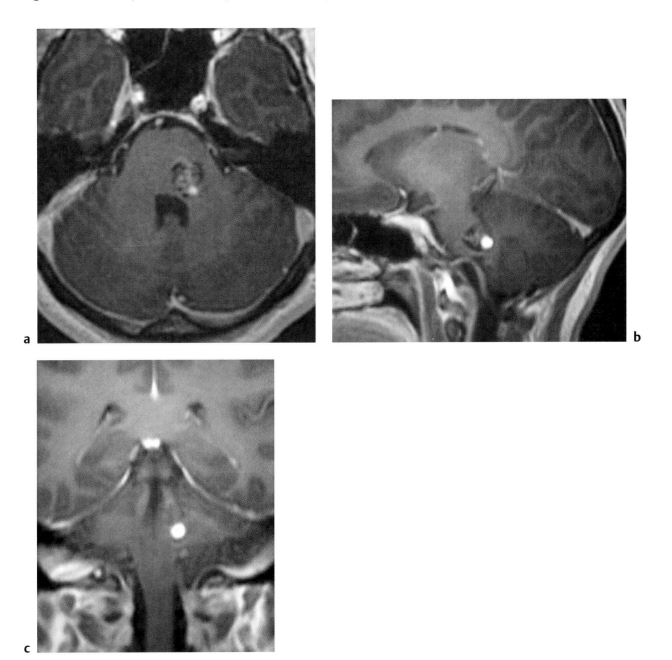

Figure 5.28. **(a)** Axial, **(b)** sagittal, and **(c)** coronal T1-weighted magnetic resonance images demonstrate a dorsal pontine cavernous malformation with evidence of prior hemorrhage.

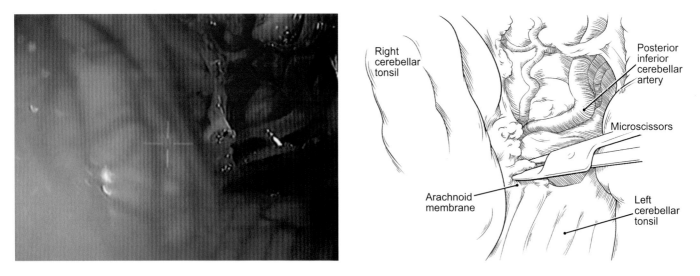

Figure 5.28. (d) This lateral dorsal pontine cavernous malformation is approached using a midline suboccipital craniotomy and telovelar dissection. Sharp dissection is used initially to mobilize the arachnoid membrane over the cerebellar hemispheres.

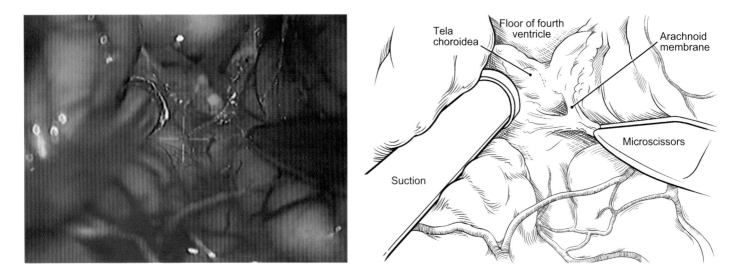

Figure 5.28. (e) Dynamic retraction of the cerebellar hemispheres, using the shaft of the suction cannula and other microinstruments such as microscissors, facilitates visualization of the floor of the fourth ventricle.

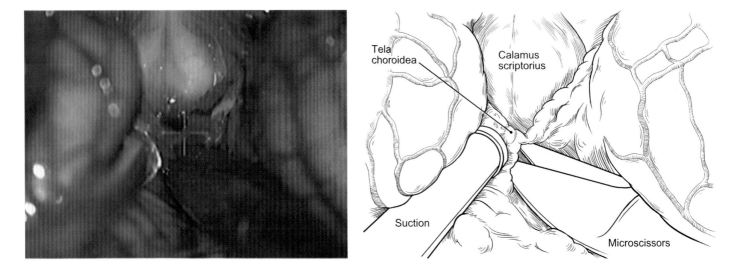

Figure 5.28. (f) Sharp dissection is used to dissect the tela choroidea to expose the foramen of Luschka.

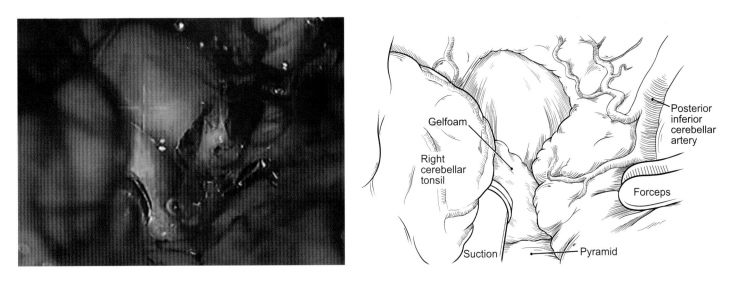

Figure 5.28. (g) Further dissection leads to development of the potential space between the cerebellar hemispheres and the dorsal brainstem. At this stage, a small piece of Gelfoam or cotton is placed into the fourth ventricle to prevent blood from pooling into the ventricular system during dissection.

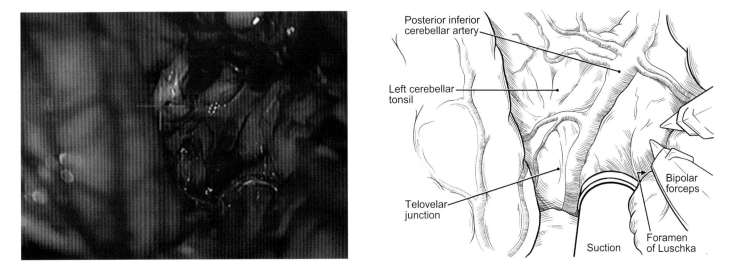

Figure 5.28. (h) Further dissection of the tela choroidea and velum facilitates visualization of the foramen of Luschka.

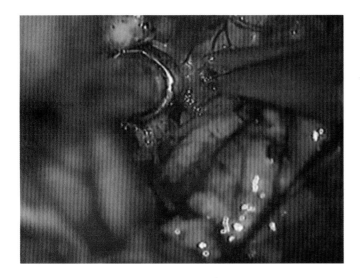
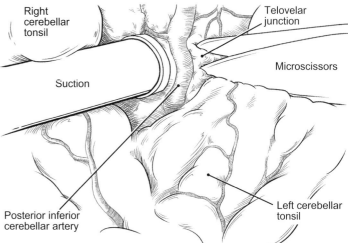

Figure 5.28. (i) Lesions in the dorsal pons can be accessed using one of four safe entry zones. These safe entry zones are divided about the facial colliculus. Lesions located above and below the colliculus in the midline can be accessed using the suprafacial and infrafacial colliculus safe entry zones. Lesions located deep in the dorsal pons at the level of the facial colliculus can be accessed safely using the superior fovea safe entry zone. Alternatively, lesions can be accessed using the median sulcus of the fourth ventricle. This lesion was approached using the superior fovea safe entry zone with the aid of neuronavigation to optimize entry. Opening the tela and velum and exposing the medial-most aspect of the foramen of Luschka provide adequate mobilization of the cerebellar hemisphere to enable the surgeon to obtain the off-midline view necessary to avoid the facial colliculus when approaching this lesion. When possible, for lesions approached dorsally at the level of the fourth ventricle, the entry into the brainstem is planned laterally instead of directly in the midline of the fourth ventricle to avoid injury to the critical nuclei in the midline. However, lesions that abut a pial or an ependymal surface are approached directly through the lesion.

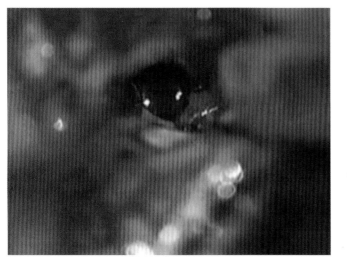
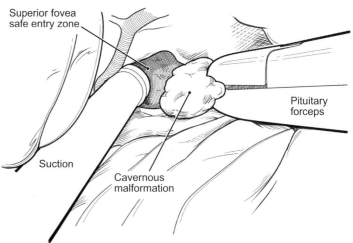

Figure 5.28. (j) The lesion is entered, internally debulked, and removed piecemeal.

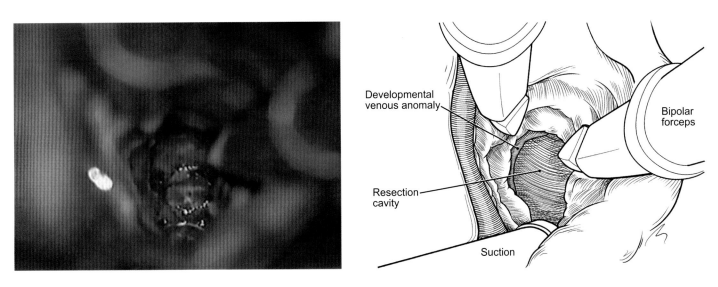

Figure 5.28. (k) The cavity is inspected, the developmental venous anomaly is kept intact, and hemostasis is obtained.

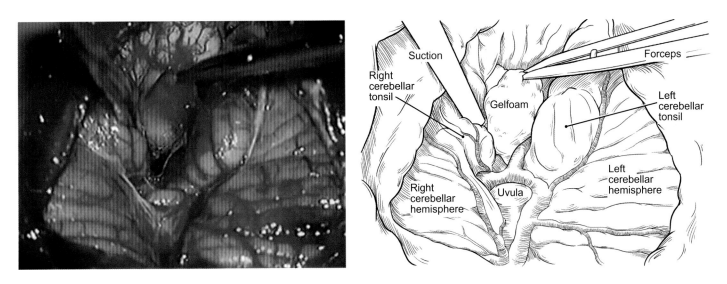

Figure 5.28. (l) The piece of Gelfoam that had been placed in the fourth ventricle to prevent the pooling of blood in the ventricular space is removed.

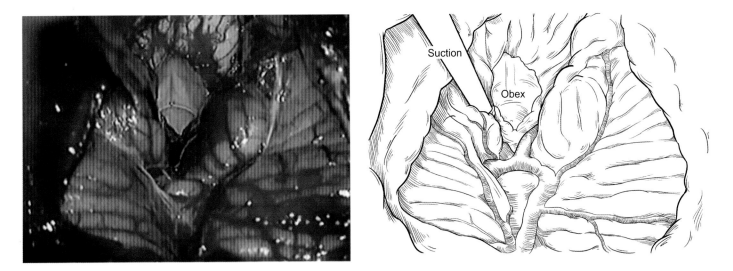

Figure 5.28. (m) Note that the floor of the fourth ventricle is completely undisturbed.

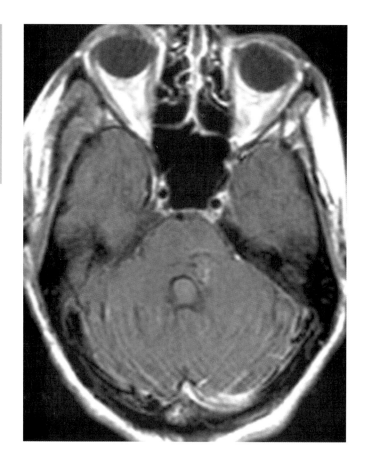

Figure 5.28. (n) Postoperative axial T1-weighted magnetic resonance image confirms complete removal of the lesion.

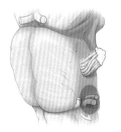

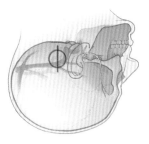

Case 5.29

- Diagnosis: Pontine cavernous malformation (related anatomy: pp. **51, 56, 62, 118–124**)

- Preoperative examination: Right-sided weakness 2–3/5; left facial nerve (CN VII) and vestibulocochlear nerve (CN VIII) deficits

- Approach: Left retrosigmoid (related approach: pp. **212–222**)

- Positioning: Supine

- Monitoring: Somatosensory evoked potentials and motor evoked potentials; trigeminal (CN V), facial (CN VII), and vestibulocochlear (CN VIII) nerves

- Outcome: Complete removal of lesion; neurologic status is unchanged.

See Video 5.29 and Animations 5.2 and 5.6

Figure 5.29. A 40-year-old man presented with right-sided weakness.

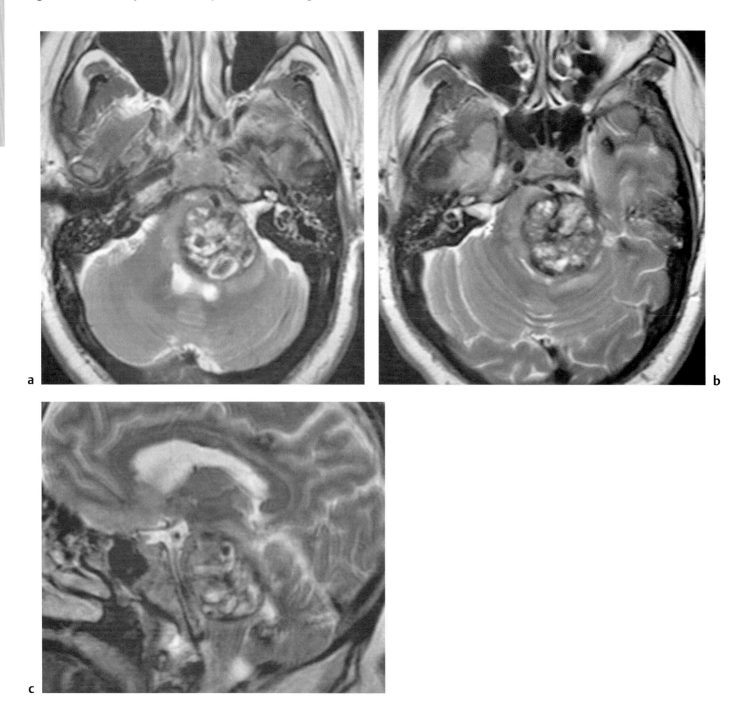

Figure 5.29. (a,b) Axial and **(c)** sagittal T2-weighted magnetic resonance images demonstrate a large pontine cavernous malformation eccentric to the left side.

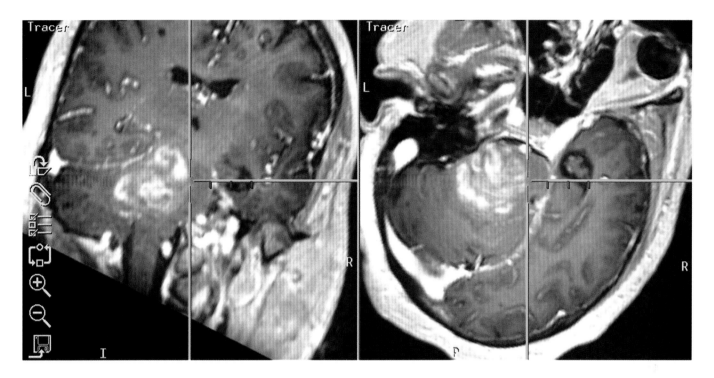

Figure 5.29. (d) Because the lesion abuts a pial surface on the left side of the pons, a left retrosigmoid approach is used to resect it. Although this lesion abuts a pial surface and is approached directly, most lateral pontine lesions should be approached through the middle cerebellar peduncle safe entry zone after generous dissection of the petrosal fissure. Neuronavigation images in the coronal (*left*) and axial (*right*) planes show the trajectory along the long axis of the lesion through the middle cerebellar peduncle.

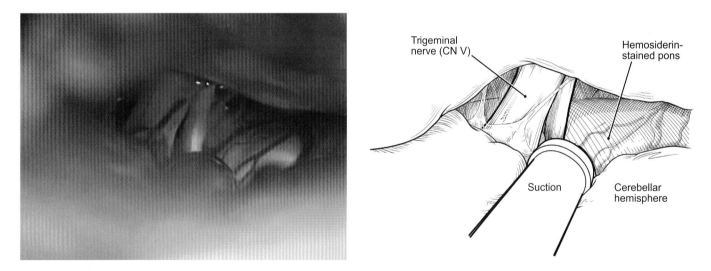

Figure 5.29. (e) A retrosigmoid craniotomy is used to access the cerebellopontine angle, and the cerebrospinal fluid is released to relax the cerebellum and to visualize the dorsolateral pons.

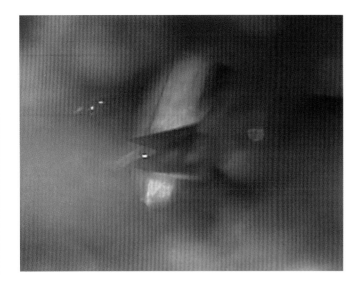
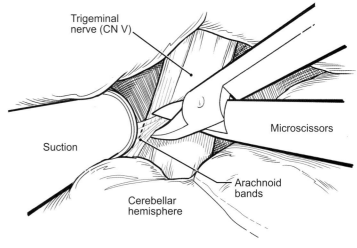

Figure 5.29. (f) Sharp dissection is used to release the arachnoid bands over the trigeminal nerve (CN V), the facial nerve (CN VII), and the vestibulocochlear nerve (CN VIII).

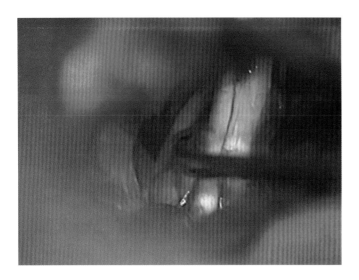

Figure 5.29. (g) Dissection of arteries and surface veins from the brainstem and cranial nerves is critical to minimize retraction of these vessels and cranial nerves during dissection. Upon dissection and exposure, several safe entry zones on the lateral pons, including the peritrigeminal, supratrigeminal, and lateral pontine (middle cerebellar peduncle) safe entry zones, can be visualized and accessed. The middle cerebellar peduncle safe entry zone is preferable for approaching deep lateral pontine lesions.

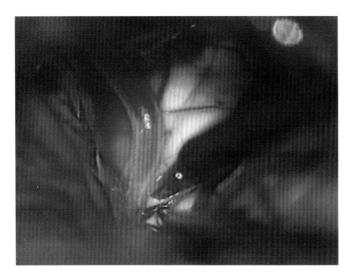
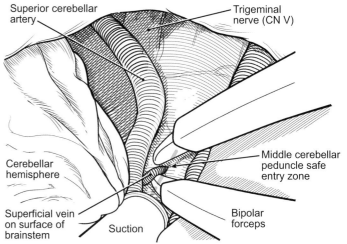

Figure 5.29. (h) Exposure of the middle cerebellar peduncle safe entry zone (*dashed line*) is enhanced by opening the petrosal fissure using a technique similar to that used for opening the sylvian fissure. Opening the petrosal fissure enables a less steep and more direct view of the middle cerebellar peduncle. Mobilization of surface veins permits entry into the brainstem at the middle cerebellar peduncle without the need to sacrifice veins.

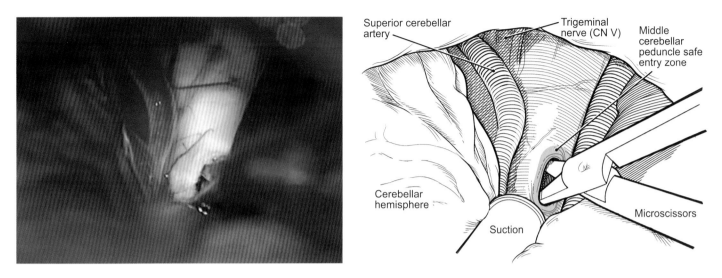

Figure 5.29. (i) The opening is carried out by sharply cutting the arachnoid membrane over the brainstem using microscissors and then using a spreading technique with microinstruments to develop a working corridor large enough for a small suction device and a second microinstrument. The direction of the opening in the middle cerebellar peduncle is not rostrocaudal but rather anteroposterior, in line with the direction of the fibers traversing the middle cerebellar peduncle.

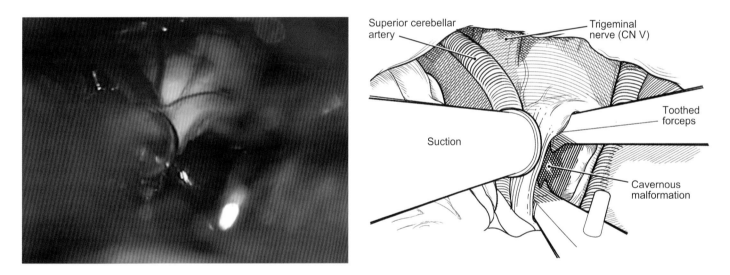

Figure 5.29. (j) Microforceps are used to expand the opening.

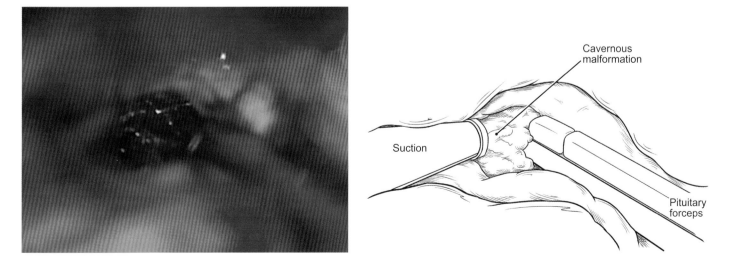

Figure 5.29. (k) The cavernous malformation is entered and removed piecemeal.

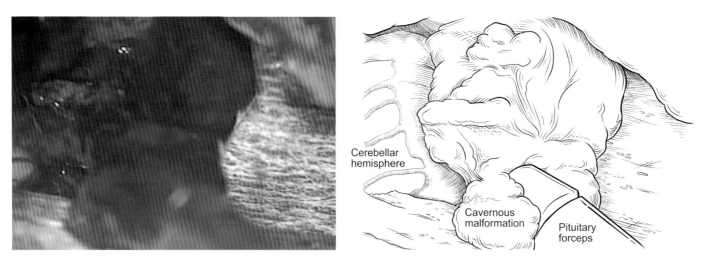

Figure 5.29. (l) The cavernous malformation is visualized as it is removed from the small opening in the brainstem.

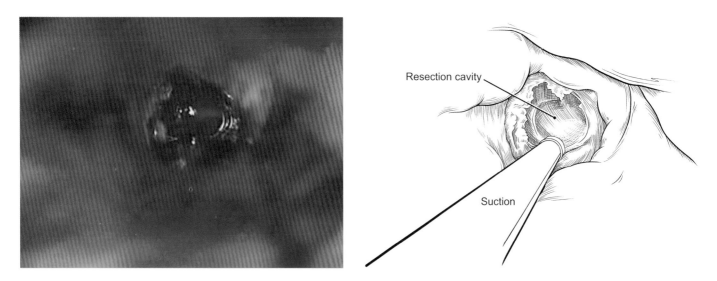

Figure 5.29. (m) The cavity is irrigated and inspected for remnants of the cavernous malformation. Care is taken to keep the developmental venous anomaly intact.

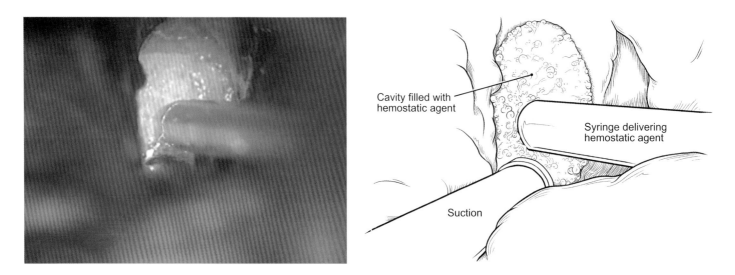

Figure 5.29. (n) When venous bleeding from the resection cavity is encountered, a small amount of hemostatic agent may be applied to the cavity and the cavity irrigated to remove it before closure.

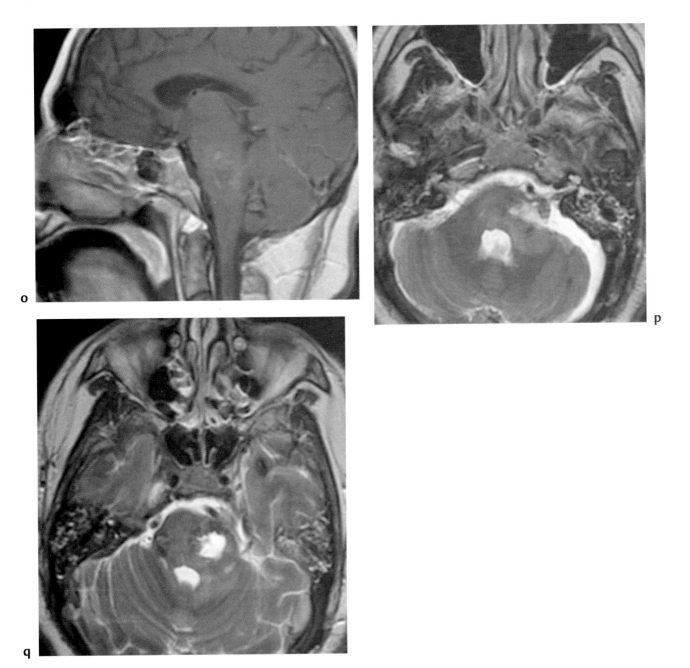

Figure 5.29. Postoperative **(o)** sagittal T1-weighted and **(p,q)** axial T2-weighted magnetic resonance images document complete removal of the lesion.

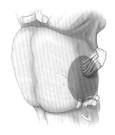

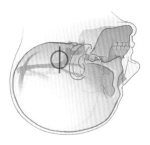

Case 5.30

- Diagnosis: Pontine cavernous malformation (related anatomy: pp. **51, 56, 62, 118–124**)

- Preoperative examination: Right-sided weakness (4/5), right facial nerve (CN VII) palsy, right arm and leg numbness

- Approach: Left retrosigmoid (related approach: pp. **212–222**)

- Positioning: Supine

- Monitoring: Somatosensory evoked potentials and motor evoked potentials; trigeminal (CN V), facial (CN VII), and vestibulocochlear (CN VIII) nerves

- Outcome: Complete removal of lesion; intranuclear ophthalmoplegia and right-sided weakness (3/5)

See Video 5.30 and Animations 5.2 and 5.6

Figure 5.30. A 37-year-old man presented with a 4-month history of right hand numbness and writing difficulty that progressed to right arm and leg weakness (4/5) and diminished sensation; two prior surgeries had been performed at another institution.

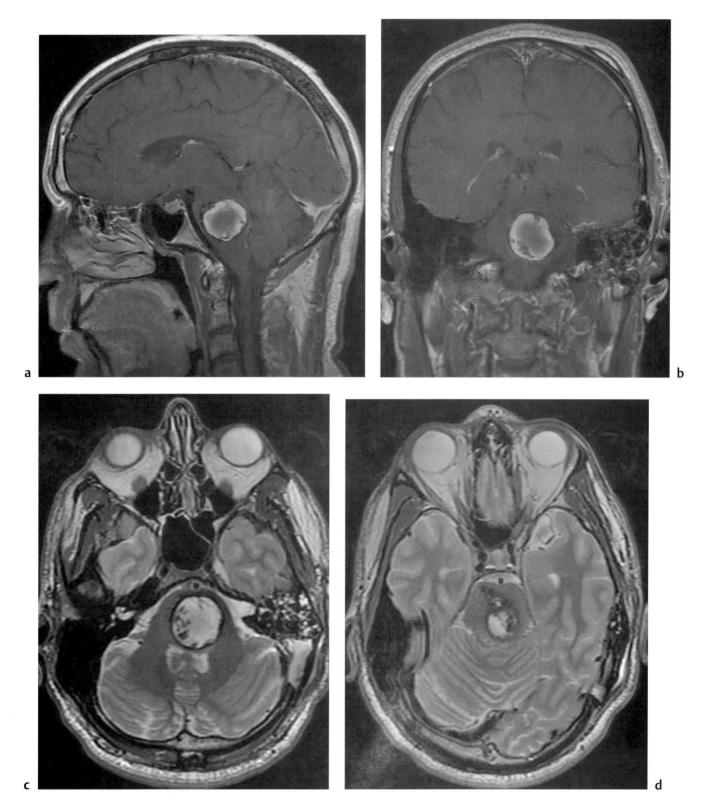

a

b

c

d

Figure 5.30. **(a)** Sagittal and **(b)** coronal T1-weighted and **(c,d)** axial T2-weighted magnetic resonance images demonstrate a large, deep pontine cavernous malformation eccentric to the left side. The patient had previously undergone a left presigmoid craniotomy at another institution. The resection was aborted due to excessive bleeding. Because the lesion was eccentric to the left side, we approached it using a left retrosigmoid craniotomy.

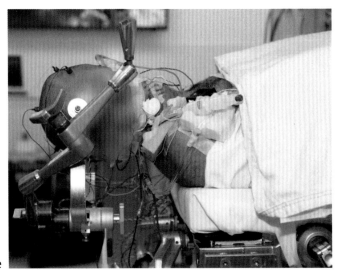

e

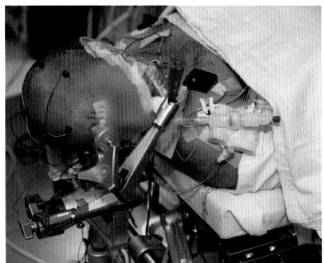

f

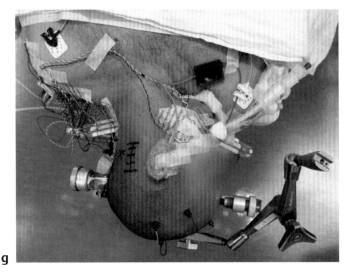

g

Figure 5.30. (e–g) Intraoperative photographs show patient positioning for the retrosigmoid craniotomy and approach. **(e)** The patient is placed supine, with the head turned to the contralateral side so that it is parallel to the floor. This head position may be possible only with young patients who have supple necks. **(f)** The chin is tucked toward the chest to open the craniocervical angle, where most of the dissection is to be performed. **(g)** The head is slightly extended toward the floor to open the angle between the head and the chest and to facilitate visualization of the brainstem up to the level

of the trigeminal nerve (CN V). Because of the deep location, the cavernous malformation is approached using the middle cerebellar peduncle safe entry zone. For improved visualization of the middle cerebellar peduncle safe entry zone from a retrosigmoid approach, the petrosal fissure is dissected. The petrosal fissure can be dissected and split in a manner akin to splitting the sylvian fissure to provide a direct path to the middle cerebellar peduncle, which is the preferred safe entry zone for accessing the brainstem to resect deep lateral pontine lesions.

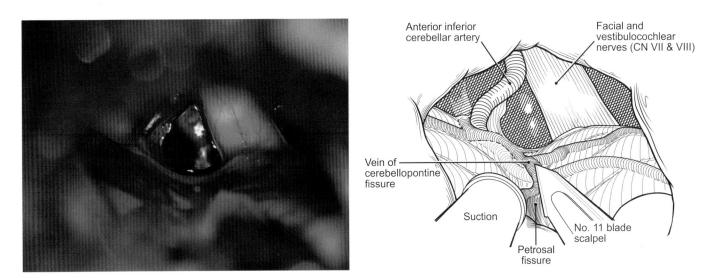

Figure 5.30. (h–p) Intraoperative photographs and illustrations show the step-by-step dissection of the petrosal and cerebellopontine fissures and the resection of the lesion. **(h)** The vein of the cerebellopontine fissure is identified and the arachnoid membrane overlying the vein is dissected to free and mobilize the vein. The lobules of the cerebellum are then separated by sharply disconnecting the arachnoid bands tethering them to expose the petrosal fissure (*shaded area*).

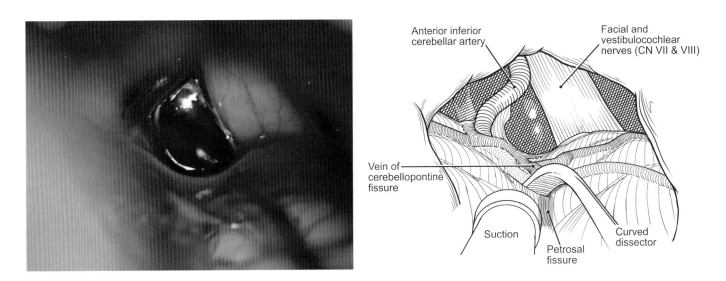

Figure 5.30. (i) The microdissector is used to expand the potential space between the cerebellar lobules; this is the petrosal fissure (*shaded area*).

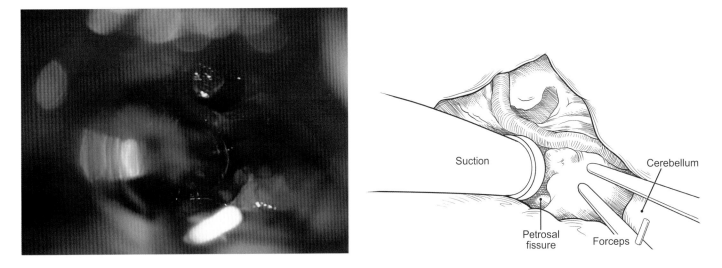

Figure 5.30. (j) The dissection is deepened to arrive at the pons, which is visualized at the tip of the suction cannula.

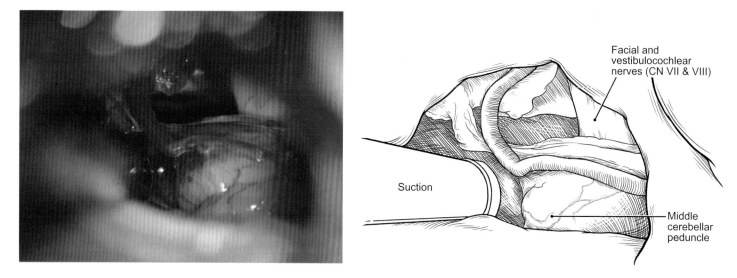

Figure 5.30. (k) Final view obtained after splitting the petrosal fissure of the cerebellum.

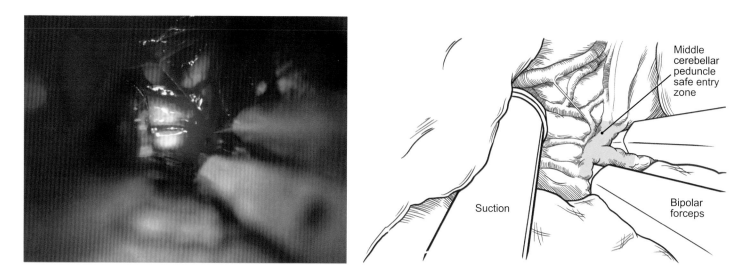

Figure 5.30. (l) A transverse opening is placed in the middle cerebellar peduncle safe entry zone (*shaded area*), parallel to the direction of fibers migrating in the middle cerebellar peduncle.

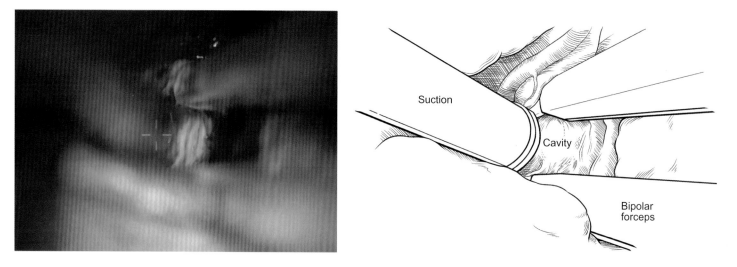

Figure 5.30. (m) The opening is expanded.

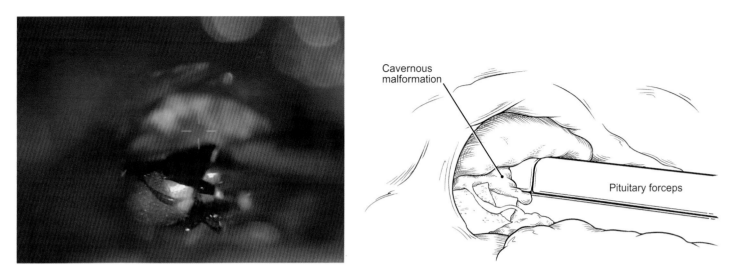

Figure 5.30. (n) The cavernous malformation is identified and mobilized using microdissectors and pituitary forceps.

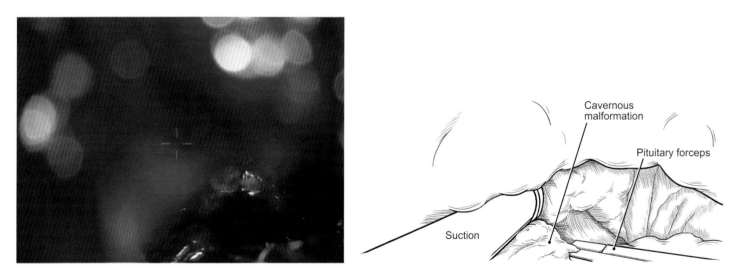

Figure 5.30. (o) Once freed, the cavernous malformation is resected piecemeal.

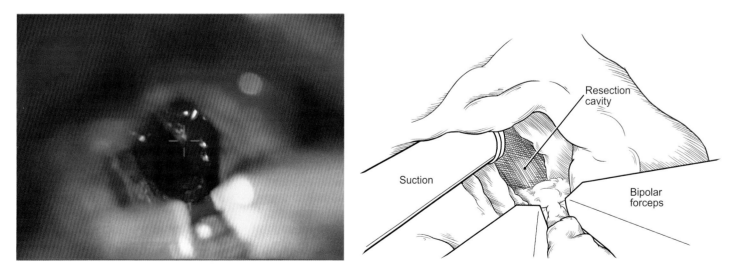

Figure 5.30. (p) Lighted microinstruments facilitate visualization at the depth of the operative bed. In this example, lighted bipolar forceps facilitate illumination and hemostasis. A small amount of hemostatic material may also be applied to the surface of the resection bed to obtain hemostasis, but the cavity should be irrigated before closure.

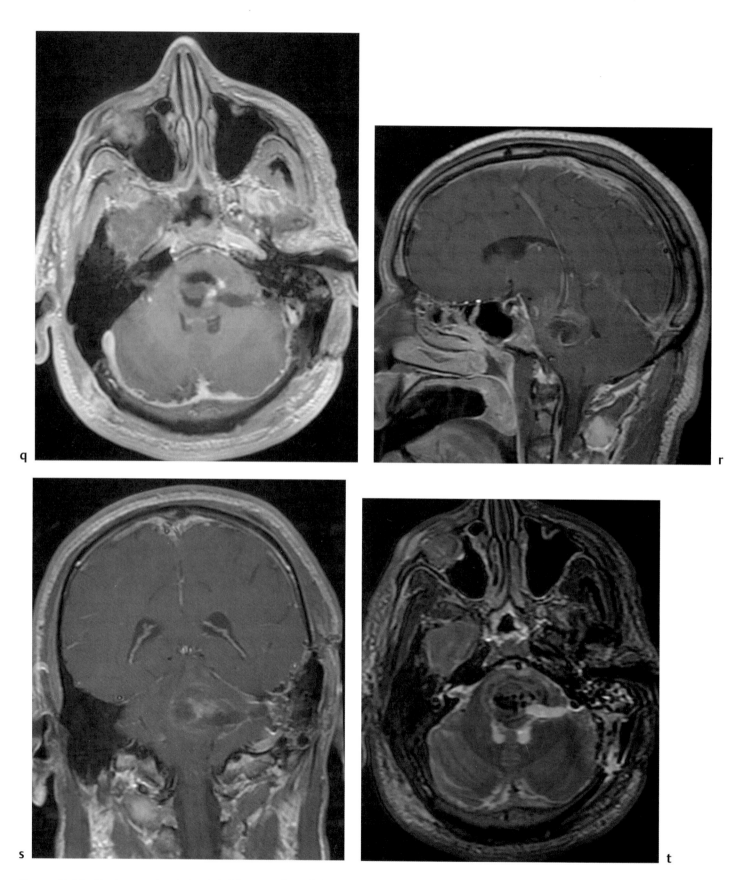

q

r

s

t

Figure 5.30. Postoperative **(q)** axial, **(r)** sagittal, and **(s)** coronal T1-weighted and **(t)** axial T2-weighted magnetic resonance images demonstrate complete removal of the lesion.

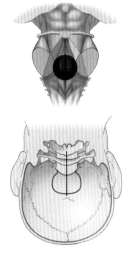

Case 5.31

- Diagnosis: Pontine cavernous malformation (related anatomy: pp. **25, 57–59**)
- Preoperative examination: Right internuclear ophthalmoplegia
- Approach: Midline suboccipital (related approach: pp. **200–211**)
- Positioning: Prone
- Monitoring: Somatosensory evoked potentials and motor evoked potentials; facial nerve (CN VII)
- Outcome: Complete removal of lesion; neurologic status is unchanged.

See Video 5.31 and Animations 5.2 and 5.5

Figure 5.31. A 56-year-old man presented with sudden-onset facial numbness and diplopia.

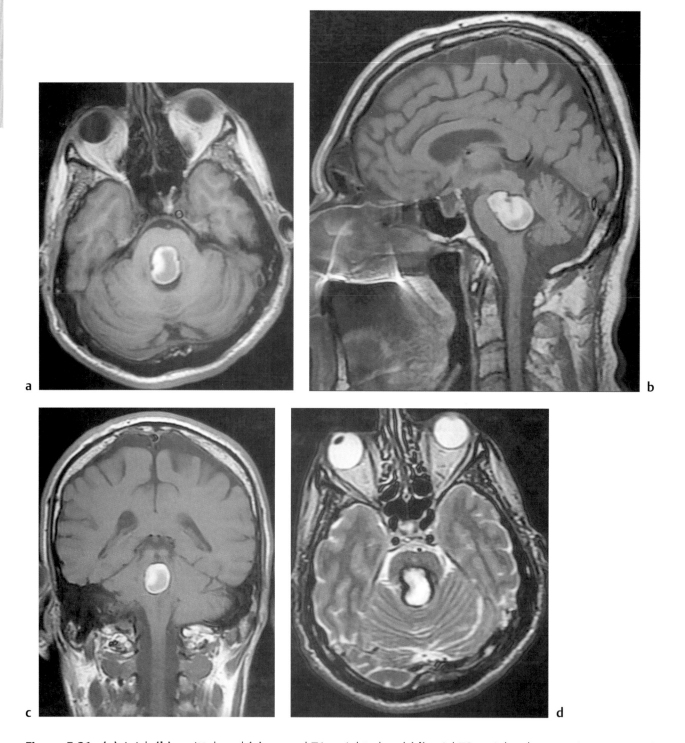

Figure 5.31. **(a)** Axial, **(b)** sagittal, and **(c)** coronal T1-weighted and **(d)** axial T2-weighted magnetic resonance images demonstrate a dorsal pontine lesion that abuts the floor of the fourth ventricle.

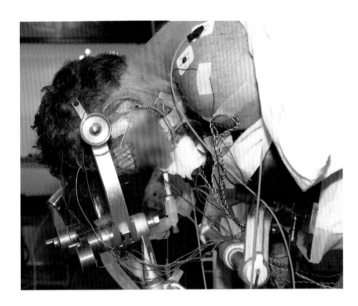

Figure 5.31. (e) The patient is positioned for a midline suboccipital craniotomy. The patient is placed prone, with the head flexed and the chin tucked to maximally expose the suboccipital region. The higher the lesion is on the floor of the fourth ventricle, the lower the craniotomy, and the skin incision should extend to provide the surgeon an unhindered approach to the lesion. In this case, although the craniotomy is a simple suboccipital opening, the skin incision should extend at least to the second cervical vertebra. However, removal of C1 and C2 posterior elements is not necessary to resect this lesion.

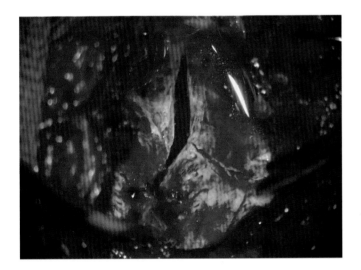
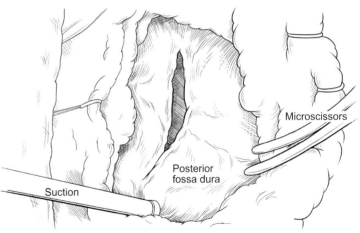

Figure 5.31. (f) The dura overlying the posterior fossa is opened in a Y fashion. Dissection of the arachnoid overlying the cerebellum enables mobilization of the loops of the posterior inferior cerebellar artery and splitting of the cerebellar hemispheres.

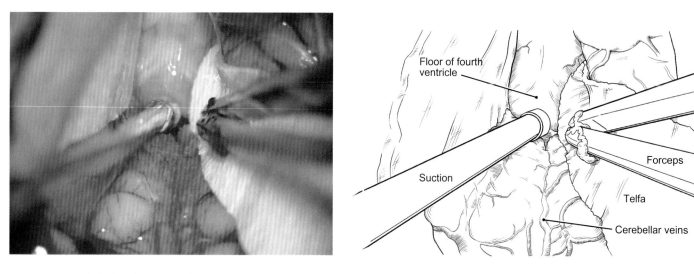

Figure 5.31. (g) Bleeding into the ventricular space is avoided by placing a small piece of Gelfoam into the fourth ventricle. Dissection is continued rostrally to expose the point where the cavernous malformation abuts the pial plane.

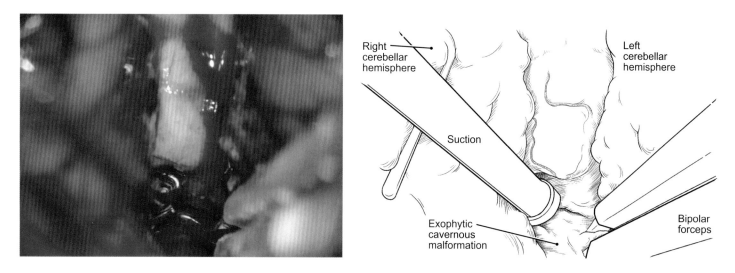

Figure 5.31. (h) The exophytic component of the cavernous malformation is readily visualized and entered to decompress the lesion.

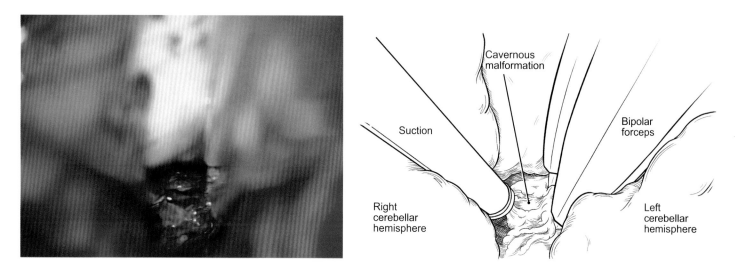

Figure 5.31. (i) Bipolar cautery is used to coagulate the cavernous malformation and to mobilize it from the brainstem.

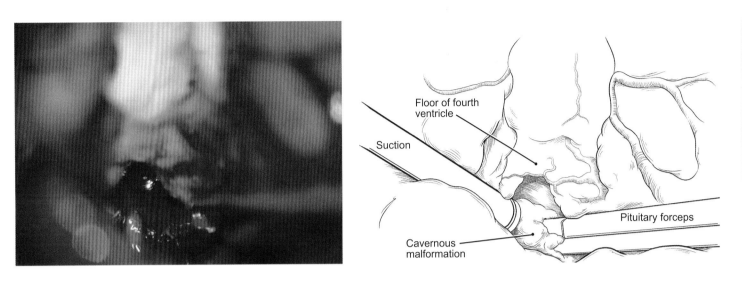

Figure 5.31. (j) Toothed forceps and pituitary forceps are used to dissect the lesion from the brainstem and to mobilize it.

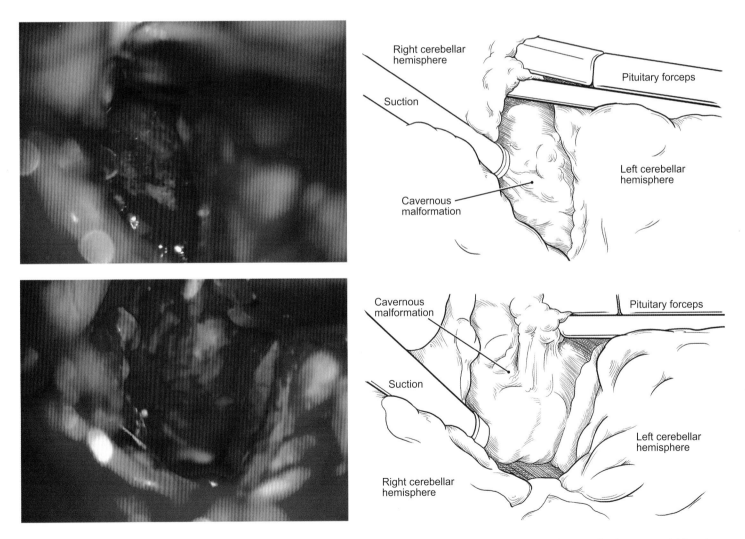

Figure 5.31. (k,l) Suction is often used as countertraction while pituitary forceps are used to elevate the lesion and bluntly dissect it free.

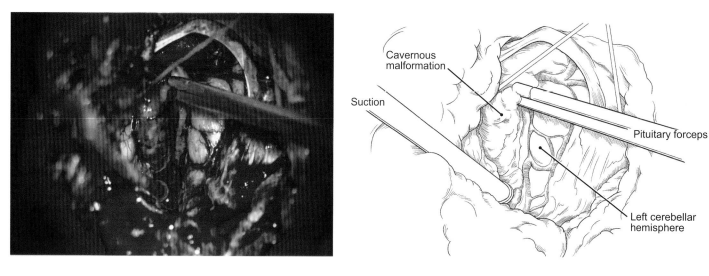

Figure 5.31. (m) Once fully mobilized, the lesion is removed.

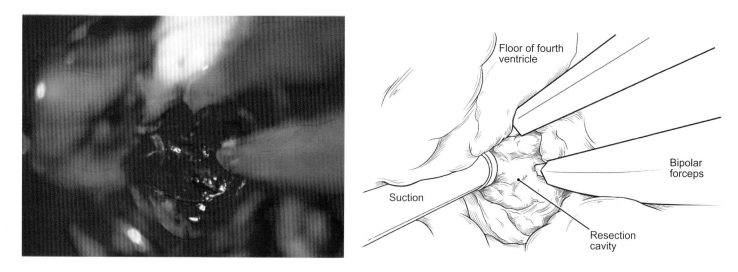

Figure 5.31. (n) A final inspection of the resection cavity is performed, and small bleeders are coagulated.

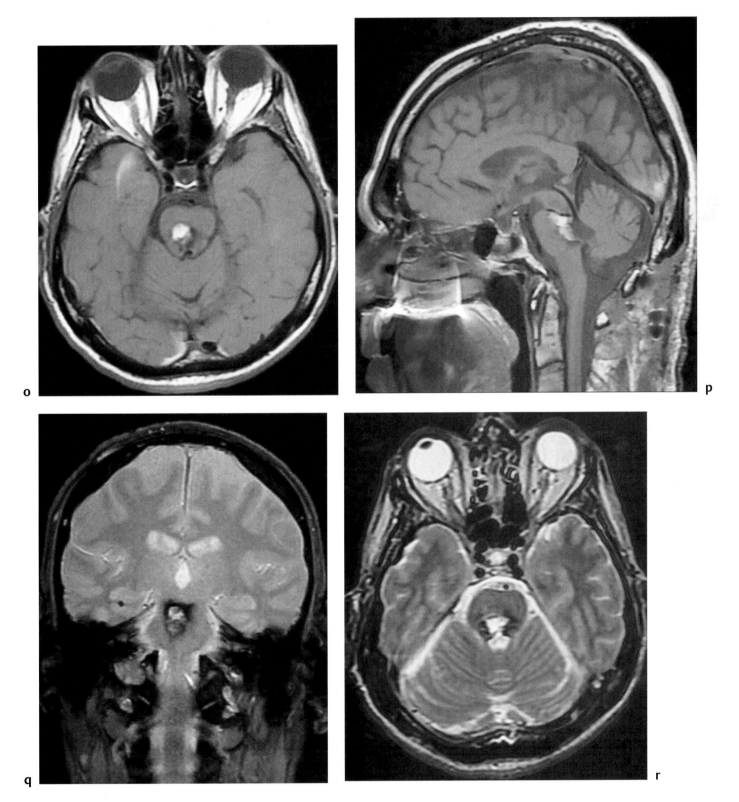

Figure 5.31. Postoperative **(o)** axial, **(p)** sagittal, and **(q)** coronal T1-weighted and **(r)** axial T2-weighted magnetic resonance images confirm complete removal of the lesion.

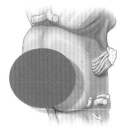

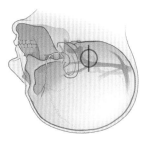

Case 5.32

- Diagnosis: Posterior fossa neuroenteric cyst (related anatomy: pp. **51, 56, 62, 118–124**)

- Preoperative examination: Neurologically intact

- Approach: Right retrosigmoid (related approach: pp. **212–222**)

- Positioning: Supine

- Monitoring: Somatosensory evoked potentials and motor evoked potentials; trigeminal (CN V), facial (CN VII), vestibulocochlear (CN VIII), glossopharyngeal (CN IX), vagus (CN X), and accessory (CN XI) nerves

- Outcome: Complete removal of lesion; patient is neurologically intact.

See Video 5.32

Figure 5.32. A 35-year-old woman presented with a history of headaches.

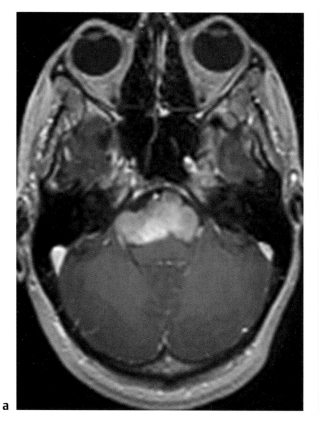

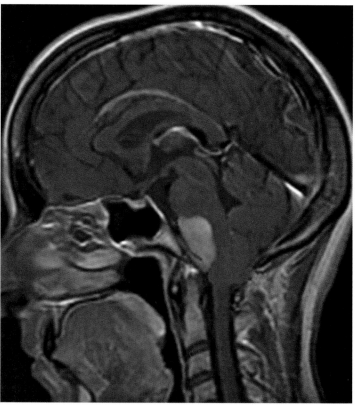

a   b

Figure 5.32. (a) Axial and **(b)** sagittal T1-weighted magnetic resonance images with contrast demonstrate a large, ventrally located, posterior fossa mass compressing and displacing the brainstem. The lesion displaces the basilar artery anteriorly, an imaging characteristic that is classic for a neuroenteric cyst.

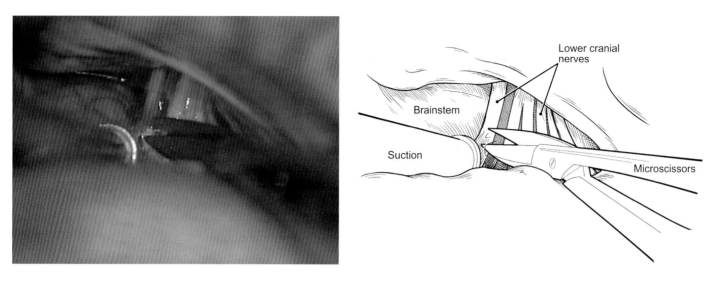

Figure 5.32. (c) The cyst is approached using a right retrosigmoid craniotomy. Upon entry to the cerebellopontine angle fissure and release of cerebrospinal fluid, the brainstem and cranial nerves are readily visualized.

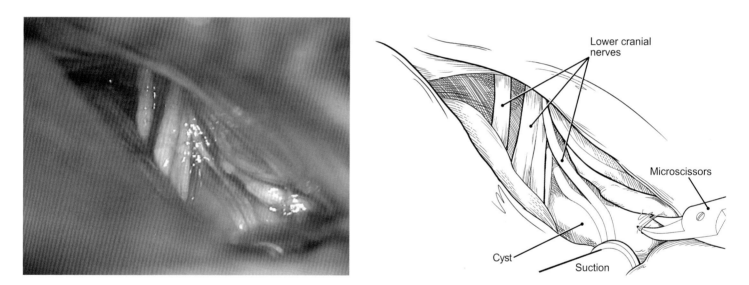

Figure 5.32. (d) Opening the arachnoid membrane over the lower cranial nerves exposes the cyst, which is deep in the surgical field.

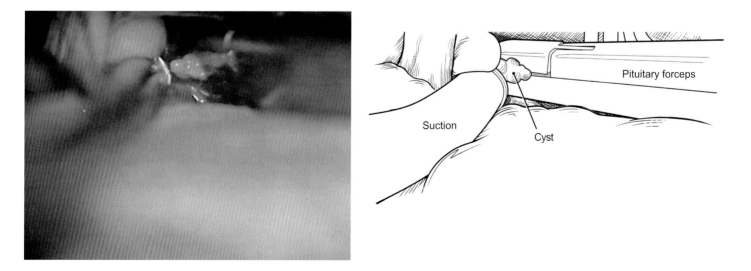

Figure 5.32. (e) The cyst is debulked internally using microforceps and pituitary forceps.

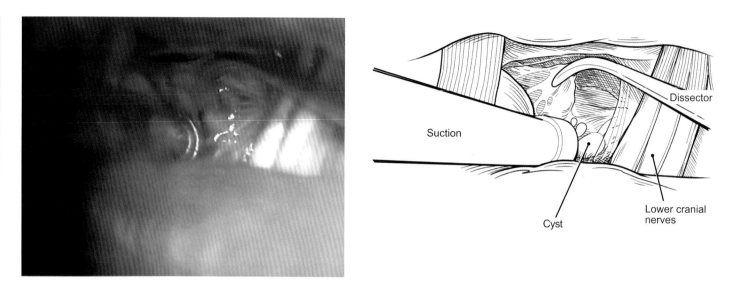

Figure 5.32. (f) The mucinous content of the cyst is removed by suction, and the cyst capsule is mobilized.

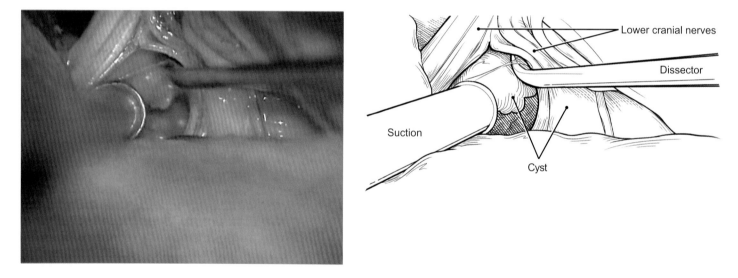

Figure 5.32. (g) Microdissectors are used to dissect the solid portion of the cyst from the brainstem and cranial nerves. Developing the potential space between the various lower cranial nerves facilitates visualizing the cyst more directly to dissect it. Therefore, generously opening the arachnoid membrane over the lower cranial nerves is essential for safe removal of these cysts.

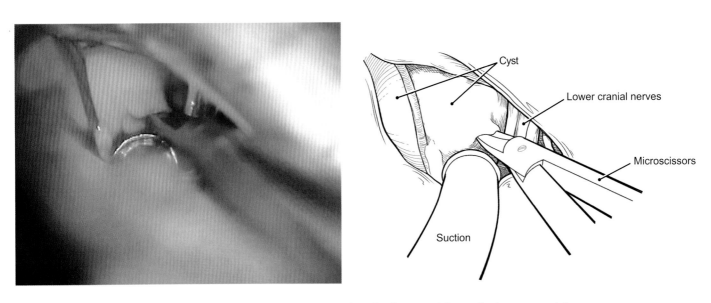

Figure 5.32. (h) After the cyst is debulked internally, it is sharply dissected from the lower cranial nerves.

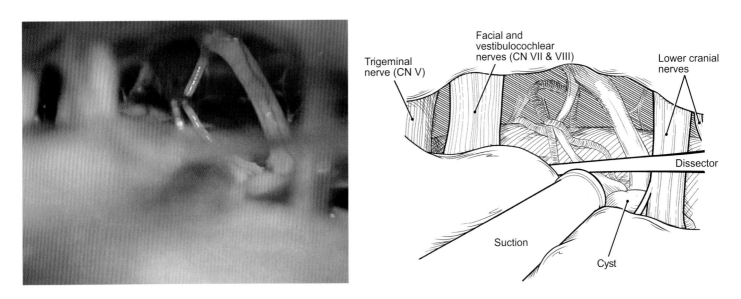

Figure 5.32. (i) When it is completely freed, the cyst capsule is rolled out and completely disconnected.

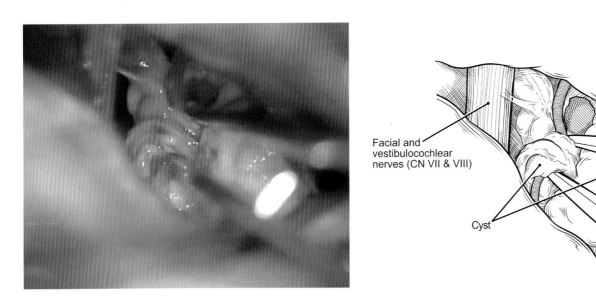

Figure 5.32. (j) Final remnants of the cyst are removed.

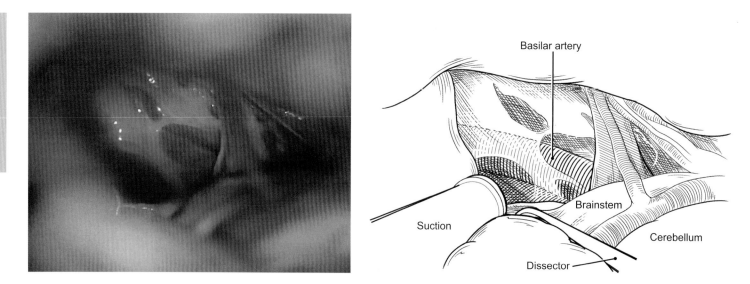

Figure 5.32. (k) Hemostasis and final inspection of the resection cavity are performed to ensure that no residual cyst is left behind. When possible, the arachnoid membrane over the cranial nerves that are not involved with the cyst should be kept in place.

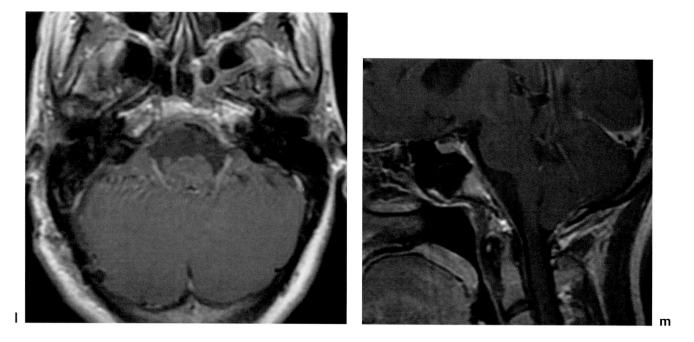

Figure 5.32. Postoperative **(l)** axial and **(m)** sagittal T1-weighted magnetic resonance images with contrast confirm complete removal of the cyst.

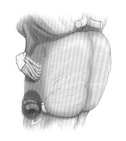

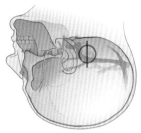

Case 5.33

- Diagnosis: Right pontine metastatic lesion (related anatomy: pp. **51, 56, 62, 118–124**)

- Preoperative examination: Neurologically intact

- Approach: Right retrosigmoid (related approach: pp. **212–222**)

- Positioning: Supine

- Monitoring: Somatosensory evoked potentials and motor evoked potentials; trigeminal (CN V), facial (CN VII), and vestibulocochlear (CN VIII) nerves

- Outcome: Complete removal of lesion; patient is neurologically intact.

See Video 5.33

Figure 5.33. A 53-year-old woman with a history of small cell lung adenocarcinoma presented with a solitary metastatic lesion.

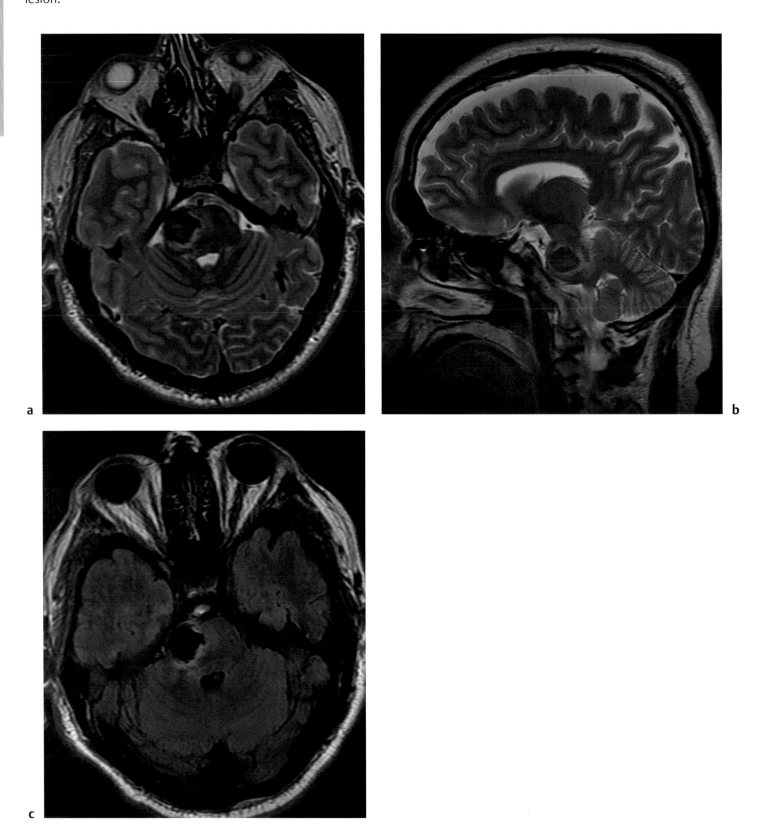

Figure 5.33. (a) Axial and **(b)** sagittal T2-weighted and **(c)** axial fluid-attenuated inversion recovery (FLAIR) magnetic resonance images demonstrate a right pontine lesion.

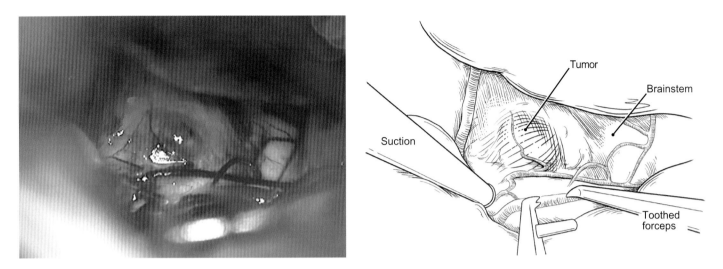

Figure 5.33. (d) The lesion is approached using a right retrosigmoid craniotomy. Release of cerebrospinal fluid from the cerebellopontine angle cistern demonstrates the lung metastasis, which is readily visible due to its discoloration of the brainstem surface.

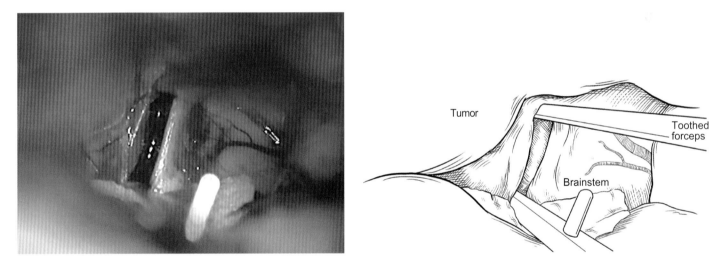

Figure 5.33. (e) Toothed forceps are used to enter the lesion, to spread the fibers of the brainstem overlying the tumor in a minimally invasive fashion, and to internally debulk the tumor.

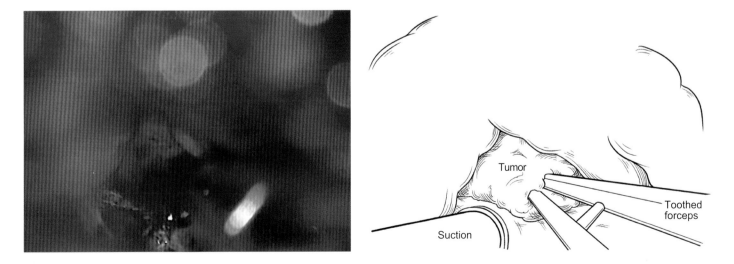

Figure 5.33. (f) A combination of toothed forceps and pituitary forceps is used to remove the tumor piecemeal.

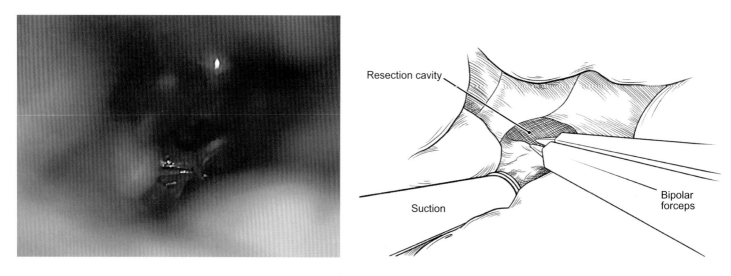

Figure 5.33. (g) Hemostasis is obtained with the judicious use of cautery to prevent injury to adjacent fiber tracts.

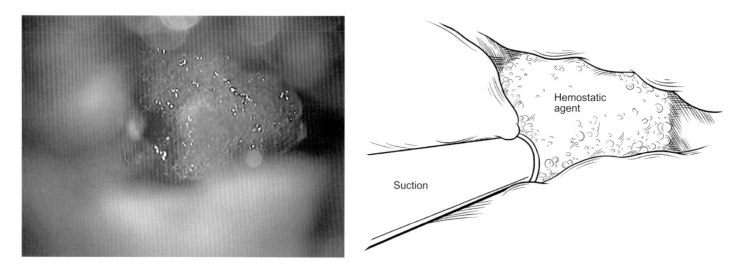

Figure 5.33. (h) At the completion of the resection, a small amount of hemostatic agent can be placed in the resection cavity to ensure hemostasis. The resection cavity is then irrigated to prevent postoperative swelling.

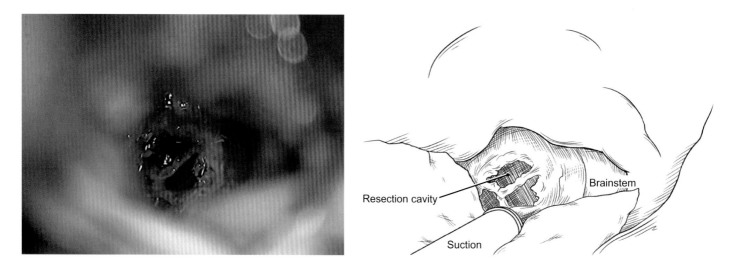

Figure 5.33. (i) A view of the resection cavity shows a dry operative field and no evidence of gross residual tumor.

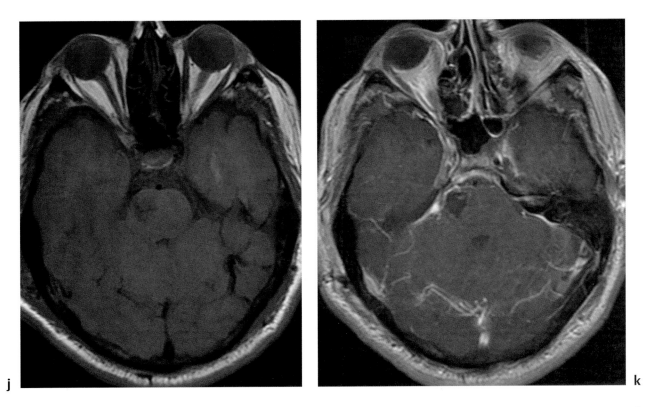

j

k

Figure 5.33. Postoperative axial T1-weighted magnetic resonance images **(j)** without and **(k)** with contrast confirm complete removal of the tumor.

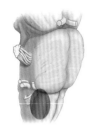

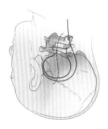

Case 5.34

- Diagnosis: Medullary cavernous malformation (related anatomy: pp. **68–71, 73, 74**)
- Preoperative examination: Neurologically intact
- Approach: Right far-lateral (related approach: pp. **223–235**)
- Positioning: Park bench
- Monitoring: Somatosensory evoked potentials and motor evoked potentials; glossopharyngeal (CN IX), vagus (CN X), accessory (CN XI), and hypoglossal (CN XII) nerves
- Outcome: Complete removal of lesion; patient is neurologically intact.

See Video 5.34 and Animations 5.2 and 5.7

Figure 5.34. A 26-year-old woman presented with a history of three prior hemorrhages.

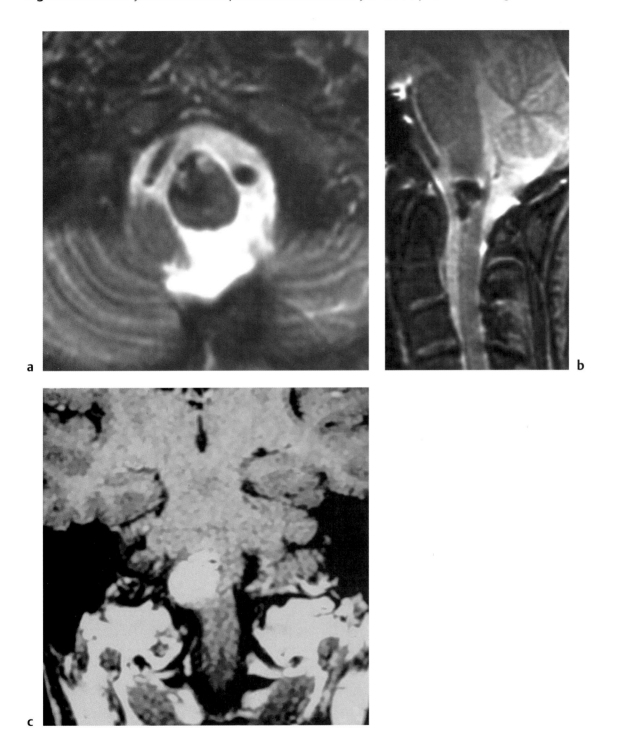

Figure 5.34. (a) Axial and **(b)** sagittal T2-weighted and **(c)** coronal gradient-echo magnetic resonance images demonstrate a lateral medullary cavernous malformation with evidence of hemorrhage in a patient with three prior hemorrhages.

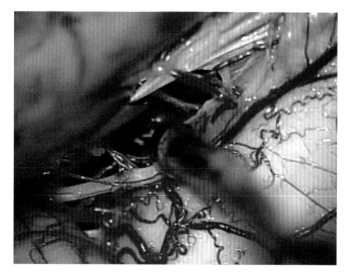

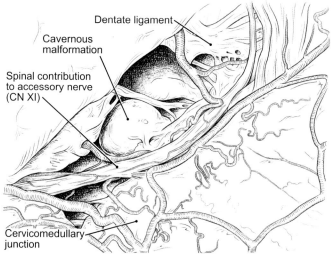

Figure 5.34. (d) The patient is placed in a park bench position for a right far-lateral craniotomy to access the lesion. The dura is opened and cerebrospinal fluid is released to expose the cervicomedullary junction. The component of this lesion in the lateral medulla is exposed by sharply cutting the dentate ligaments so that the spinal cord can be safely rotated. It is usually necessary to cut the dentate ligaments at multiple levels. Note the pearly white color of the dentate ligament, which differs from the ivory color of the nerve roots (under the suction device).

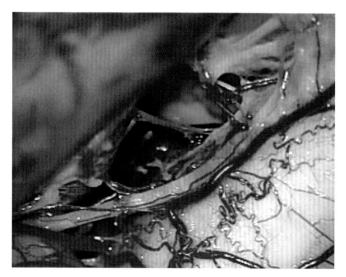

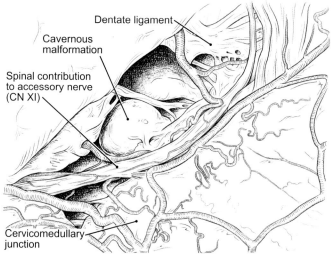

Figure 5.34. (e) Resection of the dentate ligament exposes the exophytic portion of the cavernous malformation.

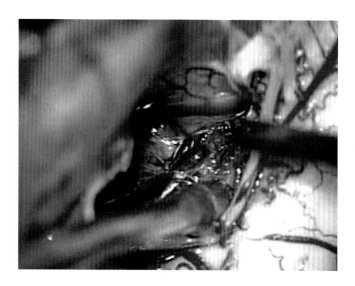

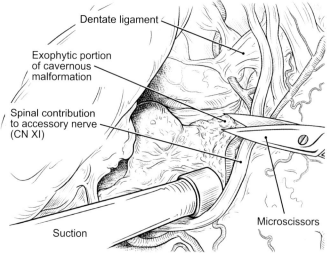

Figure 5.34. (f) Sharp dissection of the lesion from the adjacent cervicomedullary junction is critical to minimize traction morbidity to the brainstem and spinal cord. Suction is used to provide countertraction while the exophytic portion of the cavernous malformation is debulked and separated from the cervicomedullary junction.

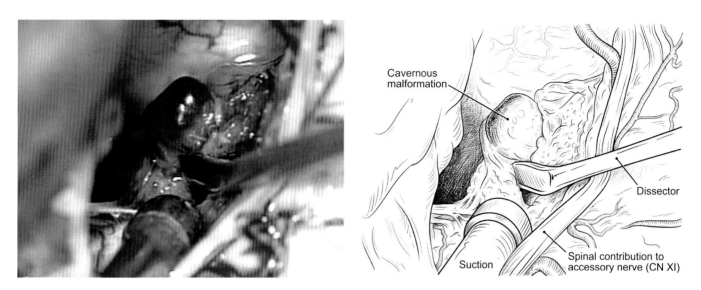

Figure 5.34. (g) Microdissectors are used to lift the cavernous malformation, further mobilizing it.

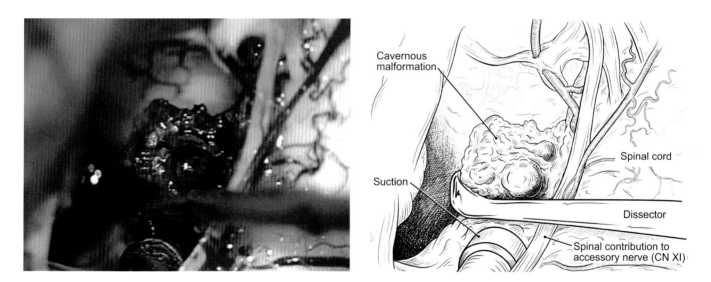

Figure 5.34. (h) Microdissectors are used to continue mobilizing the malformation, with minimal deformation of the spinal cord while the dissection proceeds.

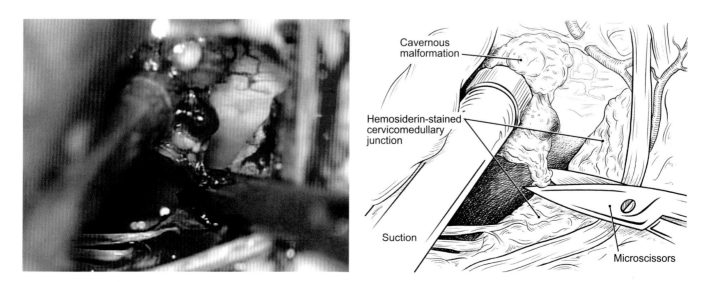

Figure 5.34. (i) The cavernous malformation is sharply cut from its pedicle. Hemosiderin-stained tissue is visible but should not be removed to minimize deficits.

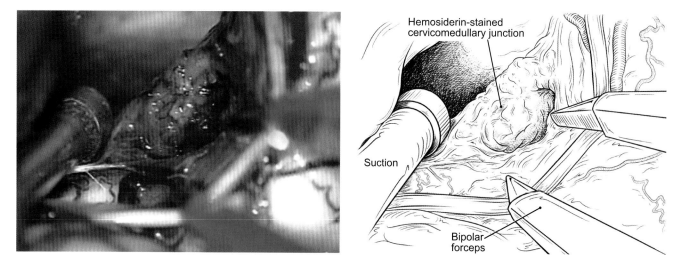

Figure 5.34. (j) The resection bed is inspected, and bipolar cautery is used to control focal points of bleeding.

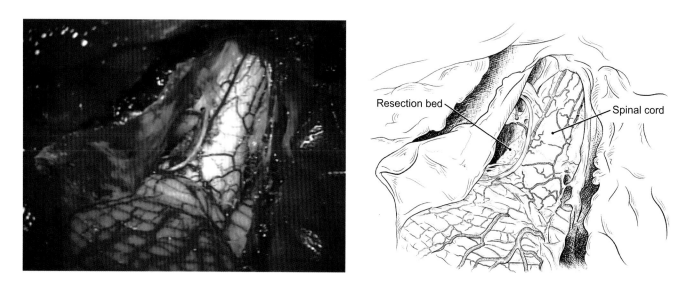

Figure 5.34. (k) Intraoperative photograph shows the final resection bed with the exposure afforded by this approach.

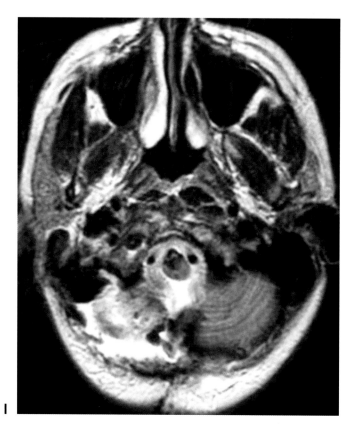

l

Figure 5.34. (l) Postoperative axial T2-weighted magnetic resonance image documents complete removal of the lesion.

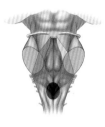
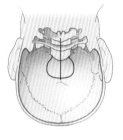

Case 5.35

- Diagnosis: Pontomedullary cavernous malformation (related anatomy: pp. **68–71, 73, 74**)

- Preoperative examination: Transient sensory disturbances

- Approach: Midline suboccipital (related approach: pp. **200–211**)

- Positioning: Prone

- Monitoring: Somatosensory evoked potentials and motor evoked potentials

- Outcome: Complete removal of lesion; postoperative worsening of sensory deficits that gradually improved

See Video 5.35 and Animations 5.2 and 5.5

Figure 5.35. A 34-year-old woman presented with transient sensory disturbances.

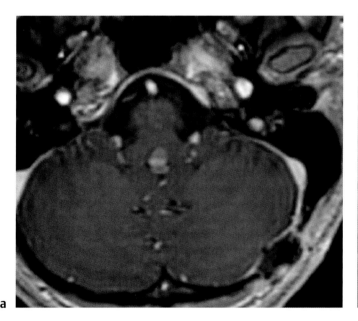
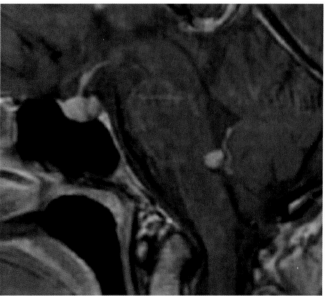

a   b

Figure 5.35. **(a)** Axial and **(b)** sagittal T1-weighted magnetic resonance images with contrast demonstrate a dorsally exophytic pontomedullary cavernous malformation.

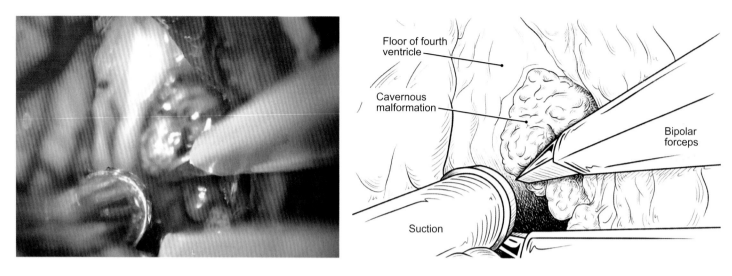

Figure 5.35. (c) The patient is positioned prone, and a midline suboccipital craniotomy is performed to expose the lesion. The exophytic cavernous malformation is readily identified.

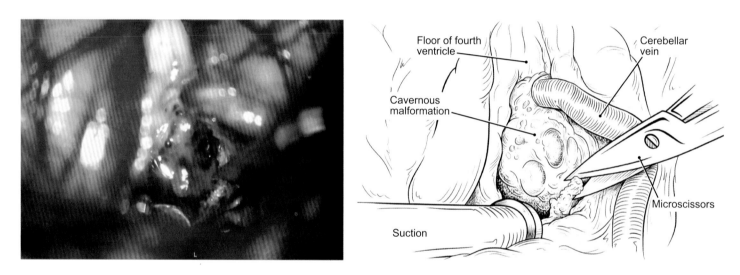

Figure 5.35. (d) The surface of the dorsal pontomedullary junction is visualized. The residual cavernous malformation, with its distinct mulberry appearance, is readily apparent. A small portion of cavernous malformation is cut sharply and removed.

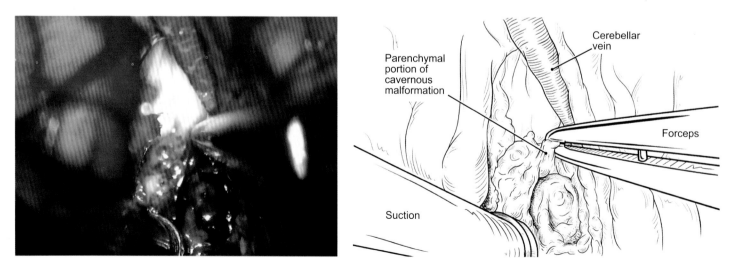

Figure 5.35. (e) Microdissectors and forceps are used to mobilize the parenchymal portion of the cavernous malformation from the underlying brainstem.

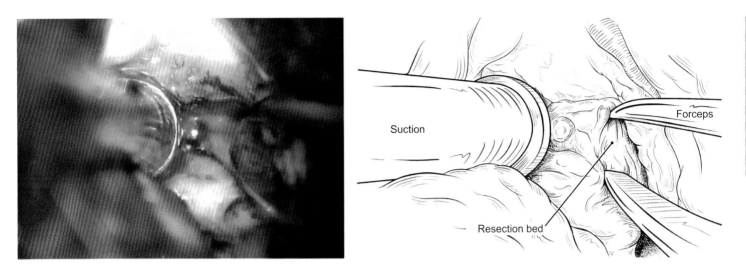

Figure 5.35. (f) After a large portion of the cavernous malformation is removed, any remnants are removed from the resection bed using microforceps.

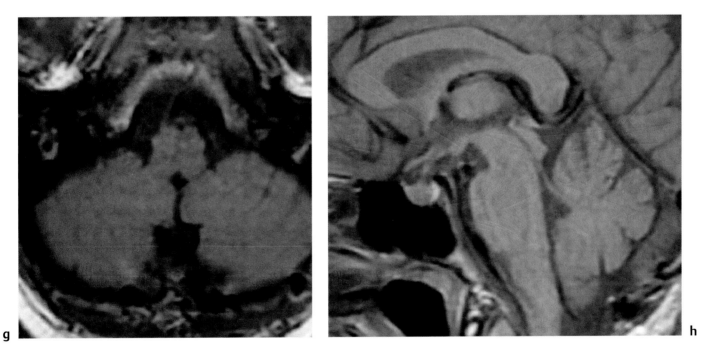

Figure 5.35. Postoperative **(g)** axial and **(h)** sagittal T1-weighted magnetic resonance images confirm complete removal of the lesion.

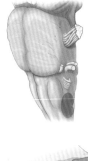

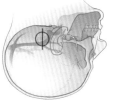

Case 5.36

- Diagnosis: Pontomedullary cavernous malformation (related anatomy: pp. **68–71, 73, 74**)
- Preoperative examination: Diffuse quadriparesis
- Approach: Left retrosigmoid (related approach: pp. **212–222**)
- Positioning: Supine
- Monitoring: Somatosensory evoked potentials and motor evoked potentials
- Outcome: Complete removal of lesion; patient is neurologically stable.

See Video 5.36 and Animations 5.2 and 5.6

Figure 5.36. A 40-year-old woman presented with bilateral arm and leg weakness.

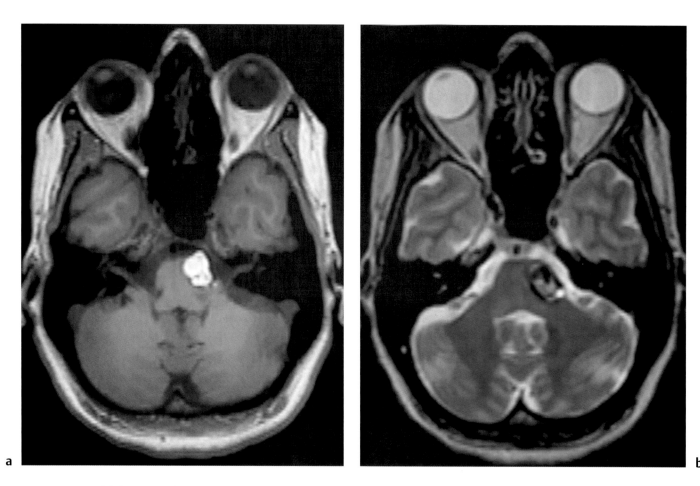

a   b

Figure 5.36 Axial **(a)** T1-weighted and **(b)** T2-weighted magnetic resonance images demonstrate a left pontomedullary cavernous malformation.

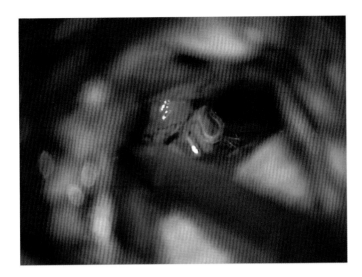

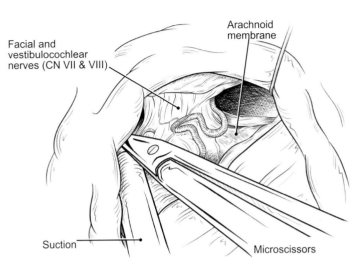

Figure 5.36. (c) The lesion is exposed using a left retrosigmoid craniotomy. The patient is placed supine with the head turned to the contralateral side and flexed to open the angle between the head and neck. In patients with a large or barrel chest, the park bench position may be used instead of the supine position. A standard retrosigmoid craniotomy is performed, but it is placed lower along the sigmoid sinus to readily reach the medullary component of the cavernous malformation. After cerebrospinal fluid is released, the contents of the cerebellopontine angle cistern are visualized. Dissection of the arachnoid membrane exposes the brainstem surface. Alternatively, a far-lateral approach may be used to reach this lesion.

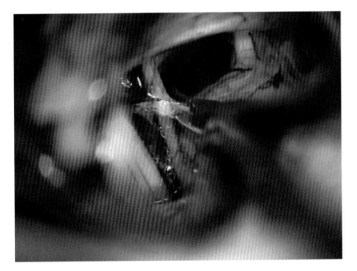

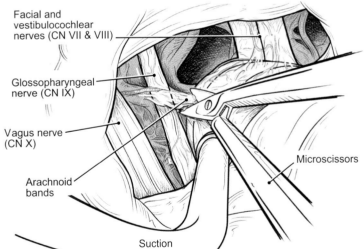

Figure 5.36. (d) Arachnoid bands over the lower cranial nerves are cut sharply to expand the exposure necessary for resection of the lesion.

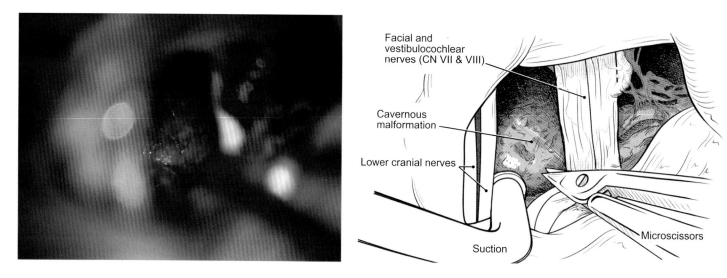

Figure 5.36. (e) The larger exposure brings the lesion into view. Note the hemosiderin-stained tissue. The cranial nerves can be gently retracted to begin dissection and mobilization of the lesion.

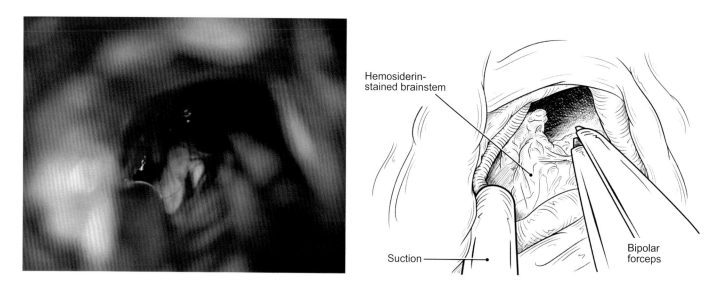

Figure 5.36. (f) Mobilization of the cavernous malformation demonstrates the hemosiderin-stained brainstem.

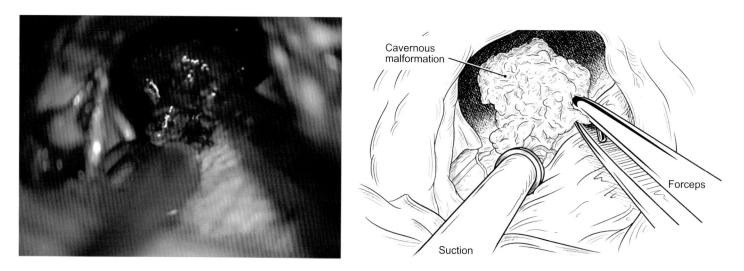

Figure 5.36. (g) The cavernous malformation is debulked, mobilized, and removed piecemeal.

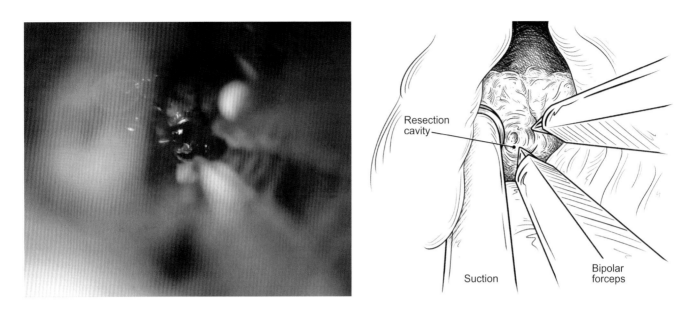

Resection
cavity

Suction

Bipolar
forceps

Figure 5.36. (h) The resection cavity is inspected to verify hemostasis.

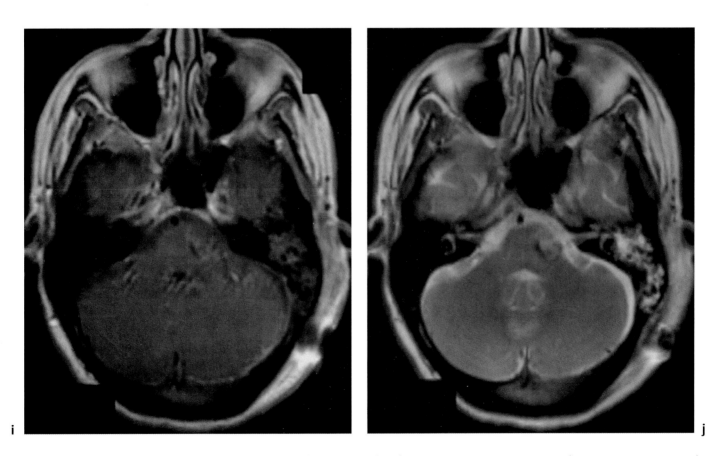

i   j

Figure 5.36. Postoperative axial **(i)** T1-weighted and **(j)** T2-weighted magnetic resonance images demonstrate gross-total resection of the lesion.

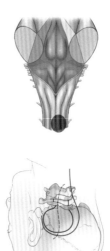

Case 5.37

• Diagnosis: Cervicomedullary hemangioblastoma (related anatomy: pp. **68–71, 73, 74**)

• Preoperative examination: Diminished sensation in all extremities

• Approach: Right far-lateral craniotomy and C1 hemilaminectomy (related approach: pp. **223–235**)

• Positioning: Park bench

• Monitoring: Somatosensory evoked potentials and motor evoked potentials

• Outcome: Complete lesion removal; patient is neurologically stable.

See Video 5.37

Figure 5.37. A 31-year-old man presented with bilateral sensory loss that was worse on the left side.

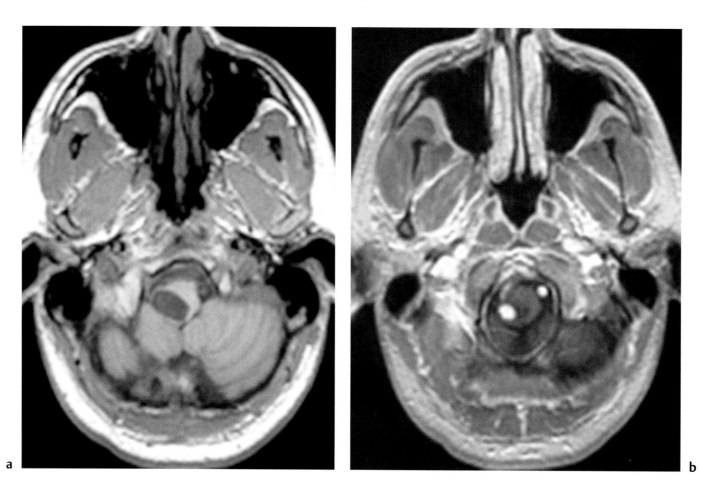

a

b

Figure 5.37. (a) Axial T1-weighted magnetic resonance image without contrast and **(b)** axial and **(c)** sagittal T1-weighted magnetic resonance images with contrast demonstrate a lesion at the lateral cervicomedullary junction consistent with a hemangioblastoma.

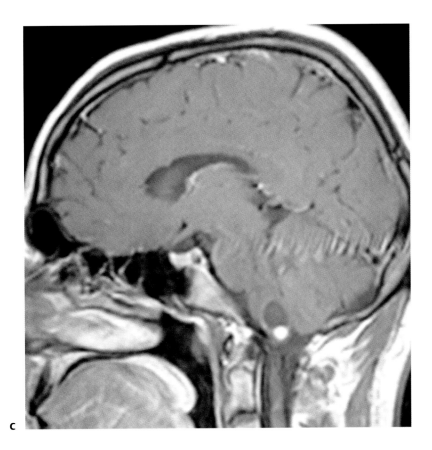

c

Figure 5.37. (Continued)

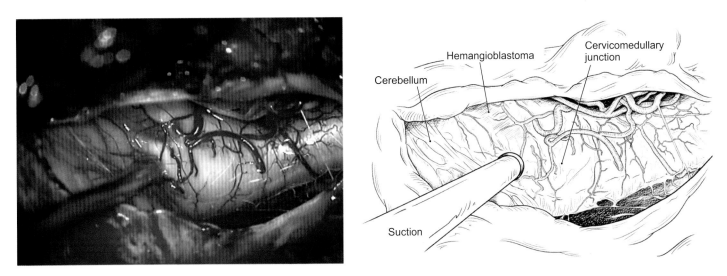

Figure 5.37. (d) The lesion was accessed using a right far-lateral approach, including a C1 laminectomy, with the patient in the park bench position. The hemangioblastoma is visible through the arachnoid membrane of the posterior fossa.

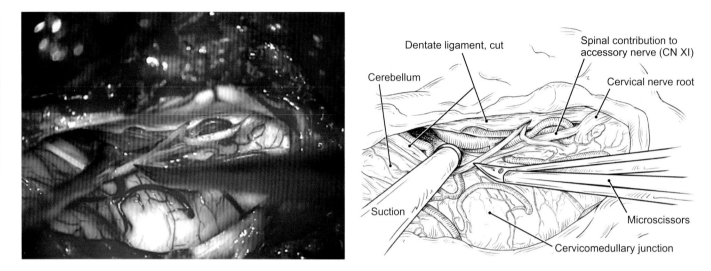

Figure 5.37. (e) The lesion is further exposed by mobilizing the rootlets of the upper cervical nerves and cutting the dentate ligaments, enabling the spinal cord to be mobilized and rotated.

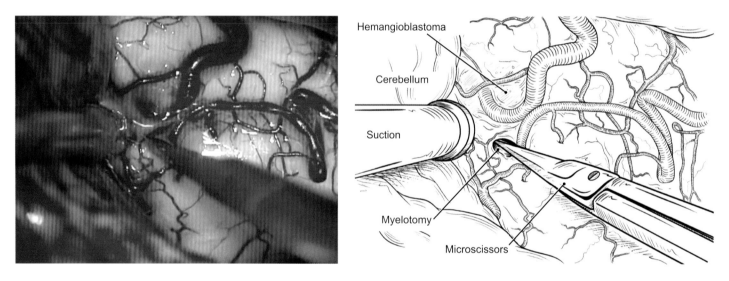

Figure 5.37. (f) Mild dynamic retraction of the cerebellum exposes the lesion, which had stained the cervicomedullary junction. Sharp dissection is used to perform a myelotomy.

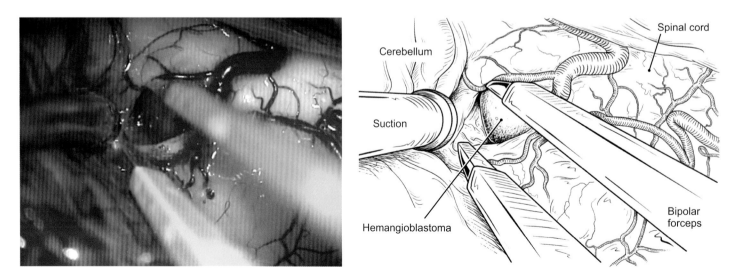

Figure 5.37. (g) The opening is expanded by spreading the tissue with bipolar forceps or microforceps.

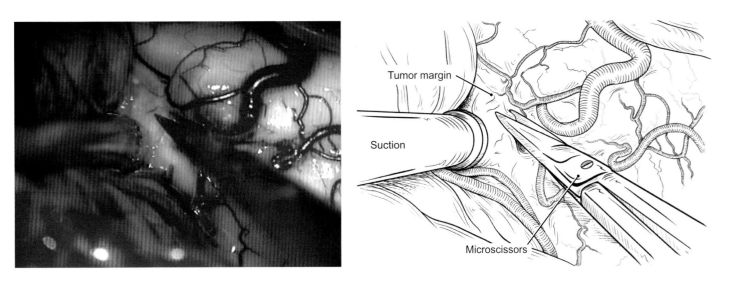

Figure 5.37. (h) The lesion is sharply dissected circumferentially using microscissors.

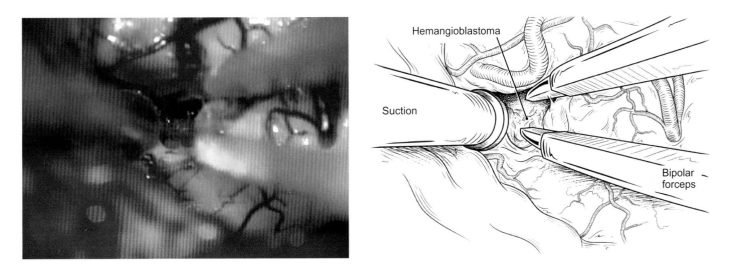

Figure 5.37. (i) The vascular supply to the tumor is cauterized.

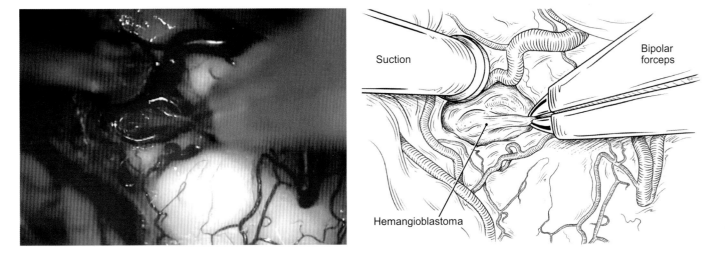

Figure 5.37. (j) The lesion is removed en bloc.

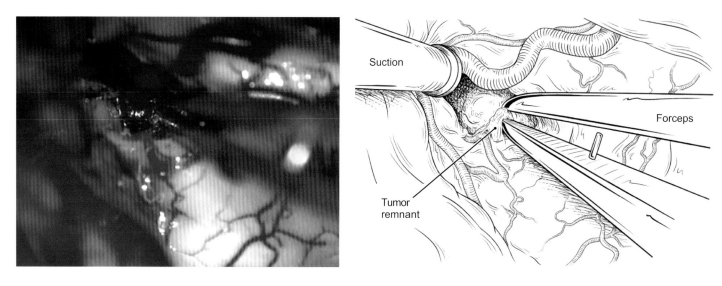

Figure 5.37. (k) Forceps are used to peel small remnants from the spinal cord.

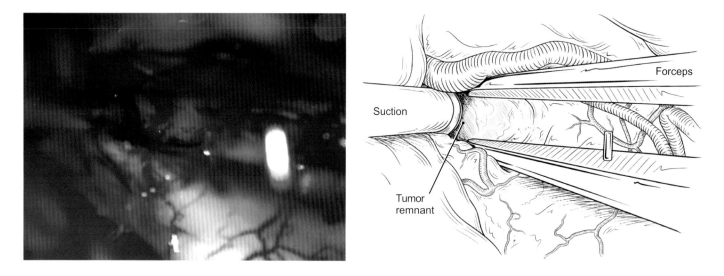

Figure 5.37. (l) Inspection of the resection cavity demonstrates a remnant of tumor at the rostral extent of the cavity.

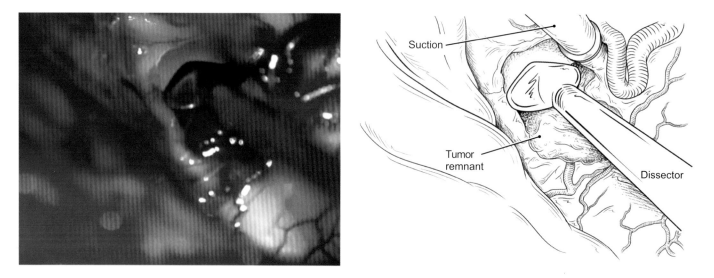

Figure 5.37. (m) A microdissector is used to remove the remnant.

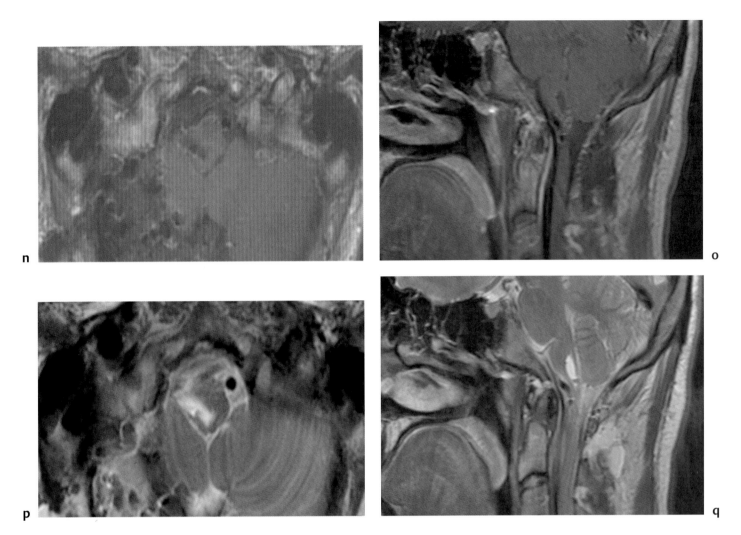

Figure 5.37. Postoperative **(n)** axial and **(o)** sagittal T1-weighted and **(p)** axial and **(q)** sagittal T2-weighted magnetic resonance images demonstrate complete resection of the lesion.

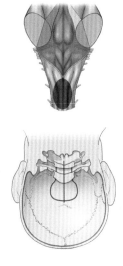

Case 5.38

- Diagnosis: Medullary glioma (related anatomy: pp. **68–71, 73, 74**)
- Preoperative examination: No sensation in left hand
- Approach: Midline suboccipital craniotomy and C1 laminectomy (related approach: p. **248**)
- Positioning: Prone
- Monitoring: Somatosensory evoked potentials and motor evoked potentials
- Outcome: Complete lesion removal; patient is neurologically stable.

See Video 5.38

Figure 5.38. A 50-year-old man presented with sensory deficit in the left hand.

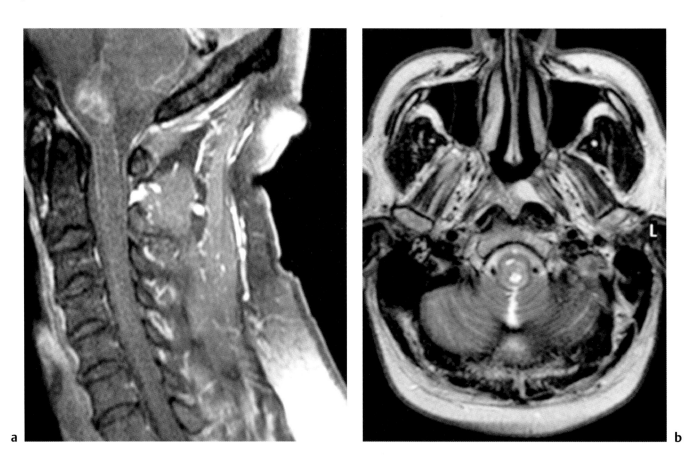

a   b

Figure 5.38. (a) Sagittal T1-weighted with contrast and **(b)** axial T2-weighted magnetic resonance images demonstrate a contrast-enhancing mass in the dorsal medulla.

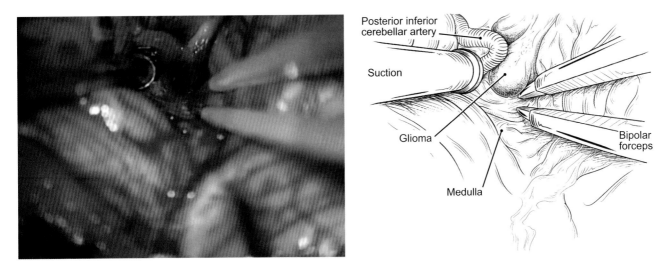

Figure 5.38. (c) The lesion, a glioma, is accessed using a midline suboccipital approach and a C1 laminectomy, with the patient in the prone position. The dorsally exophytic lesion is identifiable with minimal cerebellar retraction. Bipolar cautery is used to debulk the tumor.

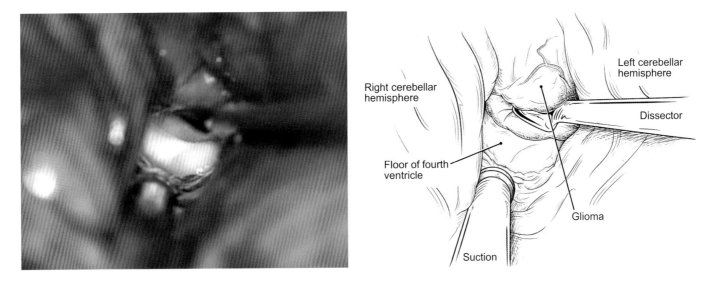

Figure 5.38. (d) A microdissector is used to mobilize the tumor from adjacent normal tissue. Although this tumor is a glioma, it has a discernible plane that may be developed.

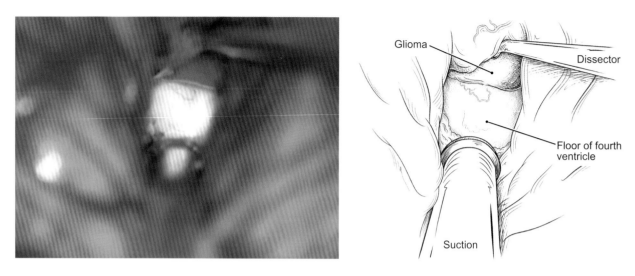

Figure 5.38. **(e)** Tumor mobilization facilitates visualization of the normal floor of the fourth ventricle.

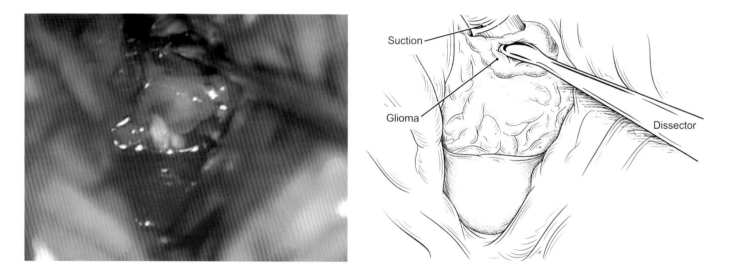

Figure 5.38. **(f)** Residual tumor is debulked from the cervicomedullary junction using a microdissector and suction.

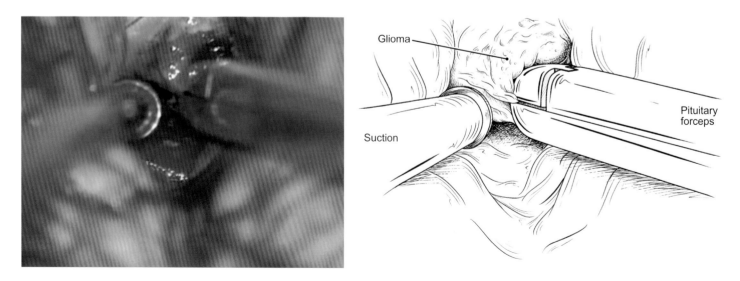

Figure 5.38. **(g)** Pituitary forceps are used to remove the tumor piecemeal.

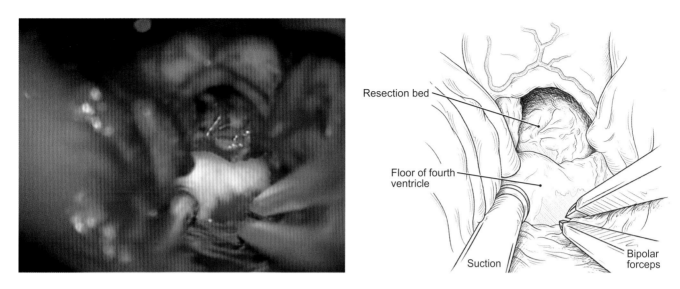

Figure 5.38. **(h)** The resection bed is inspected, and hemostasis is obtained.

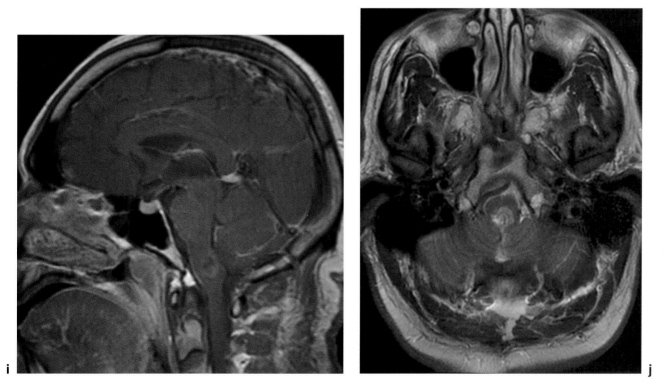

Figure 5.38. Postoperative **(i)** sagittal T1-weighted magnetic resonance image with contrast and **(j)** axial T2-weighted magnetic resonance image demonstrate complete resection of the tumor.

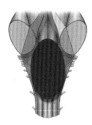

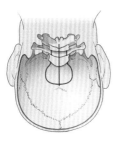

Case 5.39

- Diagnosis: Fourth ventricle ependymoma (related anatomy: pp. **25, 52, 57–59, 71, 73–75**)
- Preoperative examination: Neurologically intact
- Approach: Midline suboccipital craniotomy and C1 laminectomy (related approach: p. **248**)
- Positioning: Prone
- Monitoring: Somatosensory evoked potentials and motor evoked potentials
- Outcome: Complete lesion removal; postoperative transient palsies of glossopharyngeal nerve (CN IX) and vagus nerve (CN X), with improvement to baseline by 2-week follow-up

See Video 5.39

Figure 5.39. A 59-year-old woman presented with vertigo of 2 months' duration and headaches and nausea of 2 weeks' duration.

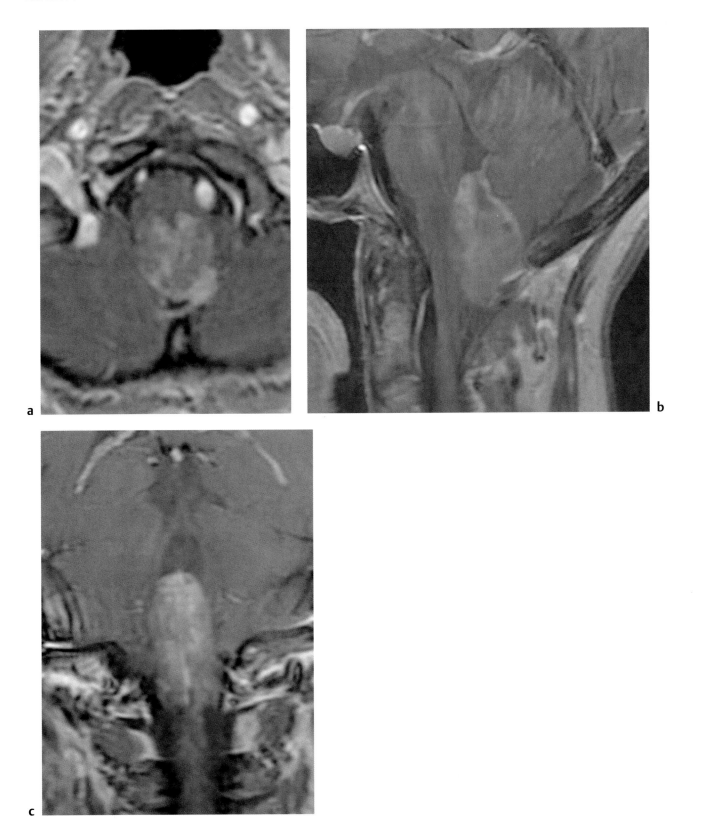

a

b

c

Figure 5.39. (a) Axial, **(b)** sagittal, and **(c)** coronal T1-weighted magnetic resonance images with contrast demonstrate a large mass in the fourth ventricle, consistent with an ependymoma.

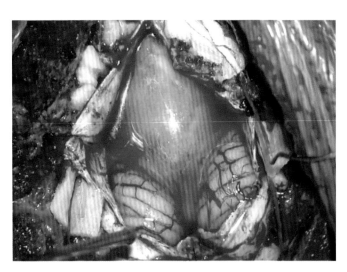
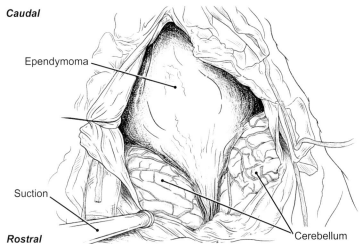

Figure 5.39. (d) The lesion is exposed using a midline suboccipital craniotomy and a C1 laminectomy. After the dura is opened, the lesion is visualized and found to be displacing the cerebellar hemispheres.

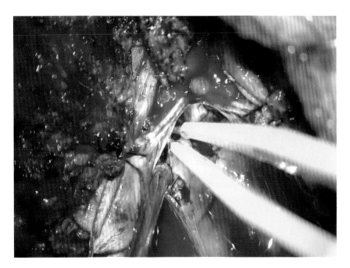
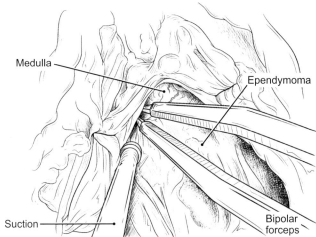

Figure 5.39. (e) The lesion is mobilized circumferentially from the adjacent structures and systematically disconnected from the arachnoid bands.

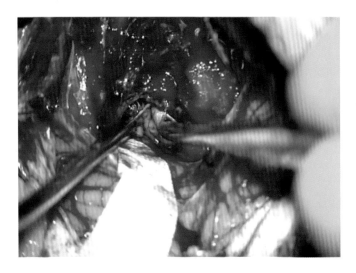
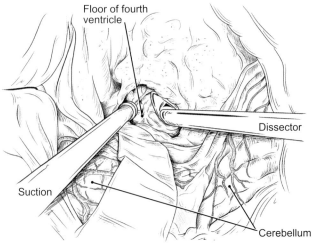

Figure 5.39. (f) The portion of the tumor adherent to the floor of the fourth ventricle is dissected with minimal manipulation of the brainstem.

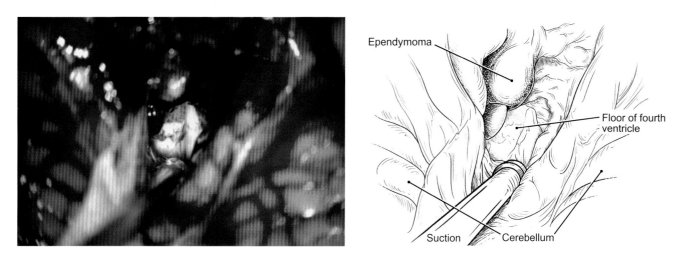

Figure 5.39. (g) Mobilization of the tumor facilitates visualization of the normal floor of the fourth ventricle.

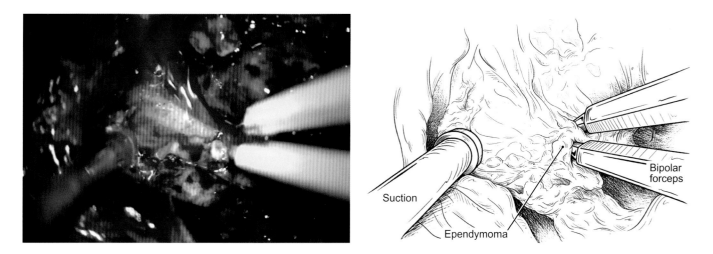

Figure 5.39. (h) After the planes between the tumor and the brainstem are defined, the tumor is internally debulked and resected.

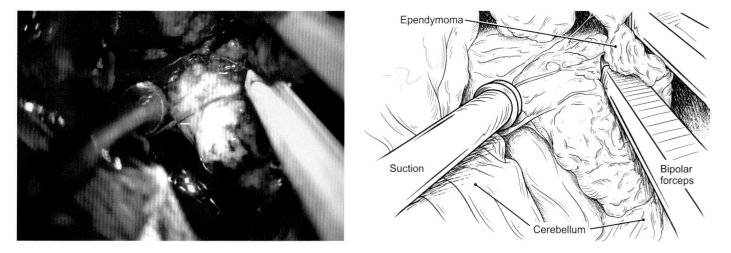

Figure 5.39. (i) The tumor is removed piecemeal using bipolar cautery and suction or an ultrasonic aspirator, depending on the consistency of the tumor.

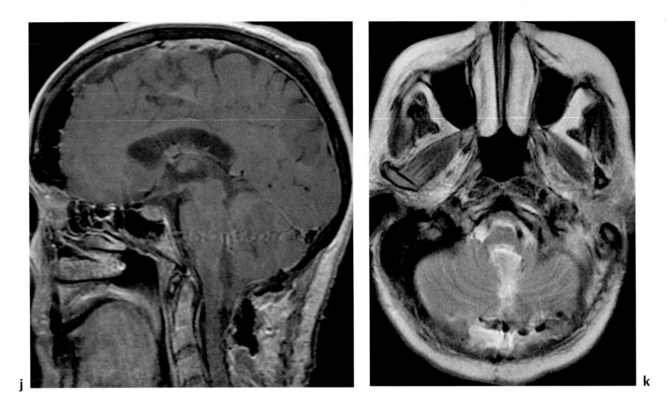

j   k

Figure 5.39. Postoperative **(j)** sagittal T1-weighted and **(k)** axial T2-weighted magnetic resonance images demonstrate complete removal of the lesion.

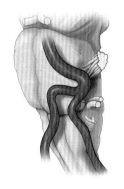

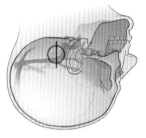

Case 5.40

- Diagnosis: Severe left V1–V2 distribution trigeminal neuralgia and refractory hypertension (related anatomy: pp. **51, 56, 62**)

- Preoperative examination: Neurologically intact

- Approach: Left retrosigmoid (related approach: pp. **212–222**)

- Positioning: Supine

- Monitoring: Somatosensory evoked potentials; trigeminal (CN V), abducens (CN VI), facial (CN VII), vestibulocochlear (CN VIII), glossopharyngeal (CN IX), vagus (CN X), accessory (CN XI), and hypoglossal (CN XII) nerves

- Outcome: Neurologically intact; V1-V2 distribution pain completely resolved; patient was weaned from one antihypertensive and is maintained on a single antihypertensive.

See Video 5.40

Figure 5.40. A 25-year-old man presented with severe left V1-V2 trigeminal neuralgia of 2 months' duration. His medical history was significant for a diagnosis of refractory essential hypertension at age 11 years. His medications included dexmedetomidine, fentanyl, ketamine, carbamazepine, hydromorphone, and lorazepam.

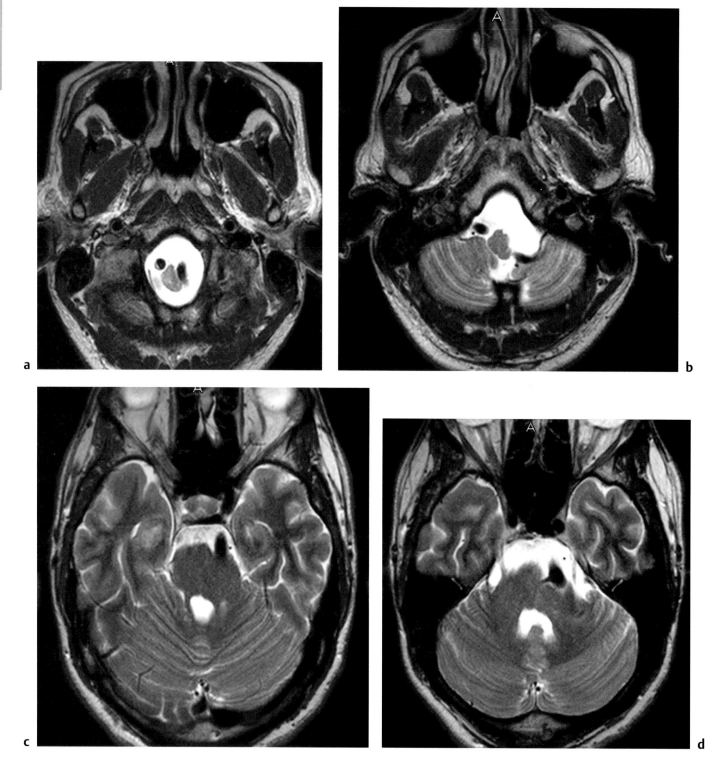

Figure 5.40. (a–d) Sequential caudal to rostral axial T2-weighted magnetic resonance images demonstrate compression of the cervicomedullary junction, the medulla, and the root entry zone of the trigeminal nerve (CN V) by a dolichoectatic vessel in the vertebrobasilar circulation in a 25-year-old man with a history of uncontrolled hypertension and severe left trigeminal neuralgia.

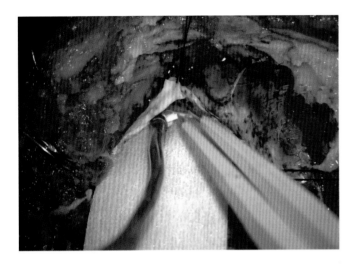

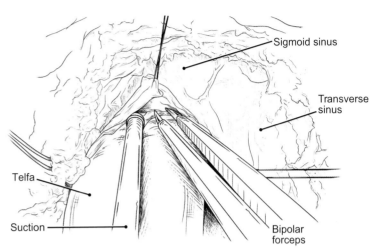

Figure 5.40. (e) Because of the complexity of this case and the need to visualize the lateral brainstem from the trigeminal nerve down to the cervicomedullary junction, a larger than usual retrosigmoid craniotomy is used to gain access to the cerebellopontine angle cistern. For most cases of microvascular decompression, a small 1- to 2-cm craniotomy at the transverse-sigmoid sinus junction is adequate. In this case, a 4-cm craniotomy is performed and the entire transverse–sigmoid sinus complex is exposed.

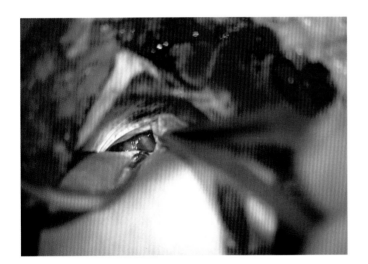

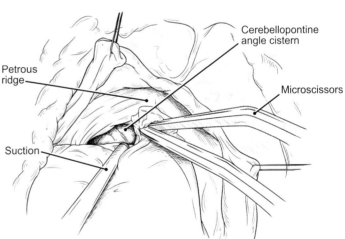

Figure 5.40. (f) After a Telfa strip is placed on the surface of the cerebellum, gentle dynamic retraction is used to gain access to and to fenestrate the arachnoid membrane over the cranial nerves to release cerebrospinal fluid and obtain cerebellar relaxation. It is important for the surgeon to be patient at this stage and to enable the release of cerebrospinal fluid to relax the contents of the posterior fossa. The cerebellum can easily be injured with aggressive retraction or the overzealous use of fixed retractors.

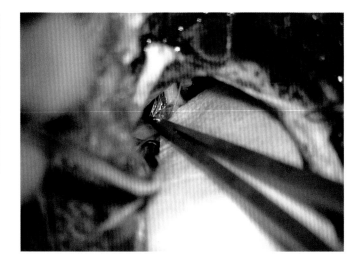

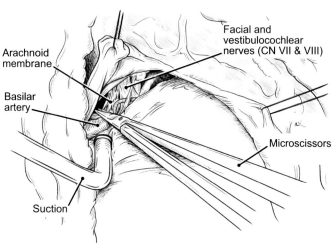

Figure 5.40. (g) After brain relaxation has been achieved, the surgeon begins by opening the arachnoid membrane over the facial nerve (CN VII) and the vestibulocochlear nerve (CN VIII) to expose them and their relationship to the basilar artery. For this case, the arachnoid membrane is exposed over the trigeminal nerve (CN V), abducens nerve (CN VI), facial nerve, vestibulocochlear nerve, and lower cranial nerves (glossopharyngeal [CN IX], vagus [CN X], accessory [CN XI], and hypoglossal [CN XII] nerves). In general, for simple cases of microvascular decompression, the surgeon should open the arachnoid membrane only over the cranial nerve or the nerves to be decompressed, as retaining the arachnoid membrane protects the other cranial nerves in the surgical field.

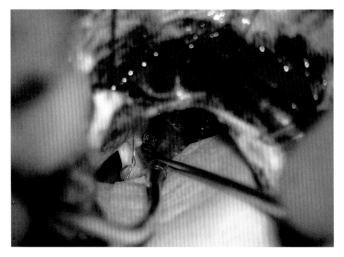

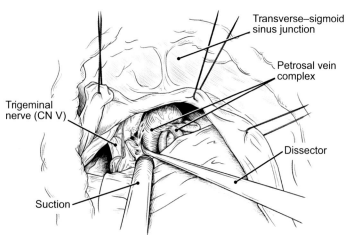

Figure 5.40. (h) In this patient, the trigeminal nerve and its root entry zone are exposed first. A large petrosal vein complex is visible. In most cases, this venous complex can be kept intact and simply mobilized. If necessary, this complex can be pruned to gain access to the trigeminal nerve.

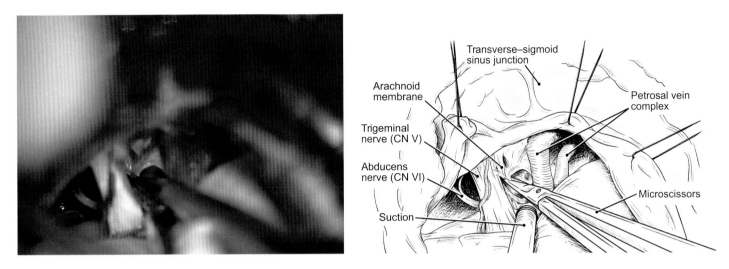

Figure 5.40. (i) Sharp dissection of the arachnoid membrane on both sides of the petrosal vein complex facilitates visualization of the basilar artery where its redundant portions course and make contact with the brainstem and the trigeminal nerve.

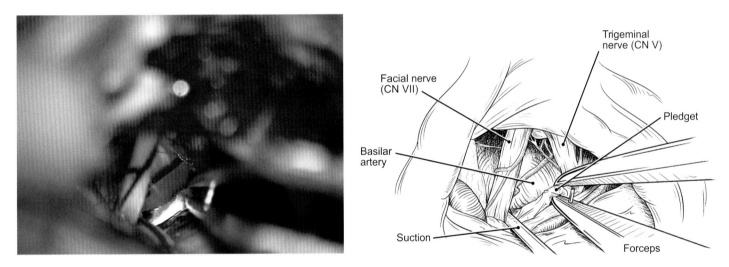

Figure 5.40. (j) After the basilar artery is mobilized from the root entry zone of the trigeminal nerve, it is buttressed away from these structures by placing Teflon pledgets between the basilar artery and the brainstem and trigeminal nerve.

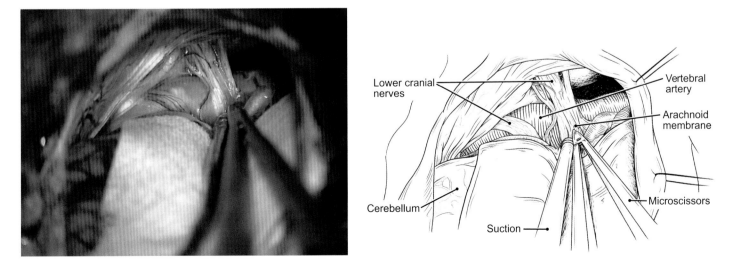

Figure 5.40. (k) Attention is turned to decompressing the cervicomedullary junction. The arachnoid membrane over the lower cranial nerves is dissected to gain access to the vertebrobasilar junction. Note that a redundant loop of the vertebral artery has stretched the lower cranial nerves.

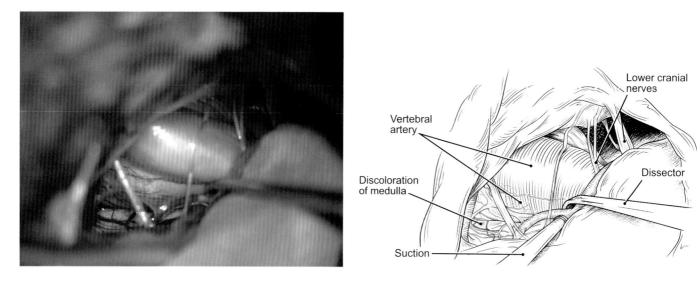

Figure 5.40. (l) The dolichoectatic nature of the vertebrobasilar system is evident. A large loop of the vertebral artery is mobilized from the cervicomedullary junction. After the vessel is mobilized, evidence of compression and discoloration of the brainstem are evident.

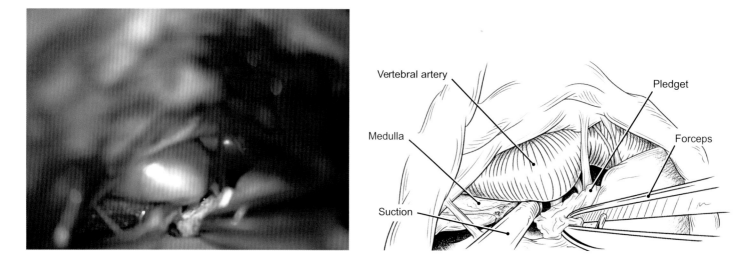

Figure 5.40. (m) Teflon pledgets are used to separate the vertebral artery from the cervicomedullary junction.

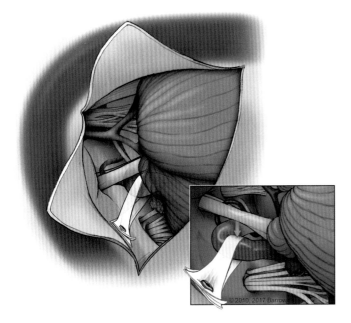

Figure 5.40. (n) Artist's illustration shows an alternative to pledgets: a sling made of synthetic material is used to mobilize the vessel (*arrow*) from the brainstem, and a screw secures the sling against the petrous bone. In this case, the significant dolichoectasia of the vertebrobasilar system precluded the use of a sling because so little room was available in the posterior fossa.

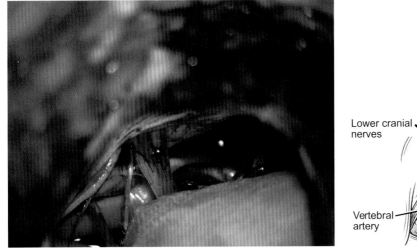
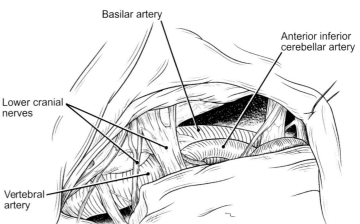

Figure 5.40. (o) Decompression of the cervicomedullary junction and mobilization of the vertebral artery alleviates the tension on the lower cranial nerves.

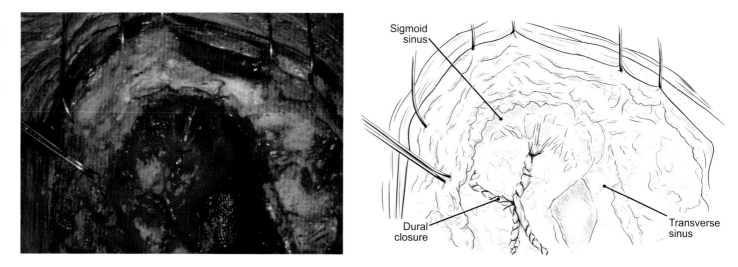

Figure 5.40. (p) Watertight closure of the dura and the application of wax to the air cells in the temporal bone are critical to avoid postoperative cerebrospinal fluid leaks.

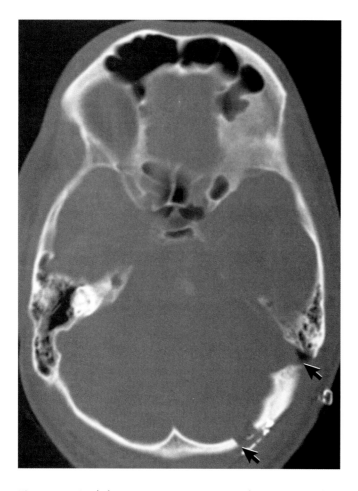

Figure 5.40. (q) Postoperative computed tomogram demonstrates the extent of the craniotomy (*arrows*).

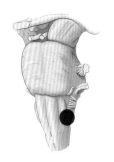

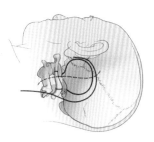

Case 5.41

- Diagnosis: Complex, previously coiled, left posterior inferior cerebellar artery calcified aneurysm (related anatomy: pp. **71, 73**)

- Preoperative examination: Left facial spasm, decreased sensation on left

- Approach: Left far-lateral (related approach: pp. **223–235**)

- Positioning: Supine

- Monitoring: Somatosensory evoked potentials and motor evoked potentials; glossopharyngeal (CN IX), vagus (CN X), accessory (CN XI), and hypoglossal (CN XII) nerves

- Outcome: Complete occlusion of the aneurysm; patent bypass; patient is neurologically intact.

See Video 5.41

Figure 5.41. A 60-year-old woman presented with left facial spasm and upper-extremity paresthesias. Her medical history was significant for a right middle cerebral artery aneurysm treated 20 years earlier, a left internal carotid artery aneurysm stented 1 year earlier, and a left posterior inferior cerebellar artery aneurysm coiled 1 year earlier.

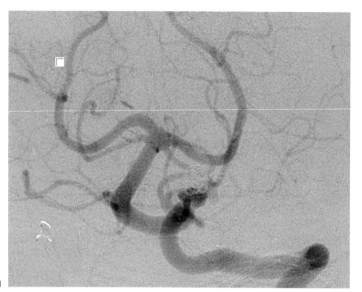

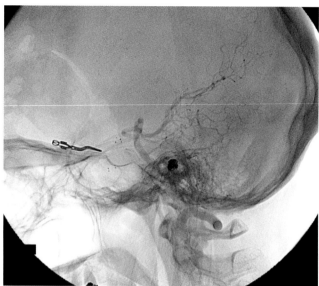

a

b

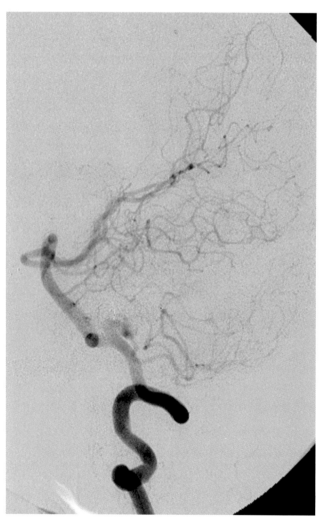

c

Figure 5.41. **(a)** Transfacial, **(b)** lateral unsubtracted, and **(c)** lateral left vertebral artery angiograms demonstrate a recurrent posterior inferior cerebellar artery aneurysm with a coil mass in a 60-year-old woman. Twenty years earlier, she had undergone clipping of a right middle cerebral artery aneurysm after a subarachnoid hemorrhage. One year earlier, she had undergone stenting of a left internal carotid artery aneurysm and coiling of a left posterior inferior cerebellar artery aneurysm. At the time of this presentation, she exhibited left facial spasm and upper-extremity paresthesias from a recurrent posterior inferior cerebellar artery aneurysm.

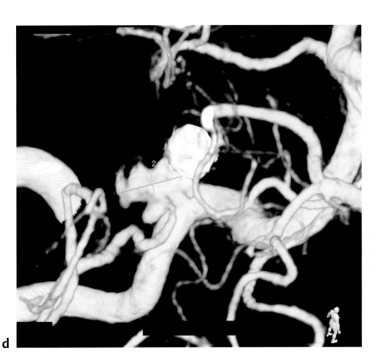
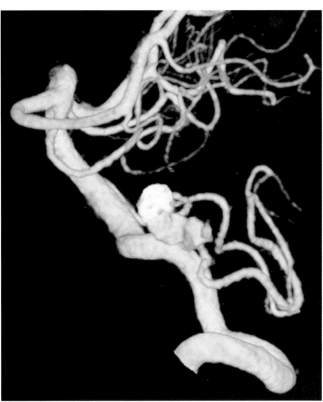

d

e

Figure 5.41. (d,e) Three-dimensional reconstructions of spin angiography show the coil mass and the left posterior inferior cerebellar artery emerging from the base of the heavily calcified aneurysm.

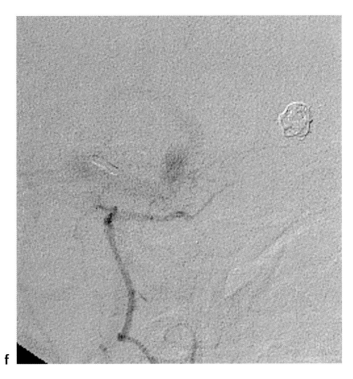
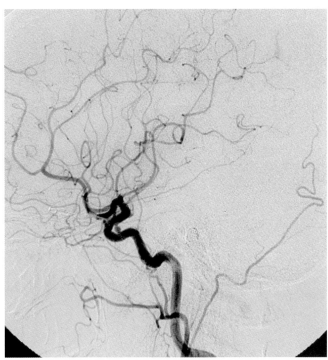

f

g

Figure 5.41. (f) Right lateral vertebral artery angiogram demonstrates that the right vertebral artery is vestigial and terminates in a posterior inferior cerebellar artery. **(g)** Left lateral common carotid artery angiogram performed during an Allcock test shows no posterior communicating artery.

The right injection also fails to demonstrate significant collaterals. Therefore, the left vertebral artery with the posterior inferior cerebellar artery aneurysm is the sole blood supply to the posterior fossa.

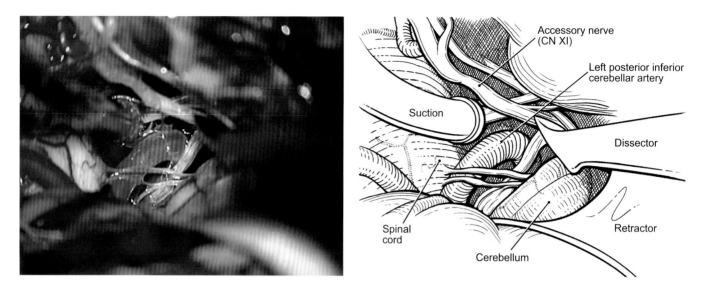

Figure 5.41. (h) The area of interest is accessed through a left far-lateral approach with the patient in the supine position. After the dura is opened, the left posterior inferior cerebellar artery is visible.

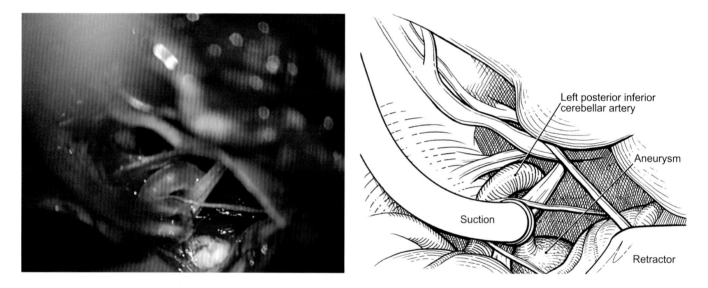

Figure 5.41. (i) After further dissection, the calcified aneurysm is visible.

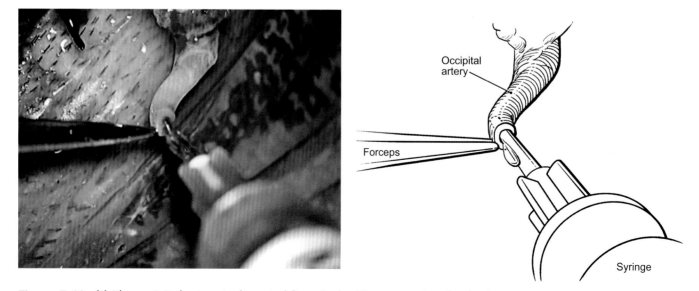

Figure 5.41. (j) The occipital artery is dissected from its bed in preparation for the bypass.

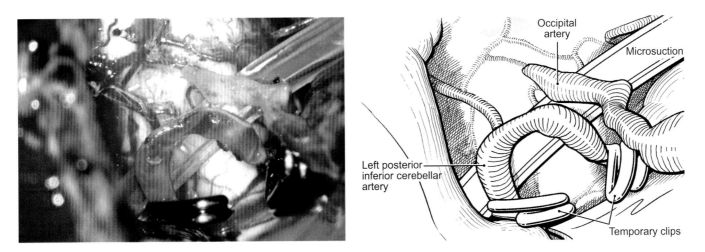

Figure 5.41. (k) Temporary clips are placed on the loop of the posterior inferior cerebellar artery distal to the aneurysm. A microsuction device is placed underneath the posterior inferior cerebellar artery, and the obliquely cut occipital artery is placed in the surgical field.

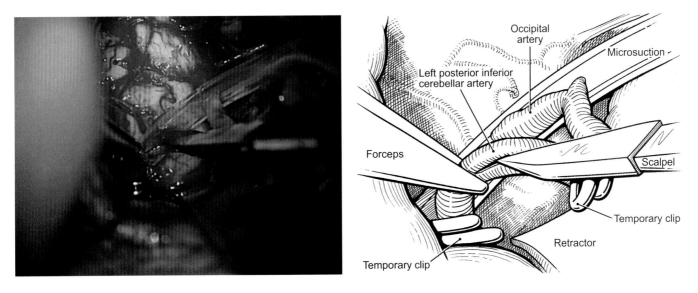

Figure 5.41. (l) An arteriotomy is made in the left posterior inferior cerebellar artery.

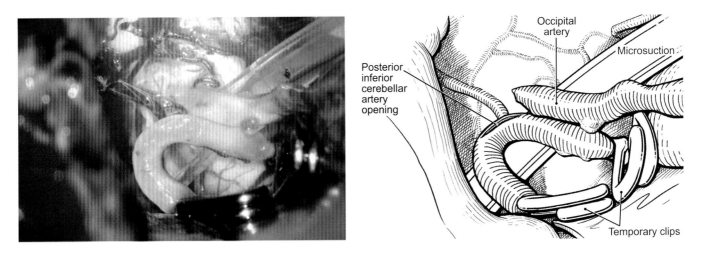

Figure 5.41. (m) The obliquely cut occipital artery is placed alongside the posterior inferior cerebellar artery in preparation for the bypass.

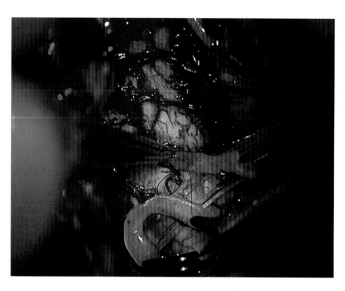 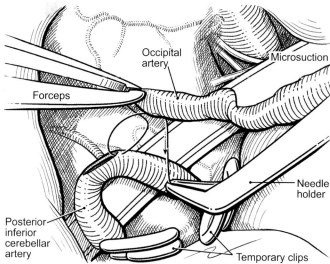

Figure 5.41. (n) A heel stitch is made in the occipital artery.

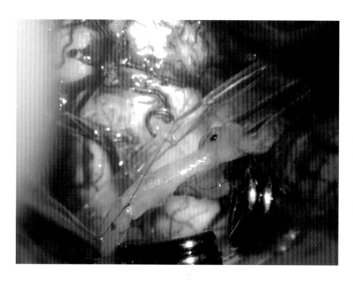 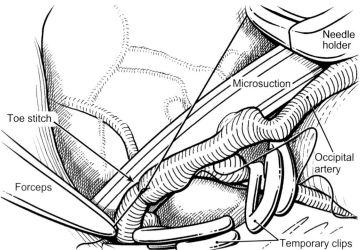

Figure 5.41. (o) A toe stitch is made.

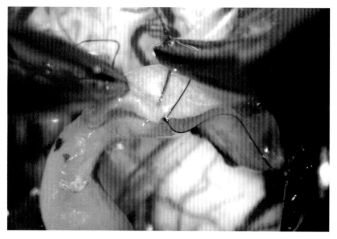 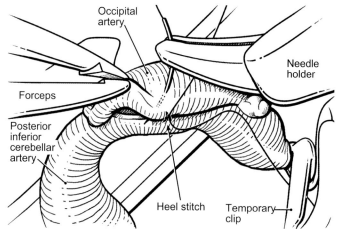

Figure 5.41. (p) A running stitch is made between the heel and the toe stitches.

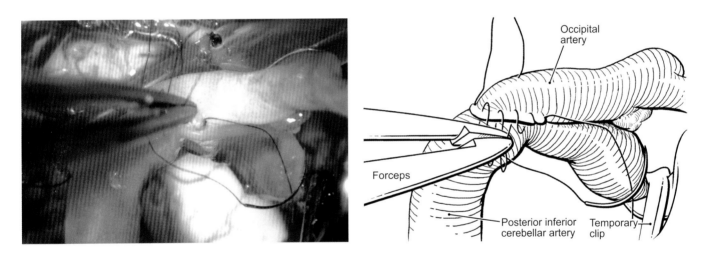

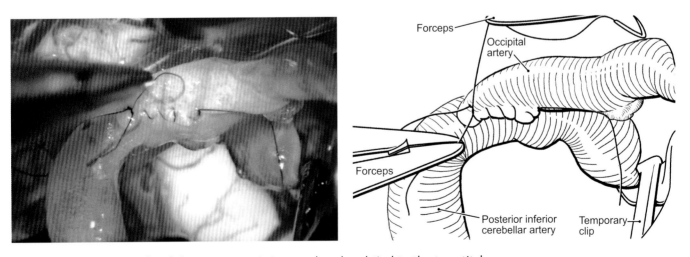

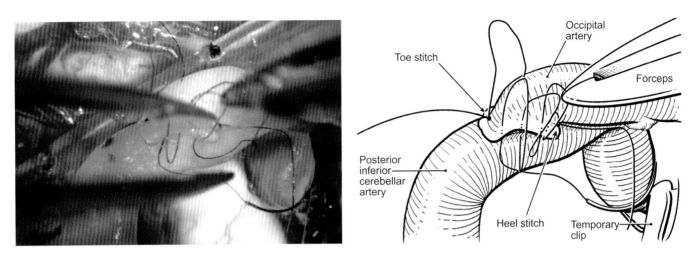

Figure 5.41. (q) The loops of the suture are sequentially tightened.

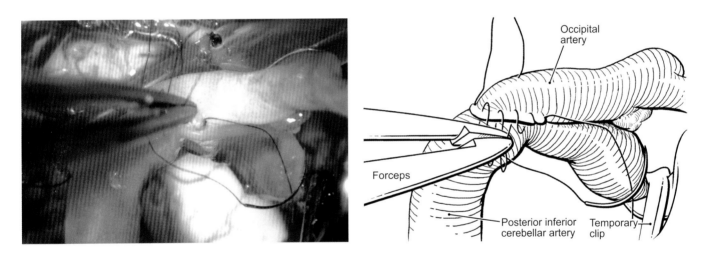

Figure 5.41. (r) The line of sutures is tightened.

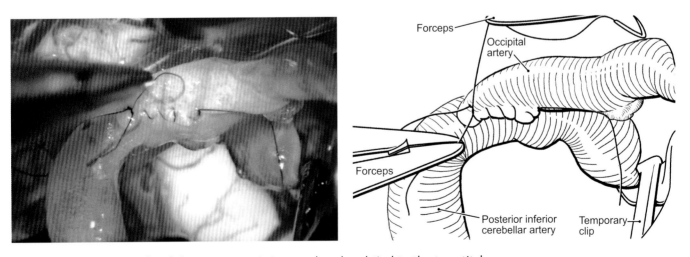

Figure 5.41. (s) One side of the anastomosis is completed and tied to the toe stitch.

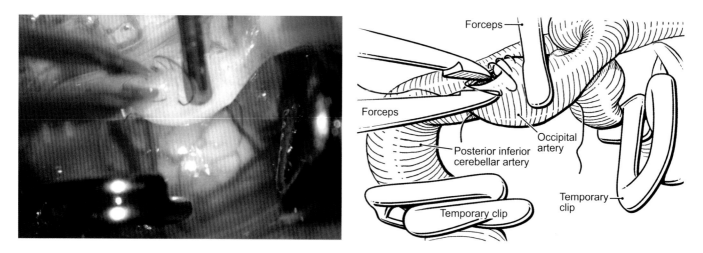

Figure 5.41. (t) The back wall of the anastomosis is stitched similarly.

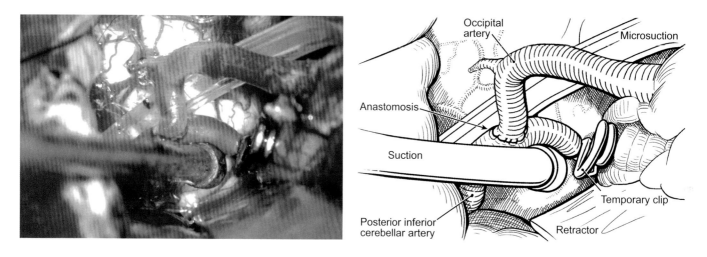

Figure 5.41. (u) The anastomosis is completed. Only one temporary clip remains in place.

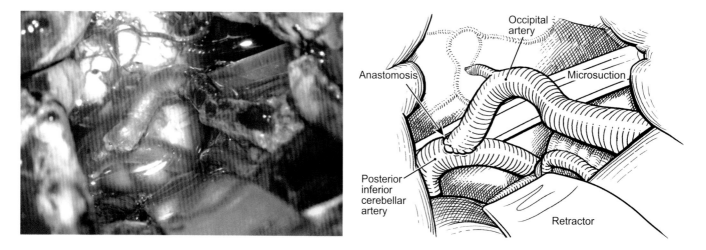

Figure 5.41. (v) The bypass is completed.

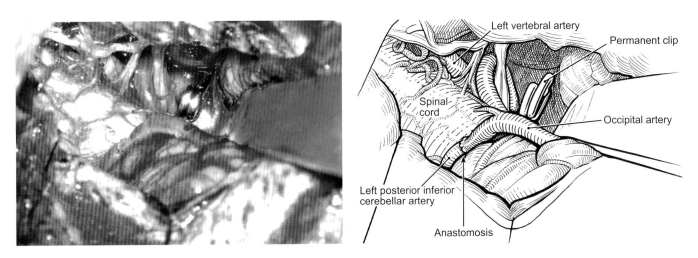

Figure 5.41. (w) A permanent clip is placed parallel to the vertebral artery to occlude the aneurysm and the origin of the posterior inferior cerebellar artery.

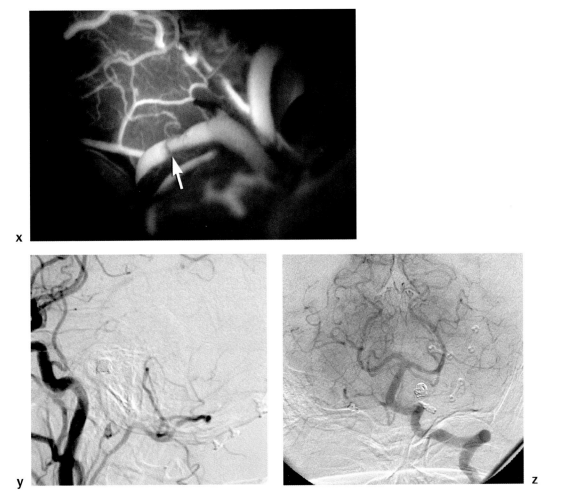

Figure 5.41. (x) Indocyanine green angiography shows good patency of the occipital artery bypass (*arrow*). **(y)** Lateral common carotid artery angiogram confirms patency of the occipital artery-to-posterior inferior cerebellar artery bypass. **(z)** Towne view vertebral artery angiogram confirms patency of the vertebral artery and exclusion of the posterior inferior cerebellar artery aneurysm.

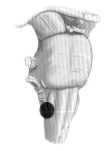

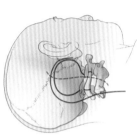

Case 5.42

- Diagnosis: Posterior inferior cerebellar artery aneurysm (related anatomy: pp. **71, 73**)
- Preoperative examination: Neurologically intact (within normal limits)
- Approach: Right far-lateral (related approach: pp. **223–235**)
- Positioning: Park bench
- Monitoring: Somatosensory evoked potentials and motor evoked potentials; glossopharyngeal (CN IX), vagus (CN X), accessory (CN XI), and hypoglossal (CN XII) nerves
- Outcome: Aneurysm is resected; bypass is patent; patient is neurologically intact.

See Video 5.42

Figure 5.42. A patient presented with headache and dizziness.

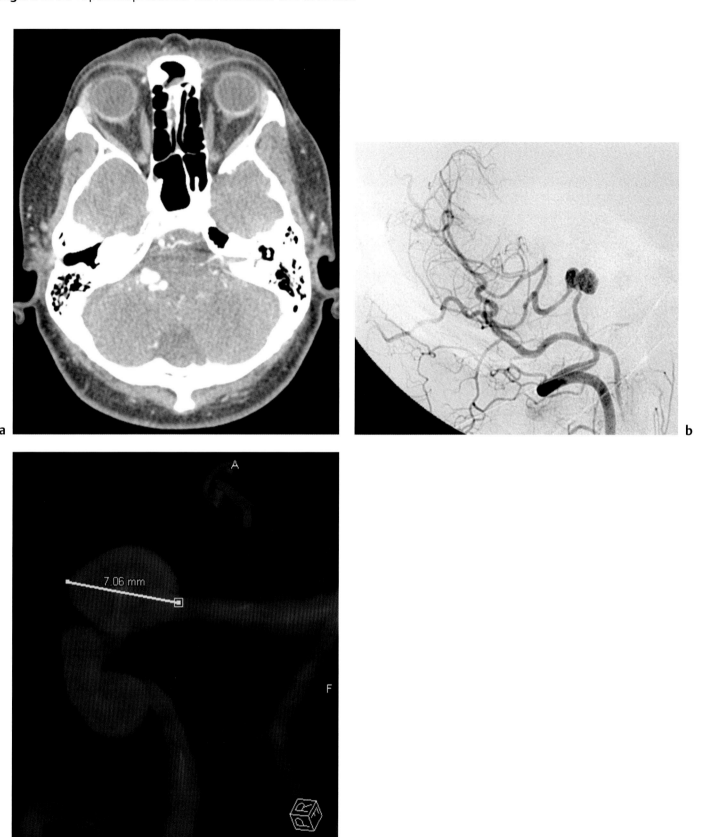

Figure 5.42. **(a)** Axial computed tomography angiogram shows a complex calcified aneurysm in the region of the right posterior inferior cerebellar artery in a patient who presented with headache and dizziness. **(b)** Lateral right vertebral artery angiogram shows the complex dissecting posterior inferior cerebellar artery aneurysm. **(c)** Three-dimensional angiographic reconstruction demonstrates the complex nature of the dissecting aneurysm.

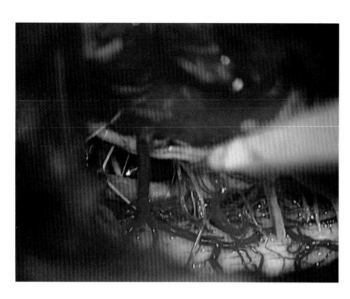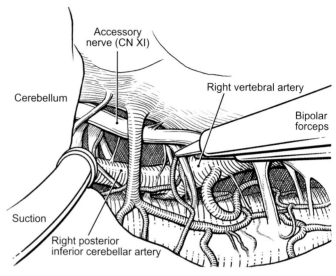

Figure 5.42. (d) The right vertebral artery and posterior inferior cerebellar artery are identified through a right far-lateral approach with the patient in the park bench position.

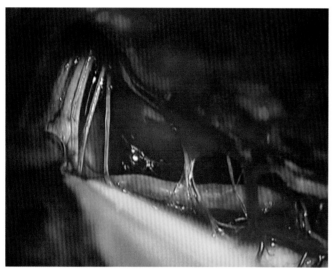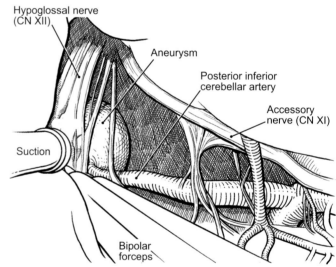

Figure 5.42. (e) The posterior inferior cerebellar artery is followed to the aneurysm.

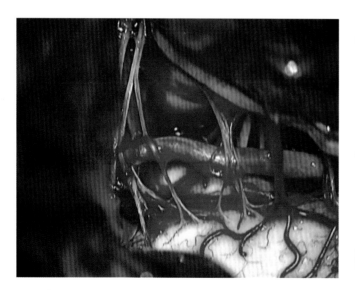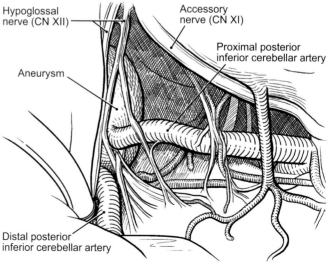

Figure 5.42. (f) The distal posterior inferior cerebellar artery is identified coursing between the rootlets of the hypoglossal nerve (CN XII).

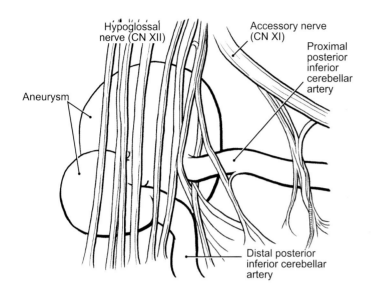

Figure 5.42. (g) The position of the complex aneurysm behind the rootlets of the hypoglossal nerve.

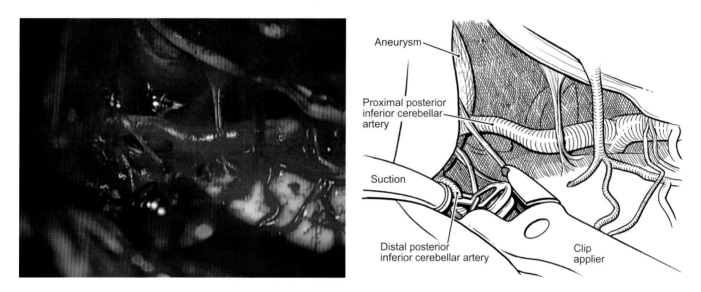

Figure 5.42. (h) A temporary clip is applied on the posterior inferior cerebellar artery outflow from the aneurysm.

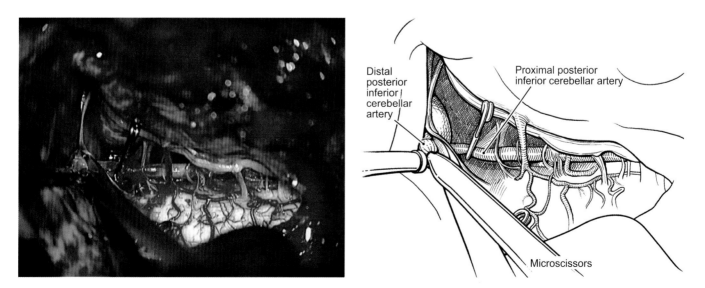

Figure 5.42. (i) After a temporary clip is placed proximal to the aneurysm, the posterior inferior cerebellar artery is cut distal to the aneurysm.

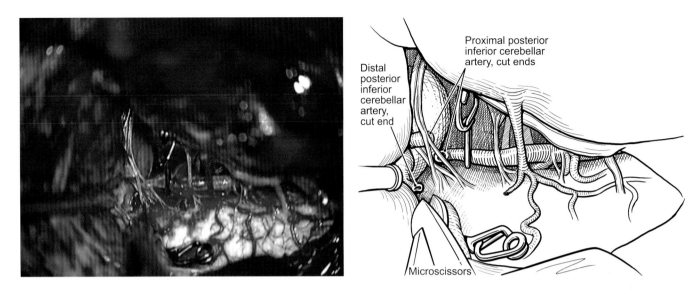

Figure 5.42. (j) The posterior inferior cerebellar artery is cut proximal to the aneurysm.

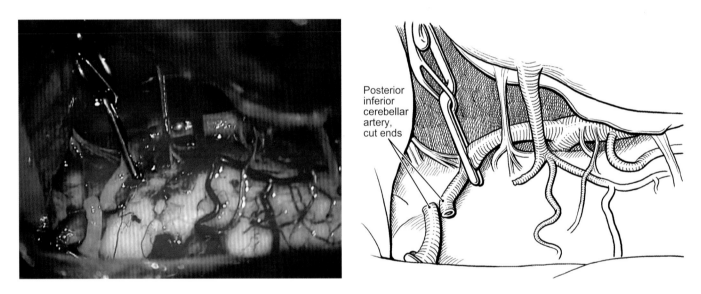

Figure 5.42. (k) The two cut ends of the posterior inferior cerebellar artery are approximated.

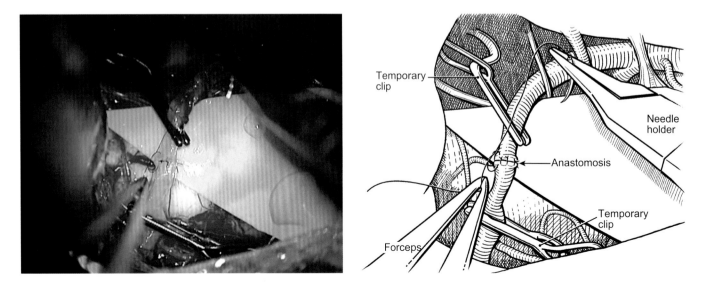

Figure 5.42. (l) The direct posterior inferior cerebellar artery-to-posterior inferior cerebellar artery reanastomosis is performed.

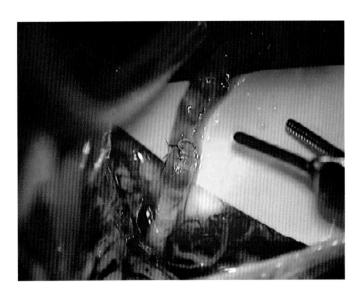
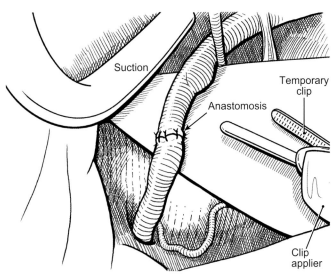

Figure 5.42. (m) The temporary clips are removed.

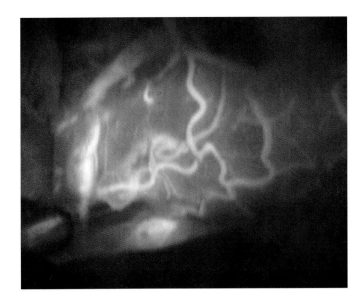

Figure 5.42. (n) Intraoperative indocyanine green angiography confirms patency of the posterior inferior cerebellar artery-to-posterior inferior cerebellar artery reanastomosis.

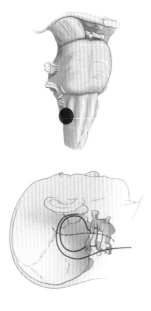

Case 5.43

- Diagnosis: Ruptured posterior inferior cerebellar artery aneurysm (related anatomy: pp. **71, 73**)

- Preoperative examination: Severe obtundation

- Approach: Right far-lateral (related approach: pp. **223–235**)

- Positioning: Park bench

- Monitoring: Somatosensory evoked potentials and motor evoked potentials; glossopharyngeal (CN IX), vagus (CN X), accessory (CN XI), and hypoglossal (CN XII) nerves

- Outcome: Aneurysm is resected; bypass is patent; patient is neurologically stable.

See Video 5.43

Figure 5.43. A 38-year-old woman presented with severe obtundation.

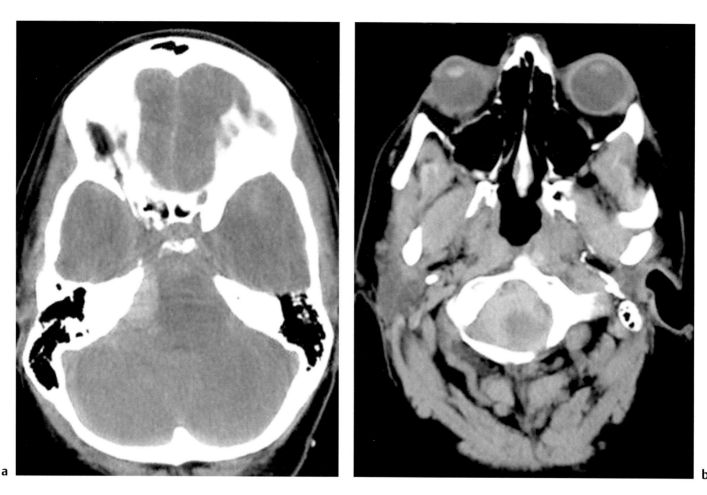

Figure 5.43. (a,b) Axial computed tomography images show diffuse subarachnoid hemorrhage in a 38-year-old woman with severe headaches and obtundation.

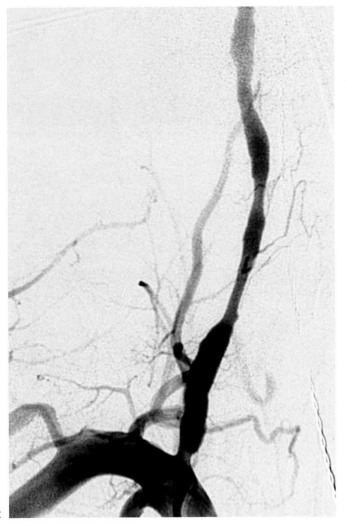

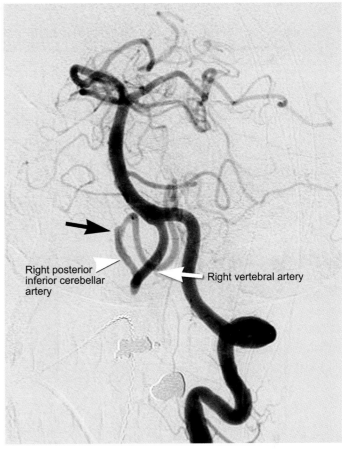

c

d

Figure 5.43. (c) Anteroposterior angiogram via a right subclavian injection shows significant right vertebral artery disease associated with dissection of the vertebral artery, which is occluded at the skull base. **(d)** Left vertebral artery angiogram demonstrates that the normal left vertebral artery feeds the right vertebral artery (*white arrow*) through retrograde flow to fill the right posterior inferior cerebellar artery (*white arrowhead*). The dissecting aneurysm (*black arrow*) is evident on the cranial loop of the distal right posterior inferior cerebellar artery.

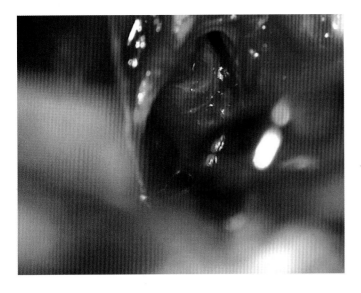

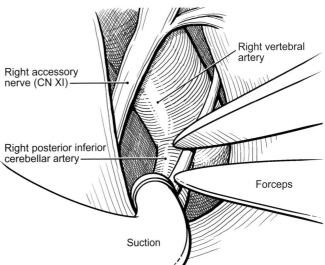

Figure 5.43. (e) Through a right far-lateral approach, the vertebral artery is identified.

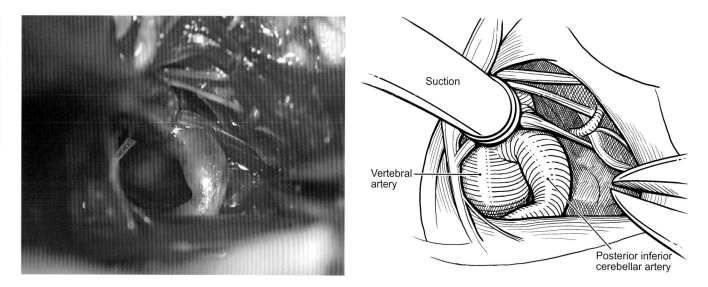

Figure 5.43. (f) The proximal portion of the posterior inferior cerebellar artery is exposed.

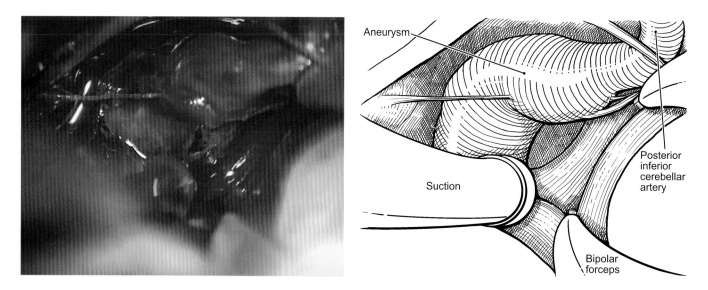

Figure 5.43. (g) The complex dissecting posterior inferior cerebellar artery aneurysm is identified.

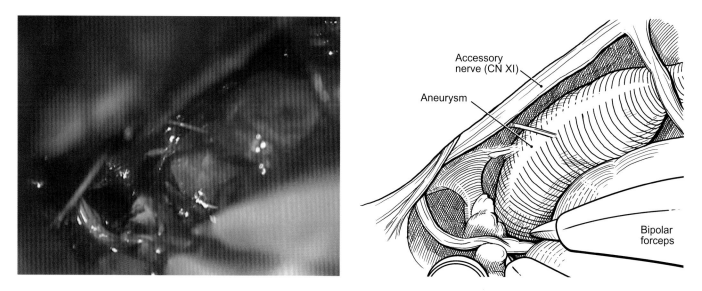

Figure 5.43. (h) The aneurysm is further exposed.

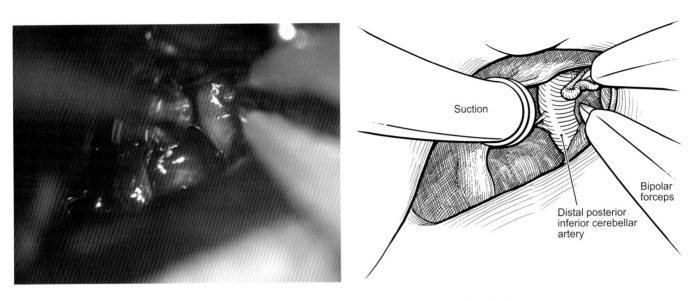

Figure 5.43. (i) The distal portion of the posterior inferior cerebellar artery is identified.

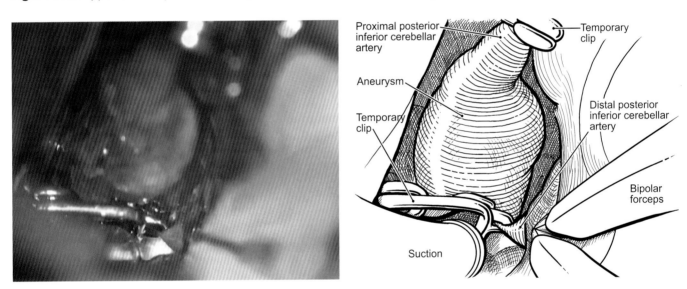

Figure 5.43. (j) Temporary clips are applied to the posterior inferior cerebellar artery proximally and to the aneurysm distally.

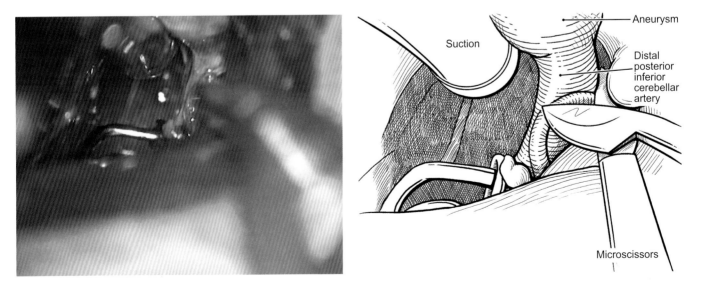

Figure 5.43. (k) The posterior inferior cerebellar artery is cut distal to the aneurysm.

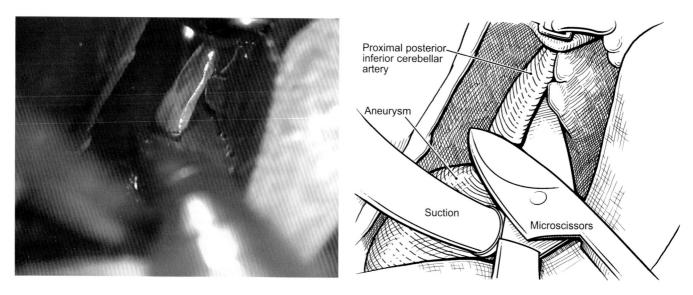

Figure 5.43. (l) The posterior inferior cerebellar artery is cut proximal to the aneurysm.

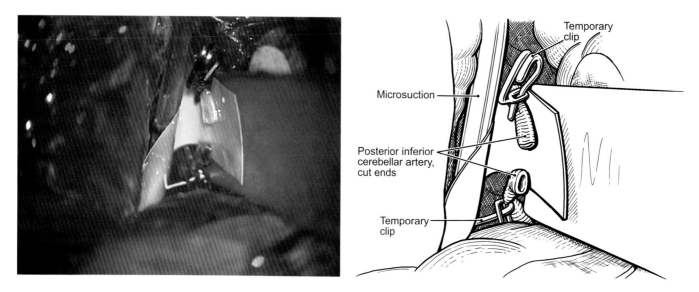

Figure 5.43. (m) The two cut ends of the posterior inferior cerebellar artery are prepared for a direct end-to-end anastomosis.

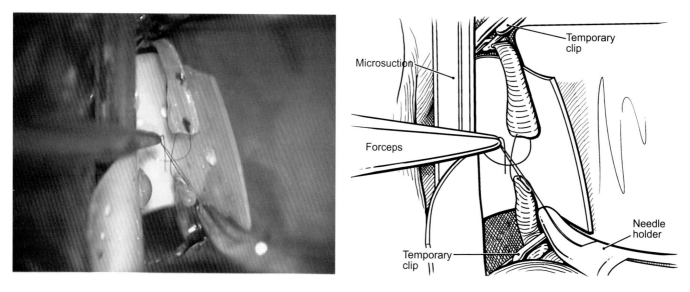

Figure 5.43. (n) The first stitch is placed.

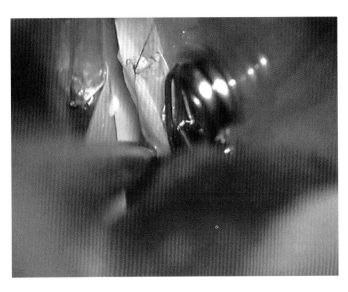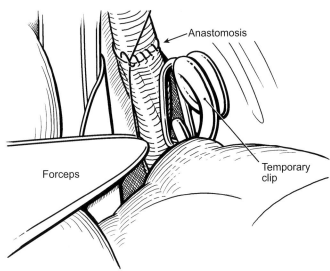

Figure 5.43. (o) The anastomosis is almost complete.

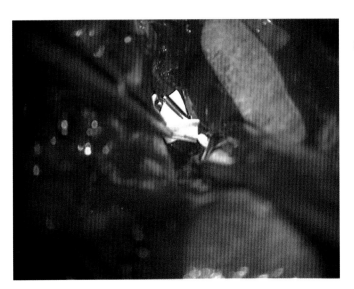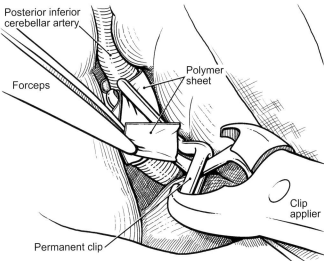

Figure 5.43. (p) Further dissection of the abnormal posterior inferior cerebellar artery is prevented by placing a polytetrafluoroethylene sheet around the anastomosis and securing it with a permanent clip.

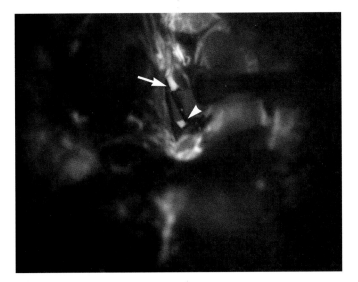

Figure 5.43. (q) Indocyanine green angiography shows the patency of the bypass proximal (*arrow*) and distal (*arrowhead*) to the wrapping.

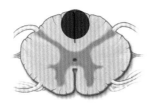

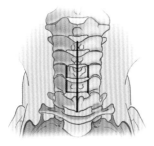

Case 5.44

- Diagnosis: C3-C4 cavernous malformation (related anatomy: pp. **32, 71, 73**)
- Preoperative examination: Neurologically intact
- Approach: Midline cervical laminectomy; via midline raphe (related approach: pp. **101, 102**)
- Positioning: Prone
- Monitoring: Somatosensory evoked potentials and motor evoked potentials
- Outcome: Complete removal of lesion; mild bilateral sensory loss; otherwise, patient is neurologically intact.

See Video 5.44

Figure 5.44. A 42-year-old man presented with a family history of cavernous malformations and fear of neurologic deterioration secondary to lesion hemorrhage.

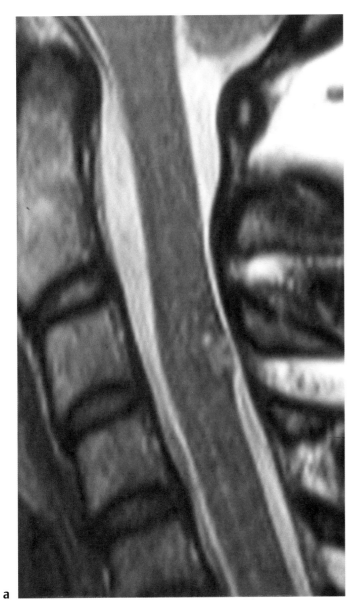

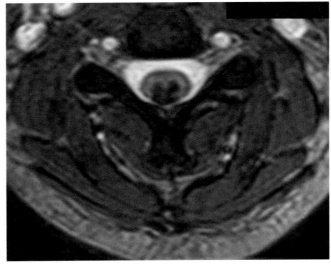

a   b

Figure 5.44. (a) Sagittal T2-weighted magnetic resonance image demonstrates a dorsal cavernous malformation at the level of C3. **(b)** Axial T2-weighted magnetic resonance image demonstrates that the lesion abuts the dorsal pial spinal cord and can be safely accessed using a posterior approach. In general, spinal cord lesions can be accessed using three well-tolerated safe entry zones. These include the midline cervical myelotomy, the dorsal root safe entry zone, and a safe entry zone located laterally between the nerve roots. Alternatively, lesions abutting a pial plane can be accessed directly through the lesion. This lesion is approached using a midline myelotomy. The patient is placed prone, and a midline laminectomy is performed at C3-C4. After subperiosteal dissection, the posterior elements can be visualized. The laminae are removed using a high-speed drill or ultrasonic bone curette. The dura is opened and tacked up with multiple stitches. The placement of the stitches enables the dura to be retracted, but also prevents soft tissue bleeding into the subarachnoid space. Placing a suction device lateral to the dura provides a clear surgical field throughout the case.

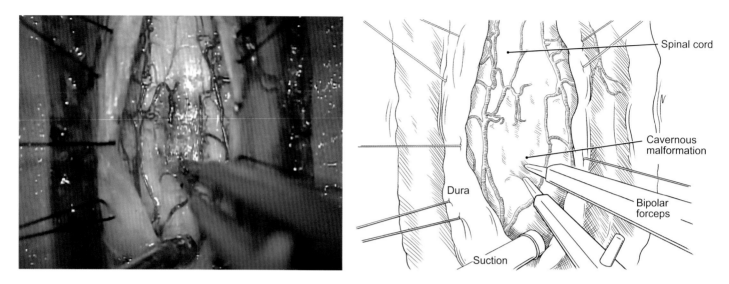

Figure 5.44. (c) The cavernous malformation is readily visible on the posterior spinal cord. The midline is devoid of vessels. This plane will be used for entering the spinal cord.

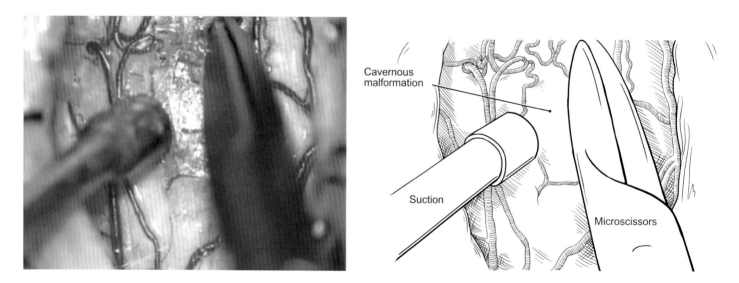

Figure 5.44. (d) The avascular plane is opened sharply using microscissors or a scalpel. In cases with a vein lying over the optimal site of entry, the vein may be dissected free from its pial connections and mobilized, thereby preserving normal spinal cord vasculature when possible. The myelotomy should be as long in the rostrocaudal direction as necessary to maximize exposure and minimize retraction on the spinal cord during resection.

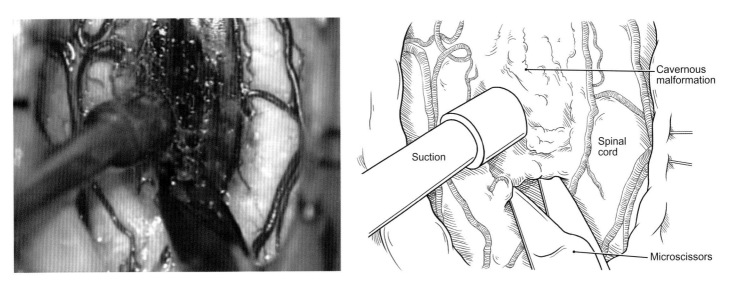

Figure 5.44. (e) Microscissors are used to mobilize the lesion and better define the plane between the cavernous malformation and the normal spinal cord. Suction can be used for countertraction in addition to helping obtain hemostasis.

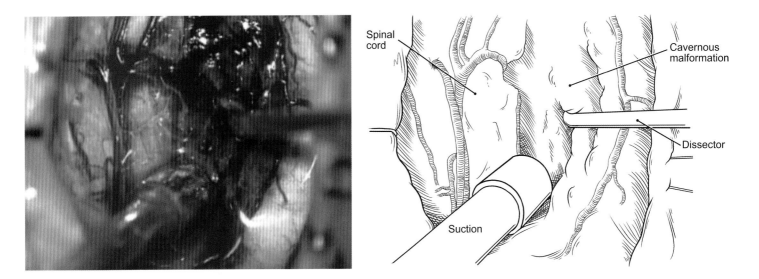

Figure 5.44. (f) The lesion is mobilized circumferentially. Suction provides countertraction while a microdissector is used to lift the lesion from the spinal cord.

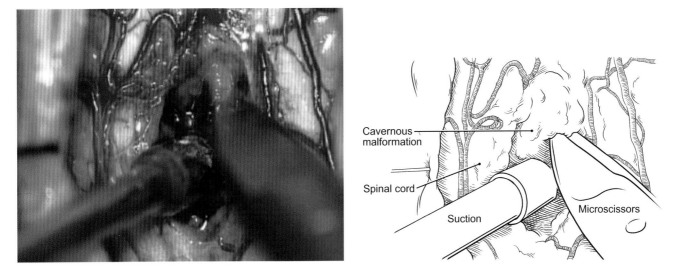

Figure 5.44. (g) Attachments between the cavernous malformation and the spinal cord are sharply resected in the deep plane.

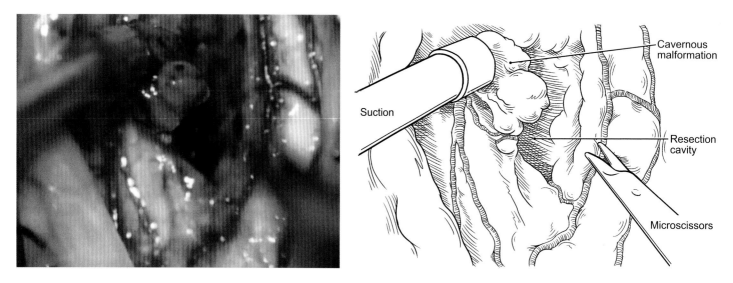

Figure 5.44. (h) The lesion is dissected free and removed from the cavity.

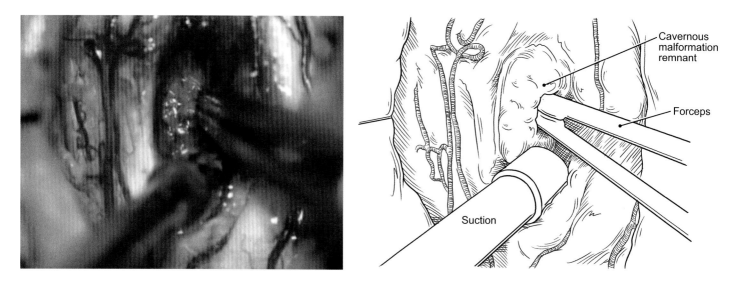

Figure 5.44. (i) Remnants of the cavernous malformation are removed using forceps and suction.

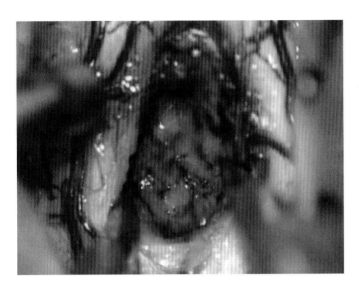

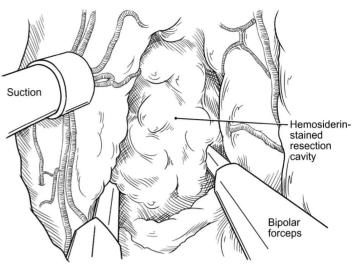

Figure 5.44. (j) The resection cavity is inspected, and bipolar cautery is set on a low setting to cauterize bleeding vessels. Use of bipolar cautery should be minimized to avoid injury to the spinal cord. After hemostasis is obtained, a final inspection of the resection cavity ensures that no remnant of cavernous malformation is left behind. Hemosiderin-stained tissue is a testament to previous episodes of hemorrhage. The dura should be closed in a watertight fashion, and the lamina should be replaced using plates and screws to minimize the likelihood of delayed kyphosis.

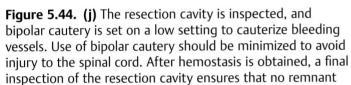

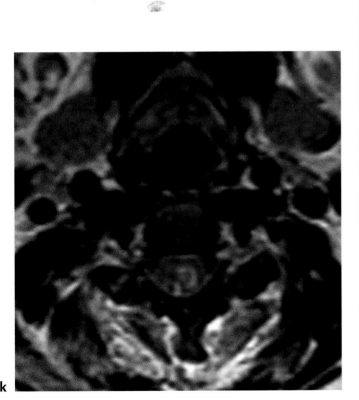

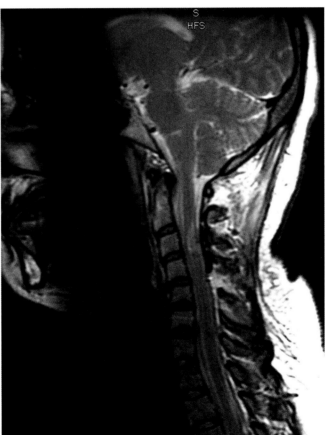

k

l

Figure 5.44. Postoperative **(k)** axial and **(l)** sagittal T2-weighted magnetic resonance images demonstrate complete resection of the lesion.

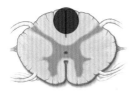

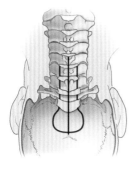

Case 5.45

- Diagnosis: C2-C3 cavernous malformation (related anatomy: pp. **32, 71, 73**)
- Preoperative examination: Quadriparesis and myelopathy
- Approach: Midline cervical laminectomy; via midline raphe (related approach: pp. **101, 102**)
- Positioning: Prone
- Monitoring: Somatosensory evoked potentials and motor evoked potentials
- Outcome: Complete removal of lesion; stable severe quadriparesis, not significantly worse than at preoperative examination

See Video 5.45

Figure 5.45. A 10-year-old boy presented with sudden-onset quadriparesis.

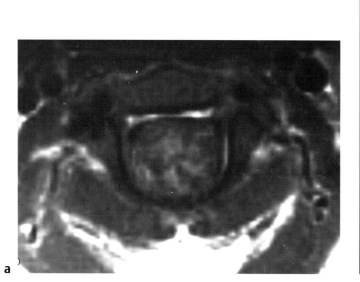

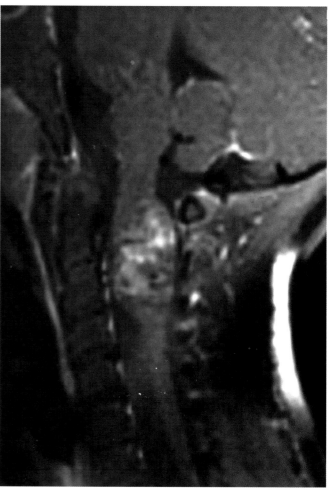

a　　　　　　　　　　　　　　　　　　　　　　　　　　　　　　　　　b

Figure 5.45. (a) Axial and **(b)** sagittal T1-weighted magnetic resonance images demonstrate a large cavernous malformation in the cervical spinal cord.

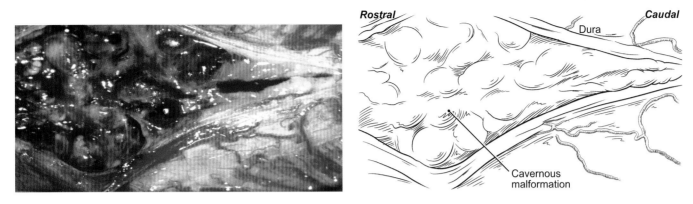

Figure 5.45. (c) The patient is placed prone and a midline incision is used to perform a laminectomy. The lesion is visualized through the layer of arachnoid membrane covering the spinal cord. A midline cervical myelotomy exposes the cavernous malformation.

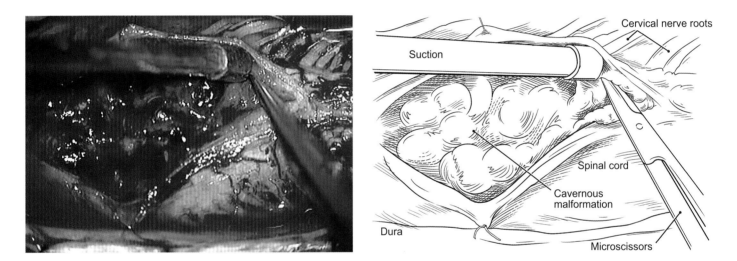

Figure 5.45. (d) A generous midline myelotomy minimizes retraction injury to the spinal cord. Microscissors are used to sharply resect the cavernous malformation from the adjacent spinal cord. The normal spinal cord is stained with hemosiderin, evidence of prior hemorrhages. Suction is used to perform dynamic retraction of the spinal cord during dissection.

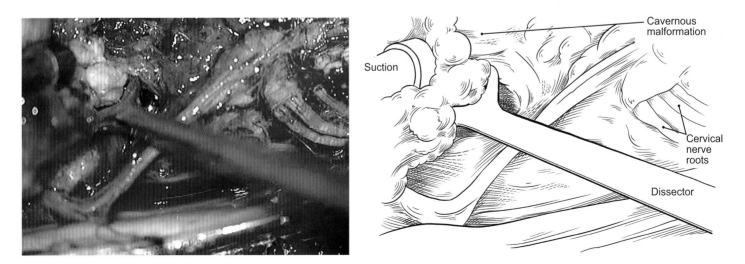

Figure 5.45. (e) A microdissector is used to mobilize the cavernous malformation and separate it from the spinal cord.

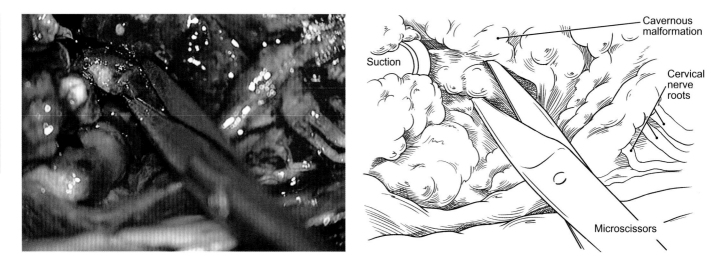

Figure 5.45. (f) After separation, sharp dissection disconnects the malformation from normal tissue.

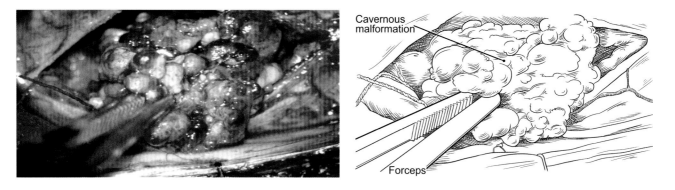

Figure 5.45. (g) The lesion is removed as one piece, but piecemeal resection is also possible with cavernous malformations or intrinsic spinal cord tumors.

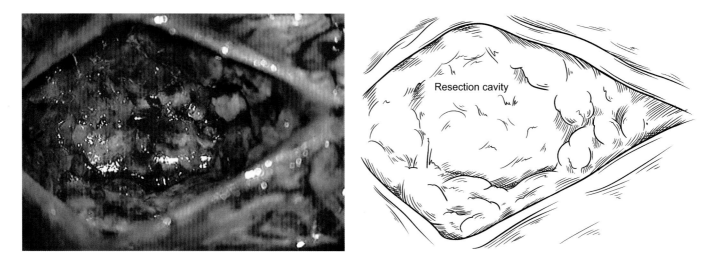

Figure 5.45. (h) Final inspection of the resection cavity ensures that remnants of the cavernous malformation are not left behind. Hemostasis can be obtained by using bipolar cautery on a low setting or by applying hemostatic agents directly to the site of bleeding.

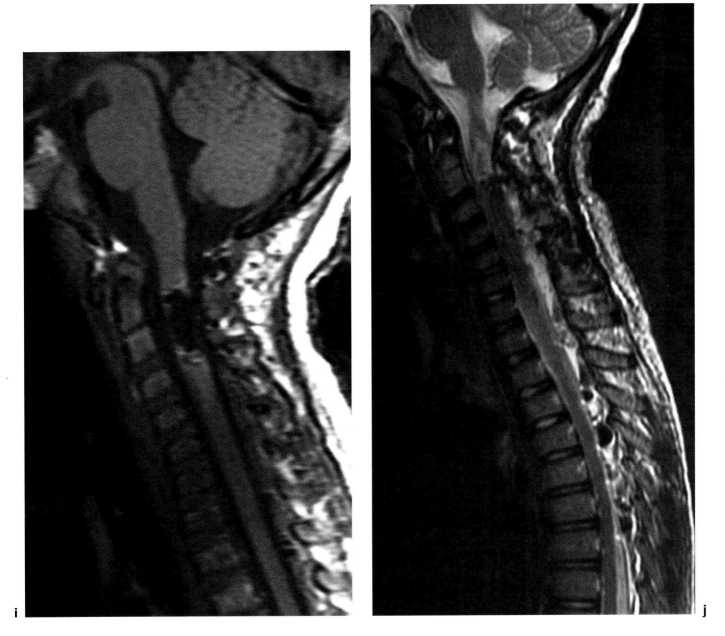

Figure 5.45. Postoperative **(i)** sagittal T1-weighted and **(j)** sagittal T2-weighted magnetic resonance images demonstrate complete resection of the lesion.

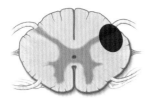

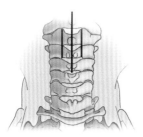

Case 5.46

- Diagnosis: Ventrolateral spinal cavernous malformation (related anatomy: pp. **32, 71, 73**)
- Preoperative examination: Neurologically intact
- Approach: Midline cervical laminectomy; via dorsal root safe entry zone (related approach: pp. **101, 102**)
- Positioning: Prone
- Monitoring: Somatosensory evoked potentials and motor evoked potentials
- Outcome: Complete removal of lesion; patient is neurologically stable.

See Video 5.46

Figure 5.46. A 59-year-old man presented with right arm and chest pain.

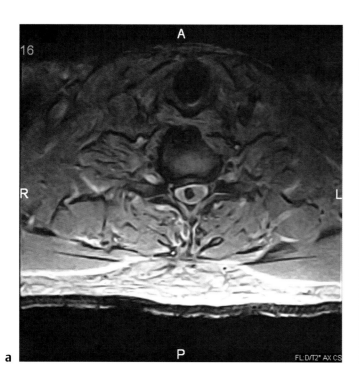

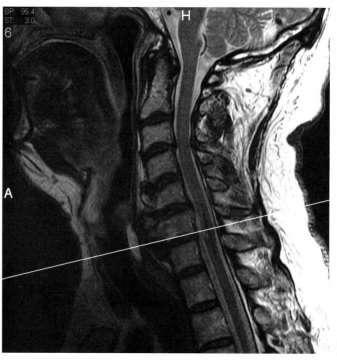

Figure 5.46. **(a)** Axial and **(b)** sagittal T2-weighted magnetic resonance images demonstrate a ventrolateral cavernous malformation at the level of C6-C7 with evidence of prior hemorrhage.

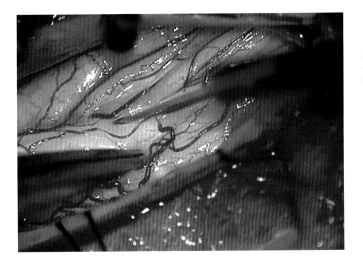

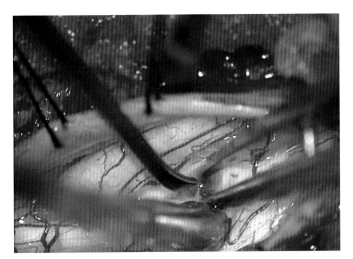

Figure 5.46. (c) The lesion is approached using a midline cervical laminectomy and opening of the spinal cord using the dorsal root safe entry zone (*dashed line*) with the patient prone. After the dura is opened and tacked up, the lateral surface of the spinal cord is visualized. Hemosiderin staining facilitates identification of the cavernous malformation. The dentate ligaments at the levels above and below the lesion, as well as at the level of the lesion, are cut to allow the spinal cord to be rotated to provide access to the ventral component of the lesion.

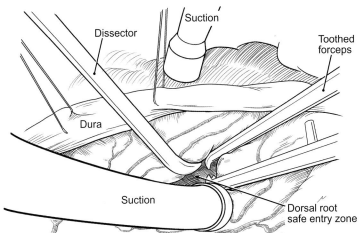

Figure 5.46. (d) After the dentate ligaments are cut, the spinal cord is rotated and the lesion is accessed. The spinal cord is opened at the dorsal root safe entry zone (*dashed line*), which is a safe entry zone for reaching dorsolateral parenchymal lesions in the spinal cord. The suction cannula and a microdissector provide countertraction, and the myelotomy is extended by using microforceps to expand the small opening.

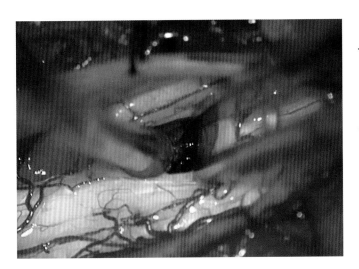

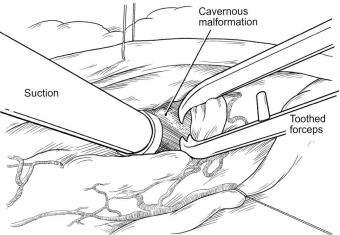

Figure 5.46. (e) The cavernous malformation is clearly visible in the resection cavity. It is debulked internally and removed piecemeal.

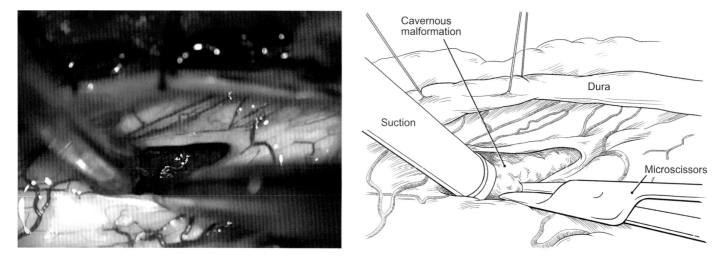

Figure 5.46. (f) Sharp dissection is used to mobilize the cavernous malformation from the spinal cord.

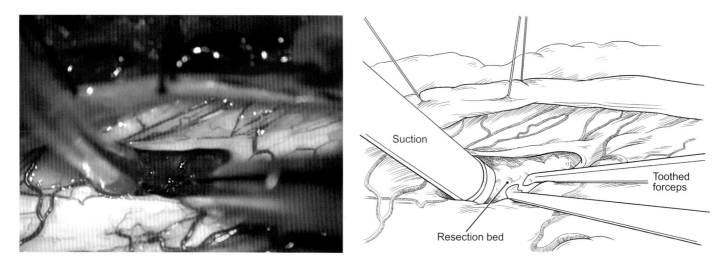

Figure 5.46. (g) The lesion is removed after being mobilized, the resection bed is inspected for any remnants of the cavernous malformation, and hemostasis is obtained. The dura is closed in a watertight fashion, and the laminae are replaced to prevent postoperative kyphosis.

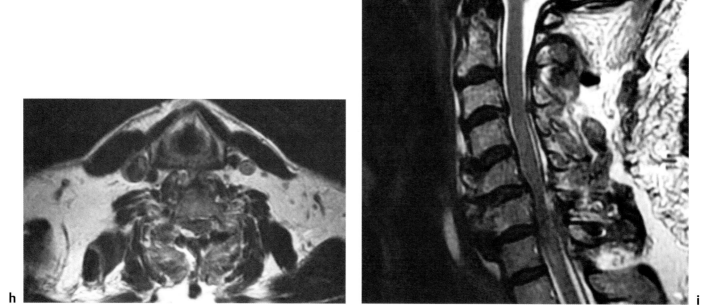

Figure 5.46. Postoperative **(h)** axial and **(i)** sagittal T2-weighted magnetic resonance images demonstrate complete resection of the lesion.

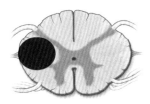

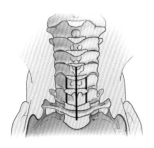

Case 5.47

- Diagnosis: Lateral ventral spinal cavernous malformation (related anatomy: pp. **32, 71, 73**)

- Preoperative examination: Right forearm and hand numbness

- Approach: Midline cervical laminectomy; lateral between dorsal and ventral nerve roots (related approach: pp. **101, 102**)

- Positioning: Prone

- Monitoring: Somatosensory evoked potentials and motor evoked potentials

- Outcome: Complete removal of lesion; patient is neurologically stable.

See Video 5.47

Figure 5.47. A 36-year-old man presented with intermittent numbness in right forearm and hand.

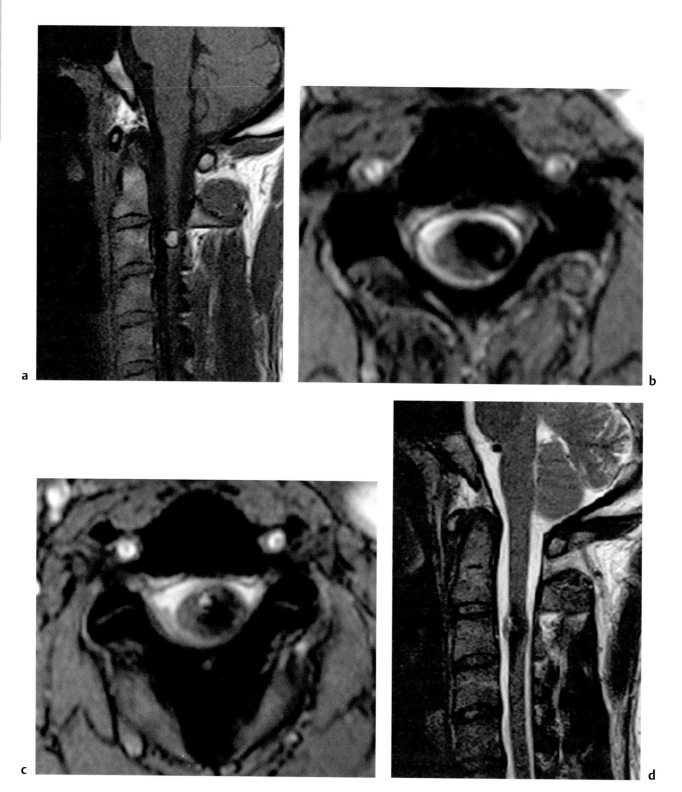

Figure 5.47. (a) Sagittal T1-weighted and **(b,c)** axial and **(d)** sagittal T2-weighted magnetic resonance images demonstrate a spinal cavernous malformation at the level of C3 with a significant ventral component.

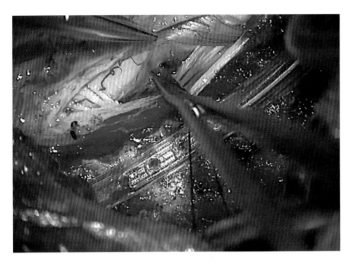
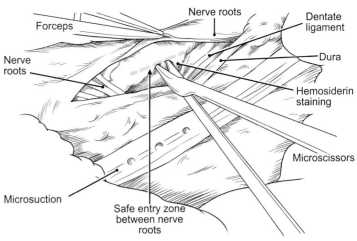

Figure 5.47. (e) This lesion is approached from a midline cervical laminectomy. Adequate visualization of the cavernous malformation is obtained by cutting the dentate ligaments (*white bands below microscissors*) at the level of the lesion, and at the levels above and below it, to mobilize the spinal cord and rotate it laterally so that the lesion can be approached using the safe entry zone between the nerve roots (*dashed line*). The area over the cavernous malformation has hemosiderin staining, proof of previous hemorrhages.

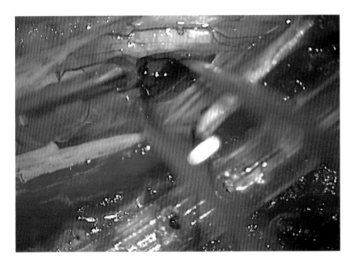
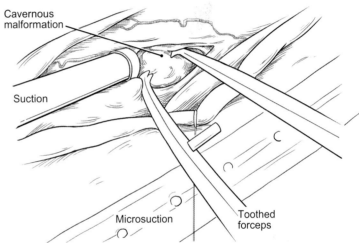

Figure 5.47. (f) A lateral myelotomy is made between the nerve roots, and forceps are used to expand the opening. The cavernous malformation is evident deep in the cavity. A suction cannula is placed in the lateral gutters and kept in position by the opened and tacked-up dura to provide a continuously clear surgical field.

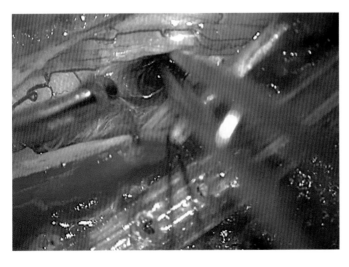
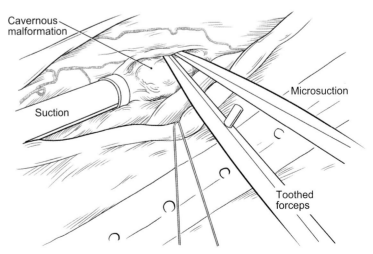

Figure 5.47. (g) The cavernous malformation is mobilized from the spinal cord using a combination of sharp dissection with microscissors and blunt dissection with microdissectors and toothed forceps.

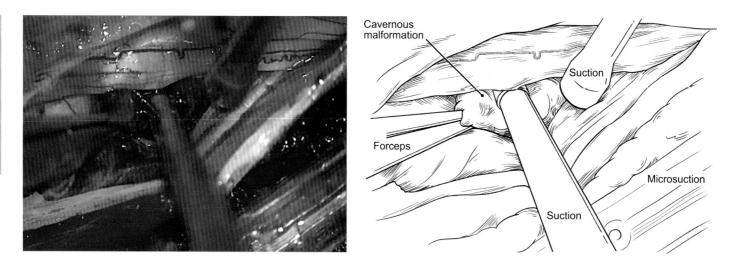

Figure 5.47. (h) Microforceps are used to remove the dissected portion of the cavernous malformation piecemeal.

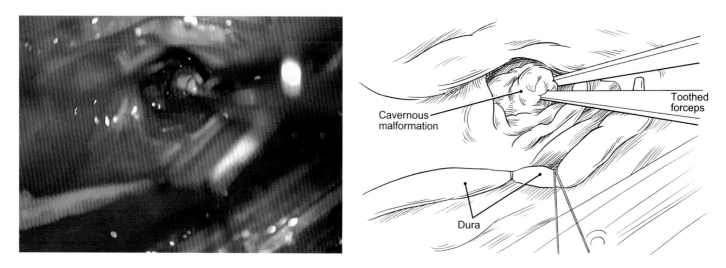

Figure 5.47. (i) The cavernous malformation is peeled from the normal spinal cord tissue.

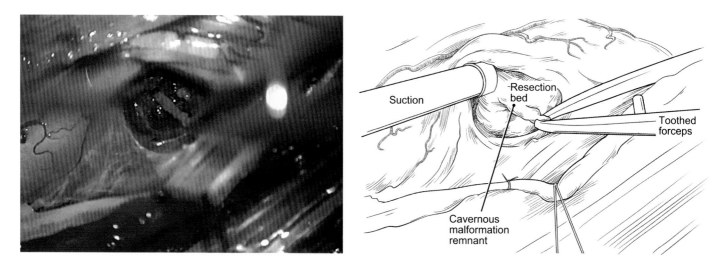

Figure 5.47. (j) After the cavernous malformation is removed, the resection bed is inspected. Any remnants of cavernous malformation that can be visualized are peeled from the cavity. These remnants often look like white flakes of tissue because venous blood has been evacuated from them, rendering them transparent. Final inspection and hemostasis are performed.

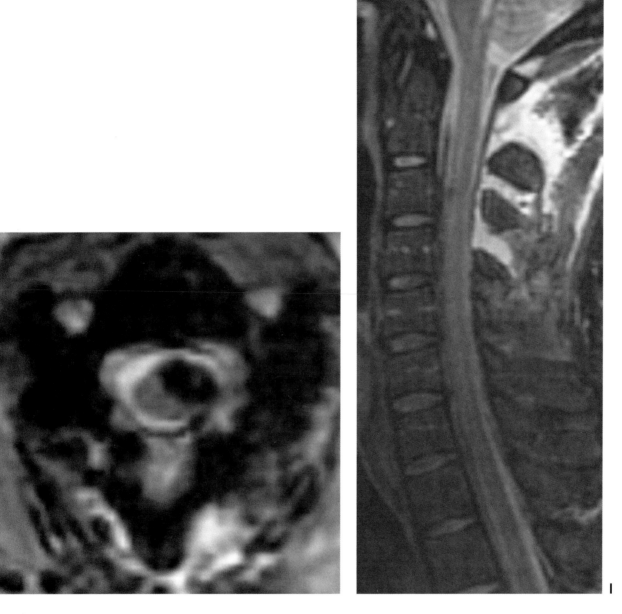

k   l

Figure 5.47. Postoperative **(k)** axial and **(l)** sagittal T2-weighted magnetic resonance images demonstrate gross-total resection of the lesion.

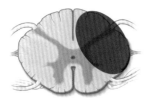

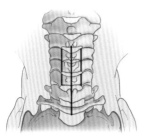

Case 5.48

- Diagnosis: Type II glomus-type spinal arteriovenous malformation (related anatomy: pp. **32, 71, 73**)

- Preoperative examination: Left hemiparesis

- Approach: Midline cervical laminectomy

- Positioning: Prone

- Monitoring: Somatosensory evoked potentials and motor evoked potentials

- Outcome: Complete removal of lesion; postoperative recovery over 1 year to neurologic baseline

See Video 5.48

Figure 5.48. A 51-year-old woman who was diagnosed at birth with cerebral palsy presented with new-onset urinary incontinence.

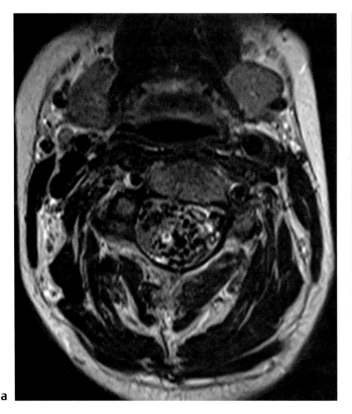

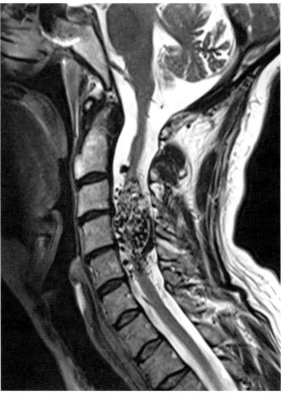

a   b

Figure 5.48. (a) Axial and **(b)** sagittal T2-weighted magnetic resonance images demonstrate flow voids at the level of C3-C5 consistent with a type II glomus-type spinal arteriovenous malformation.

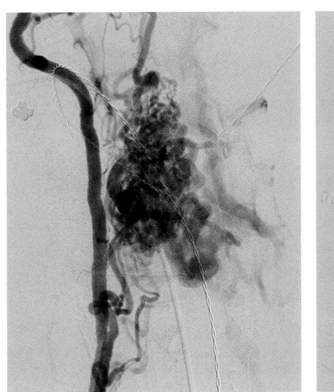
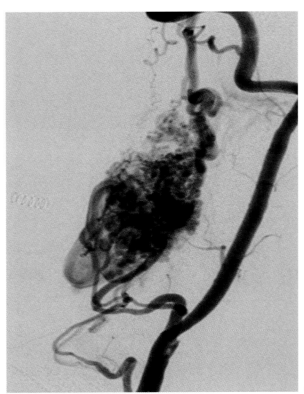

c   d

Figure 5.48. (c) Anteroposterior and **(d)** lateral angiograms of a right vertebral artery injection demonstrate the vascular blush of the arteriovenous malformation with contributions from the vertebral arteries.

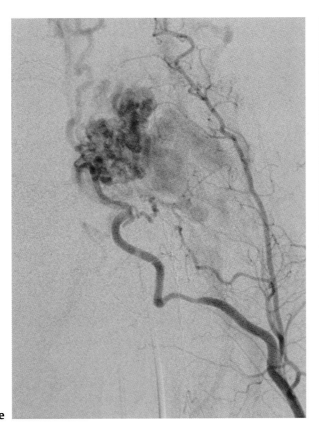
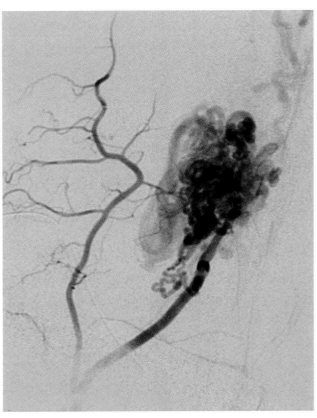

e   f

Figure 5.48. (e) Anteroposterior and **(f)** lateral angiograms of thyrocervical artery injections demonstrate further contribution to the spinal arteriovenous malformation from this vascular pedicle. The malformation is embolized in a multistage procedure using a combination of Onyx and n-butyl cyanoacrylate.

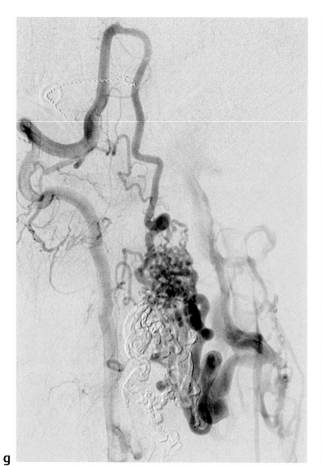
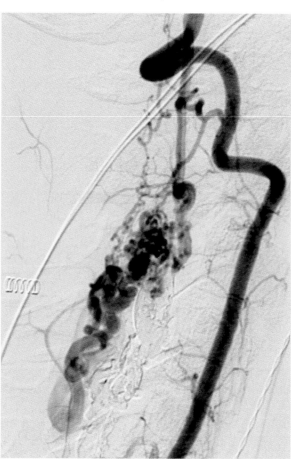

g

h

Figure 5.48. (g) Anteroposterior and **(h)** lateral angiograms of the right vertebral artery demonstrate diminished blood flow through the arteriovenous malformation after embolization of some of the vascular pedicles.

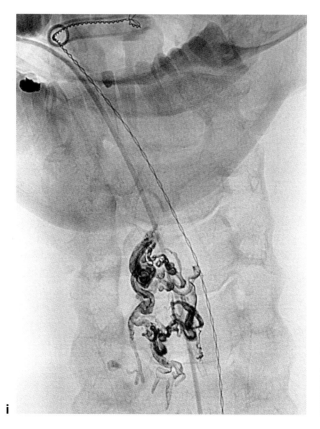
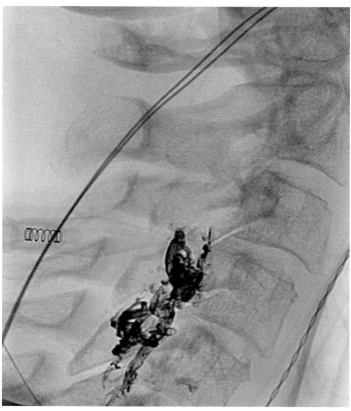

i

j

Figure 5.48. (i) Anteroposterior and **(j)** lateral unsubtracted images demonstrate the embolisate casts, which can be used during surgery to localize the lesion.

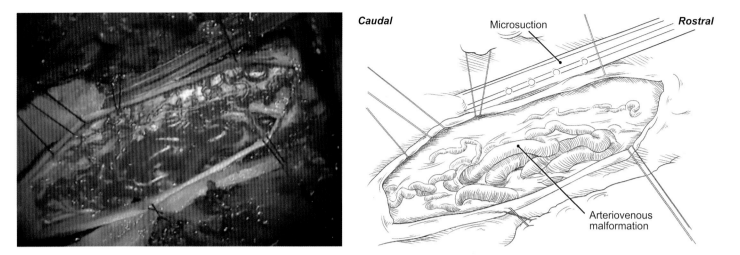

Caudal Microsuction Rostral

Arteriovenous malformation

Figure 5.48. (k) The arteriovenous malformation is approached using a midline cervical laminectomy (dorsal approach). After laminectomies are performed at C3-C5, the dura is opened and tacked up using sutures. Placement of a microsuction cannula in the lateral gutter enables continual clearing of blood from the surgical field.

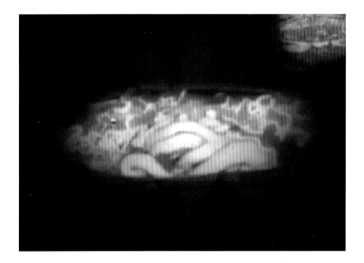

Figure 5.48. (l) Indocyanine green angiography is a useful intraoperative adjunct for defining the angioarchitecture of these arteriovenous malformations, especially when they are superficial.

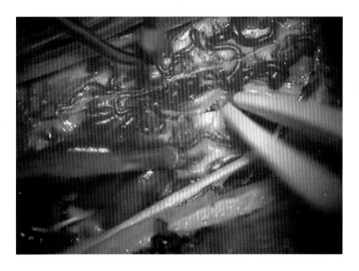

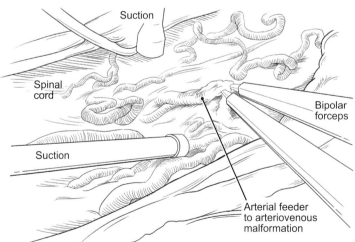

Suction

Spinal cord

Bipolar forceps

Suction

Arterial feeder to arteriovenous malformation

Figure 5.48. (m) Unlike intracranial arteriovenous malformations, spinal cord arteriovenous malformations can be resected by removing the exophytic portion and cutting across loops of vessels that enter the parenchyma of the spinal cord. Bipolar cautery is used to coagulate prominent vessels that enter the spinal cord. This technique, known as the pial resection technique, appears to result in less morbidity than that caused by chasing each vascular loop into the spinal cord, without any significant change in the rate of postoperative hemorrhage in the spinal cord arteriovenous malformation. It is not known why cutting across an arteriovenous malformation is tolerated in the spinal cord but not in the brain.

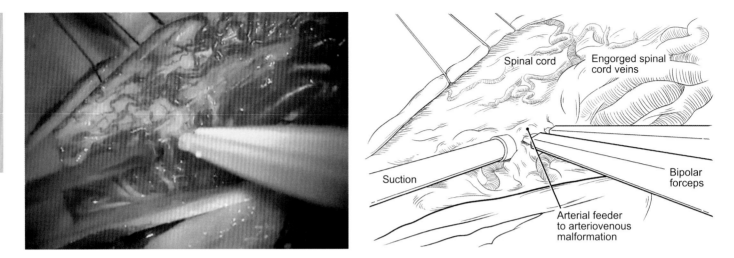

Figure 5.48. (n) Additional vascular pedicles are devascularized where they enter the spinal cord. Suction is used to provide gentle countertraction against the exophytic component of the malformation.

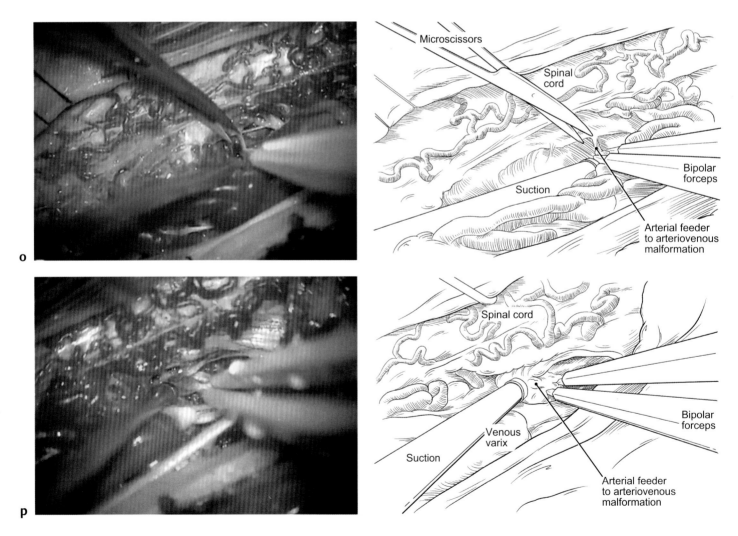

Figure 5.48. (o,p) After being coagulated, the vascular loops are cut sharply. Further devascularization of inflow vessels is achieved by cutting the dentate ligaments to mobilize and then rotate the spinal cord.

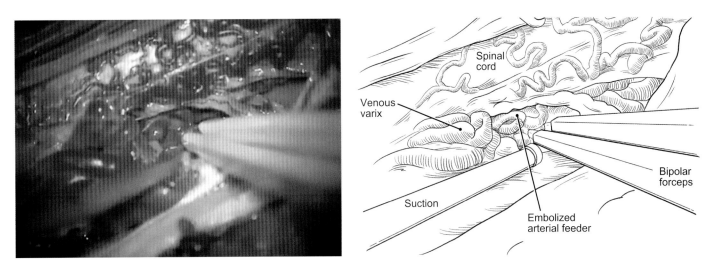

Figure 5.48. (q) Onyx embolisate can be visualized in the vessels draining into the malformation. These vessels are further coagulated and cut sharply. Despite the presence of Onyx, there can still be some flow in these highly pressurized vessels.

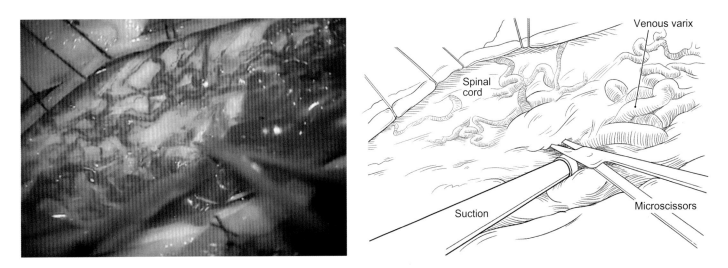

Figure 5.48. (r) Sharp dissection of the arteriovenous malformation enables further disconnection from the spinal cord without violating the pia.

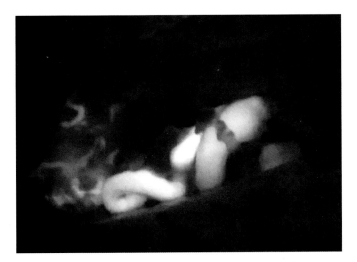

Figure 5.48. (s) Indocyanine green angiography after partial disconnection of the arterial pedicles to the malformation demonstrates the arrest of shunting from the arteriovenous malformation in the spinal cord and continued flow in the draining vein.

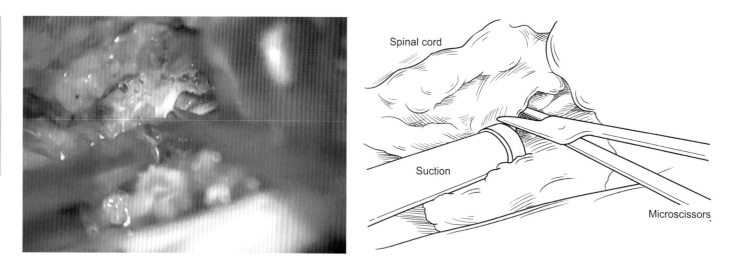

Figure 5.48. (t) The vascular loops are freed before coagulating and sharply cutting the draining vein without violating the pia.

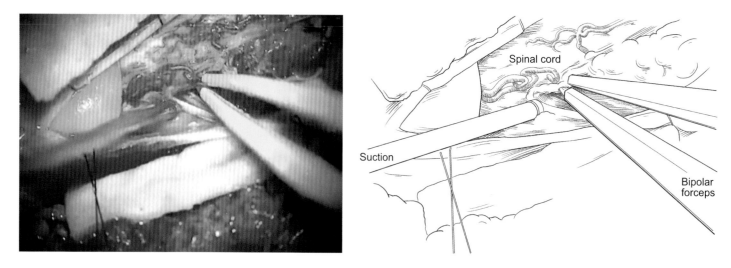

Figure 5.48. (u) After removal of the arteriovenous malformation, the resection bed is inspected to identify and safely remove any remnants. Injury to the spinal cord is minimized by leaving vascular loops that perforate the spinal cord.

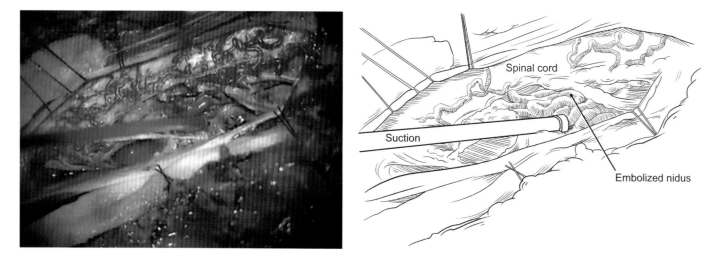

Figure 5.48. (v) A final inspection of the resection cavity is performed.

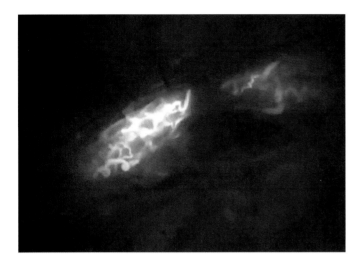

Figure 5.48. (w) Indocyanine green angiography after resection of the arteriovenous malformation confirms not only its complete removal but also the restoration of normal blood flow to the spinal cord.

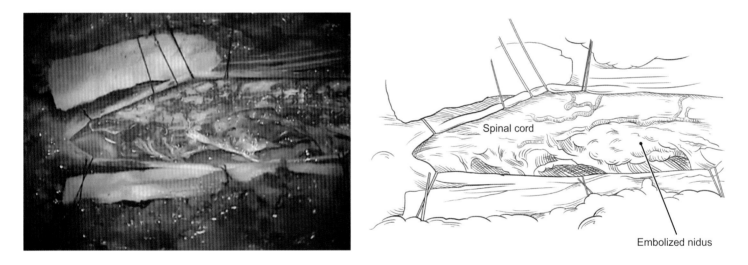

Spinal cord

Embolized nidus

Figure 5.48. (x) Hemostasis is obtained before closure, and the laminae are replaced.

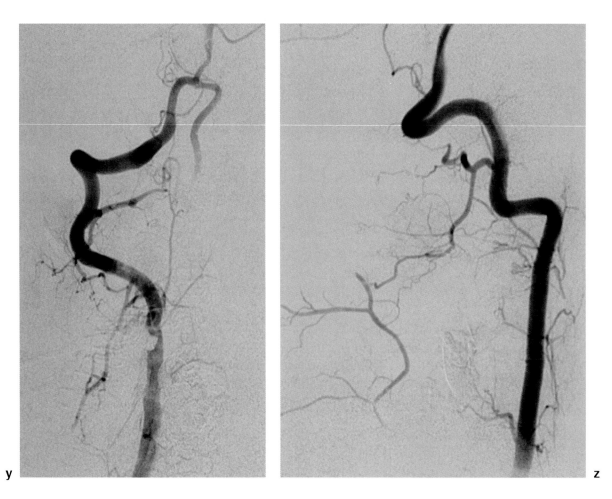

y

z

Figure 5.48. **(y)** Anteroposterior and **(z)** lateral right vertebral artery angiograms demonstrate obliteration of the vertebral artery's contribution to the arteriovenous malformation.

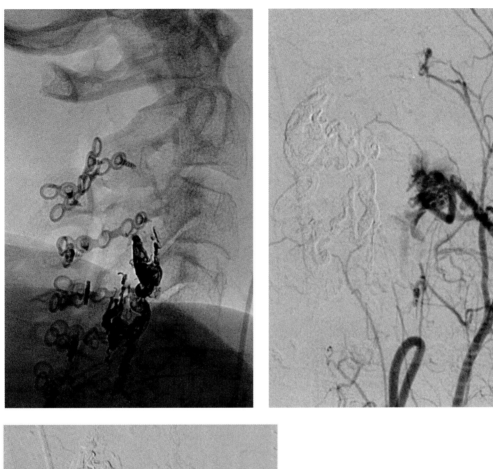

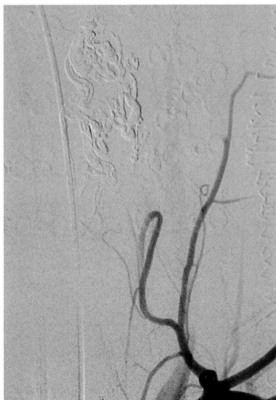

Figure 5.48. (aa) Lateral unsubtracted radiograph demonstrates the residual Onyx cast. **(bb)** A small residual pedicle fed by the left thyrocervical trunk is identified and treated with n-butyl cyanoacrylate. **(cc)** Left thyrocervical injection after treatment with n-butyl cyanoacrylate confirms complete occlusion of the arteriovenous malformation.

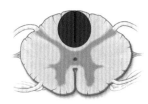

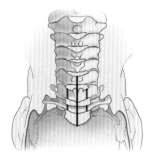

Case 5.49

- Diagnosis: Cervicomedullary ependymoma (related anatomy: pp. **32, 71, 73**)
- Preoperative examination: Left arm and hand weakness
- Approach: Midline cervical laminectomy; via midline raphe (related approach: pp. **101, 102**)
- Positioning: Prone
- Monitoring: Somatosensory evoked potentials and motor evoked potentials
- Outcome: Complete removal of lesion; neurologic status is unchanged.

See Video 5.49

Figure 5.49. A 19-year-old man with a diagnosis of neurofibromatosis 2 and an enlarging cervicomedullary ependymoma presented with weakness of the left arm and hand.

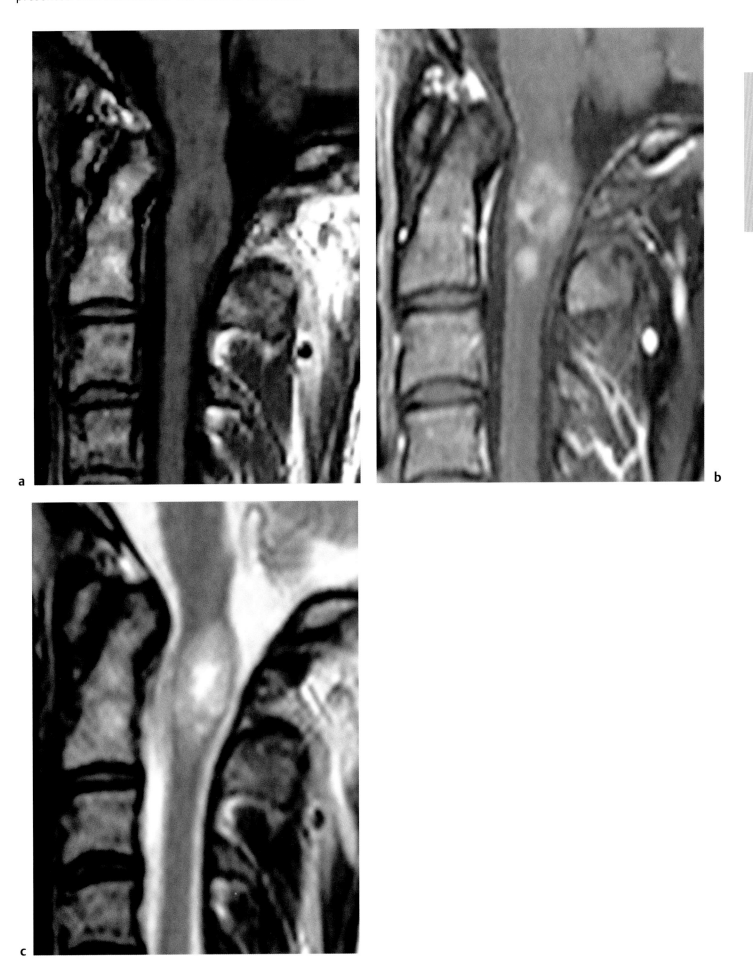

a

b

c

Figure 5.49. Sagittal T1-weighted magnetic resonance images **(a)** without and **(b)** with contrast and **(c)** sagittal T2-weighted magnetic resonance image demonstrate a large lesion at the cervicomedullary junction, consistent with ependymoma.

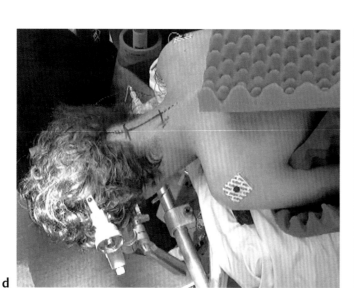
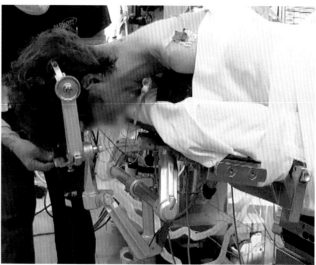

d

e

Figure 5.49. (d) Intraoperative photograph shows patient positioning for a midline approach to the cervicomedullary junction. **(e)** Intraoperative photograph shows a lateral view of the patient positioning.

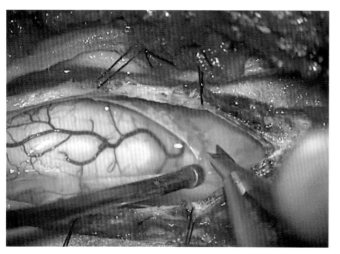
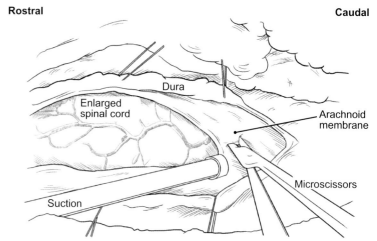

Figure 5.49. (f) After a midline cervical approach and laminectomy, the dura is opened and the arachnoid membrane overlying the spinal cord is sharply cut.

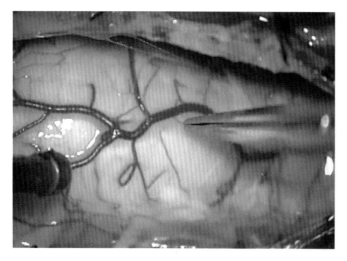
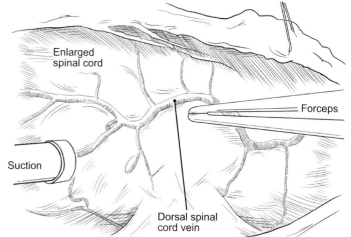

Figure 5.49. (g) The spinal cord appears enlarged and discolored. A prominent vein over the midline is identified and mobilized in preparation for a midline myelotomy.

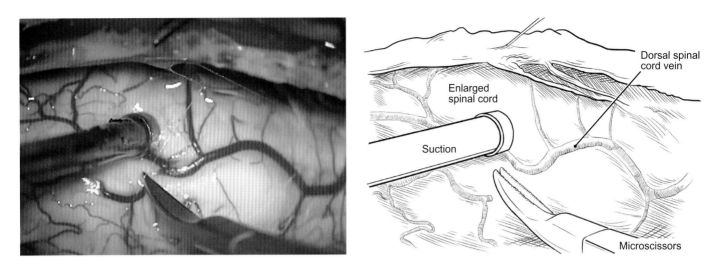

Figure 5.49. (h) Because of the large size of the vein, every attempt should be made to preserve this important outflow from the spinal cord. Veins can usually be dissected from the arachnoid membrane and the pia overlying the spinal cord and then mobilized. Microscissors are used to sharply release arachnoid bands and mobilize the vein, thereby preserving it.

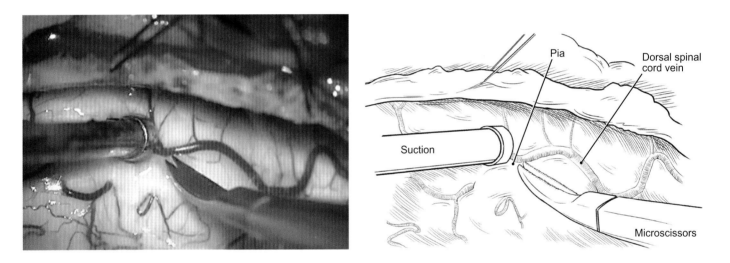

Figure 5.49. (i) The vein is then mobilized from the midline using microscissors.

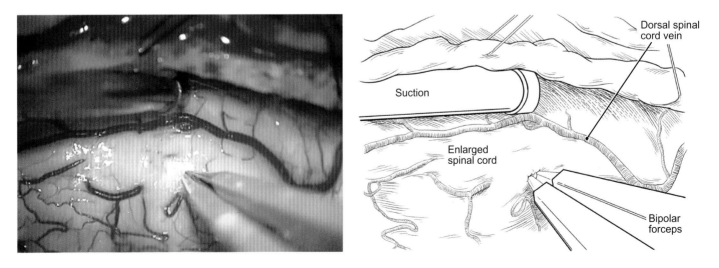

Figure 5.49. (j) After mobilization of the vein, a midline myelotomy is performed. Midline myelotomies should be generously long rostrocaudally to minimize compression and traction on the spinal cord. Bipolar forceps are used to initiate the myelotomy; for opening the spinal cord, the cautery power setting should be decreased to 20 to 30 watts.

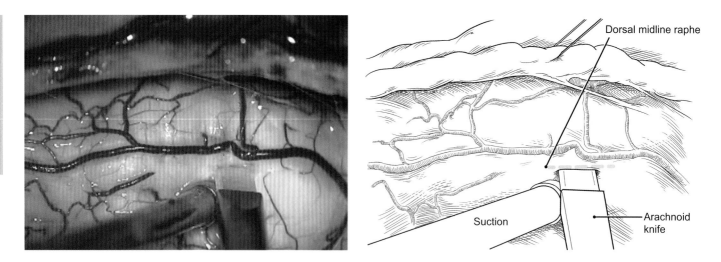

Figure 5.49. (k) After cauterization of the pia, a sharp blade is used to complete the midline myelotomy (*dashed line*).

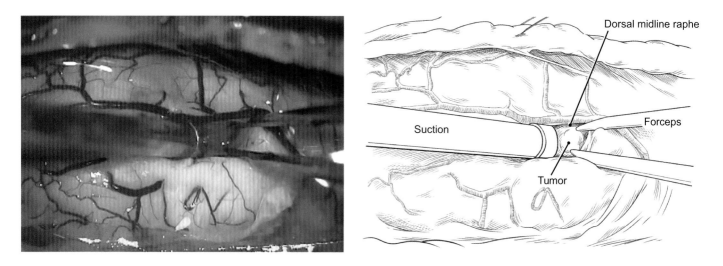

Figure 5.49. (l) Forceps are used to expand the myelotomy to arrive at the tumor.

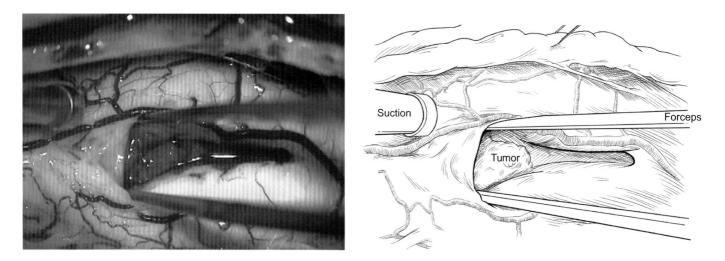

Figure 5.49. (m) The opening is further expanded to visualize the entirety of the ependymoma. Gently spreading the fibers produces minimal disruption of the ascending and descending tracts.

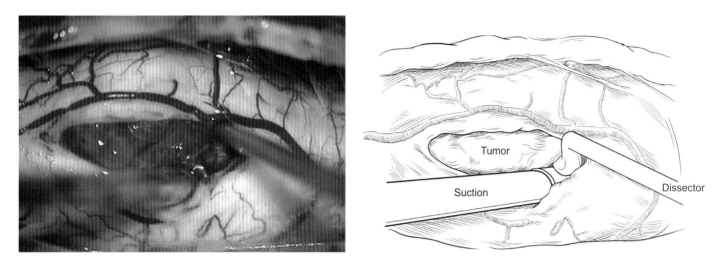

Figure 5.49. (n) The tumor is mobilized from the adjacent normal spinal cord using a combination of sharp and blunt dissection. An angled microdissector is used to develop a plane between the ependymoma and the spinal cord.

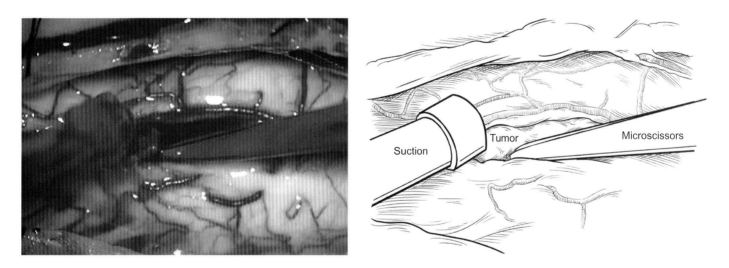

Figure 5.49. (o) Microscissors are used to sharply detach the tumor from the spinal cord.

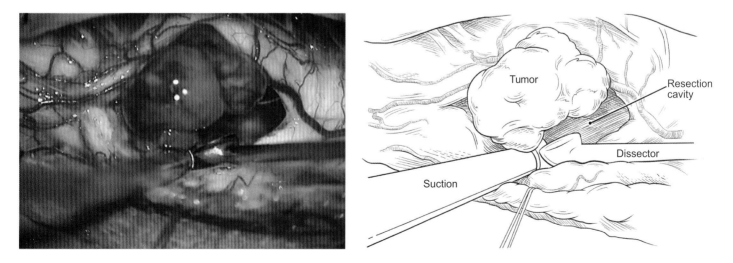

Figure 5.49. (p) Final steps in the dissection facilitate the removal of the tumor. Internal debulking of the tumor generally enables it to be safely mobilized and removed.

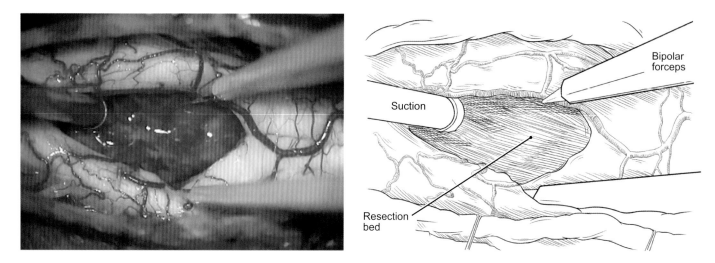

Figure 5.49. (q) Final inspection of the resection bed ensures that no remnants are left behind. Bleeding in the resection bed can be controlled using cautery with bipolar forceps on a low setting. Indiscriminate cauterization should be avoided.

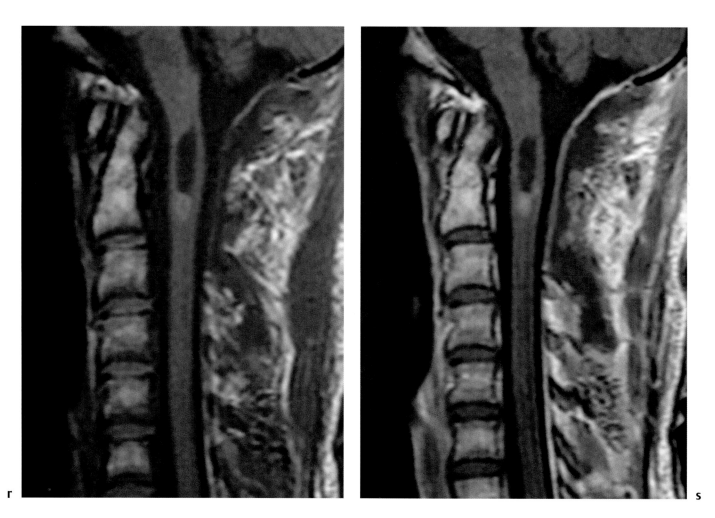

Figure 5.49. Postoperative sagittal T1-weighted magnetic resonance images **(r)** without and **(s)** with contrast confirm complete resection of the tumor with a small amount of blood product in the resection cavity.

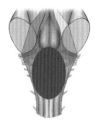
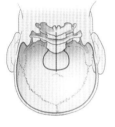

Case 5.50

- Diagnosis: Fourth ventricular epidermoid tumor (related anatomy: pp. **25, 52, 57–59, 71, 73–75**)
- Preoperative examination: Neurologically intact
- Approach: Midline suboccipital (related approach: pp. **200–211**)
- Positioning: Prone
- Monitoring: Somatosensory evoked potentials
- Outcome: Patient is neurologically stable.

See Video 5.50

Figure 5.50. A 35-year-old woman presented with headaches and diplopia.

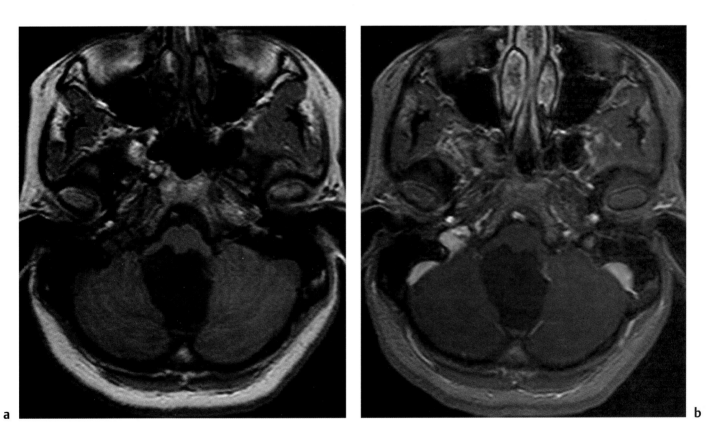

a   b

Figure 5.50. (a) Axial T1-weighted magnetic resonance image without contrast and **(b)** axial and **(c)** sagittal T1-weighted magnetic resonance images with contrast demonstrate a lesion in the fourth ventricle causing displacement of the brainstem and cervicomedullary junction.

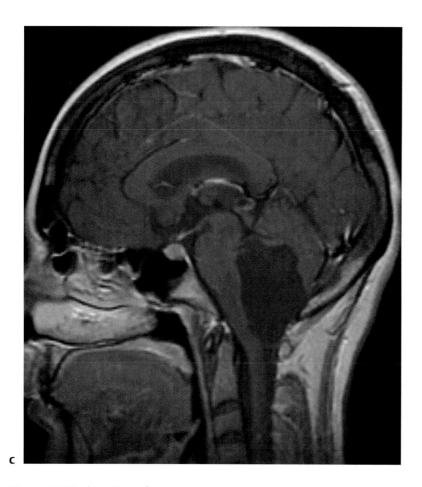

c

Figure 5.50. (*Continued*)

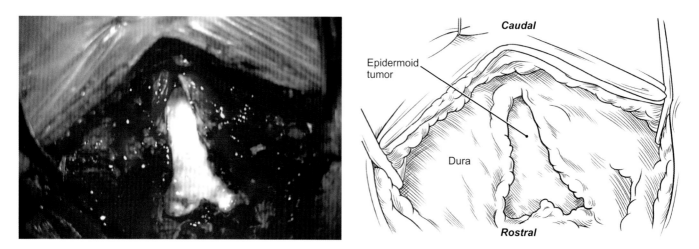

Figure 5.50. (d) The lesion, an epidermoid tumor, is accessed using a midline suboccipital approach. When the dura is opened, the glistening white surface of the epidermoid tumor is immediately evident.

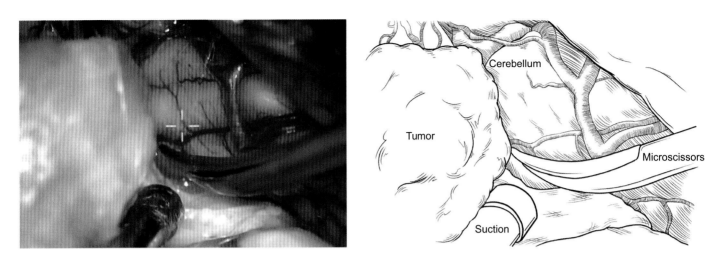

Figure 5.50. (e) Sharp dissection can be used to easily mobilize epidermoid tumors from adjacent structures. In some cases, the tumor capsule is densely adherent to adjacent structures and should be left in situ to minimize injury to them, especially the lower cranial nerves. Leaving tumor capsule remnants increases the likelihood of tumor recurrence, but it also avoids injury to critical structures.

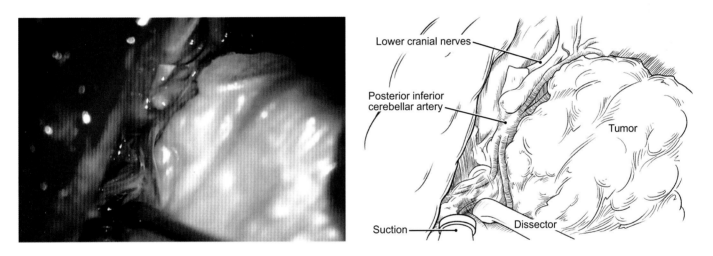

Figure 5.50. (f) A small branch of the posterior inferior cerebellar artery that is adherent to the tumor is carefully mobilized using sharp dissection.

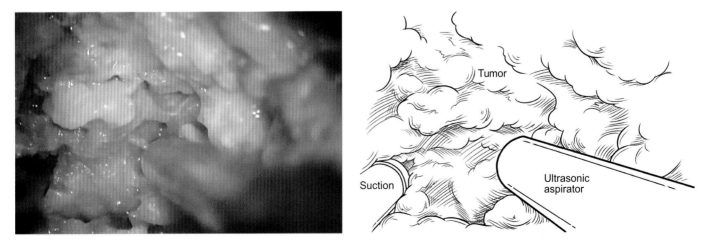

Figure 5.50. (g) An ultrasonic aspirator is used to internally debulk the tumor.

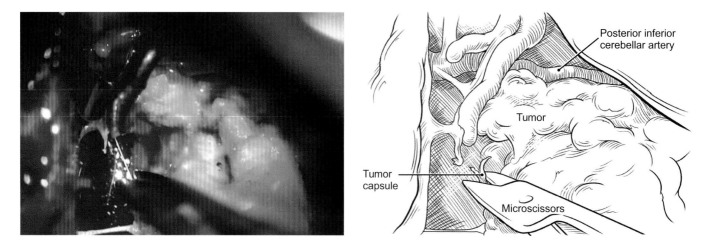

Figure 5.50. **(h)** After the tumor is internally decompressed, it is mobilized and sharply resected from adjacent structures.

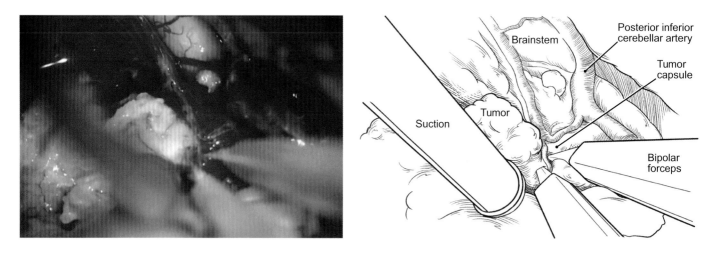

Figure 5.50. **(i)** Small vascular pedicles feeding the tumor capsule are coagulated.

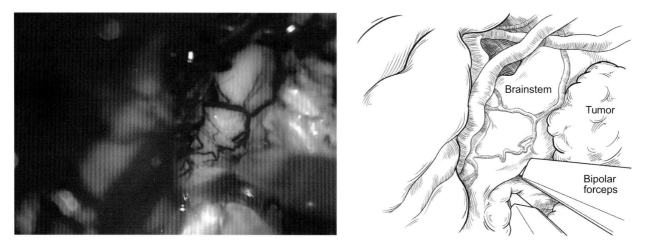

Figure 5.50. **(j)** The tumor capsule is dissected from the dorsal brainstem. When a tumor capsule is densely adherent, it should be left in place to avoid injury.

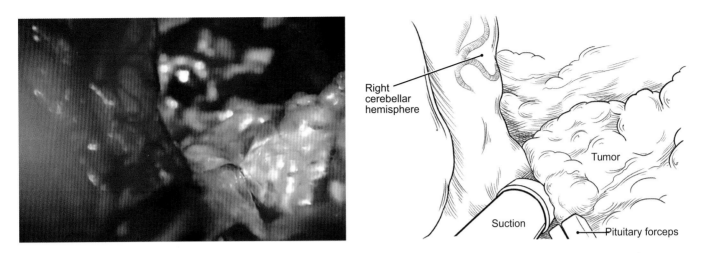

Figure 5.50. (k) The mobilized tumor and tumor capsule are peeled from the brainstem surface.

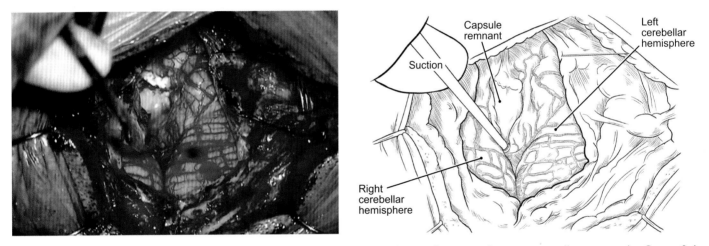

Figure 5.50. (l) The resection bed is inspected, and hemostasis is obtained. A capsule remnant adherent to the floor of the fourth ventricle was left in place.

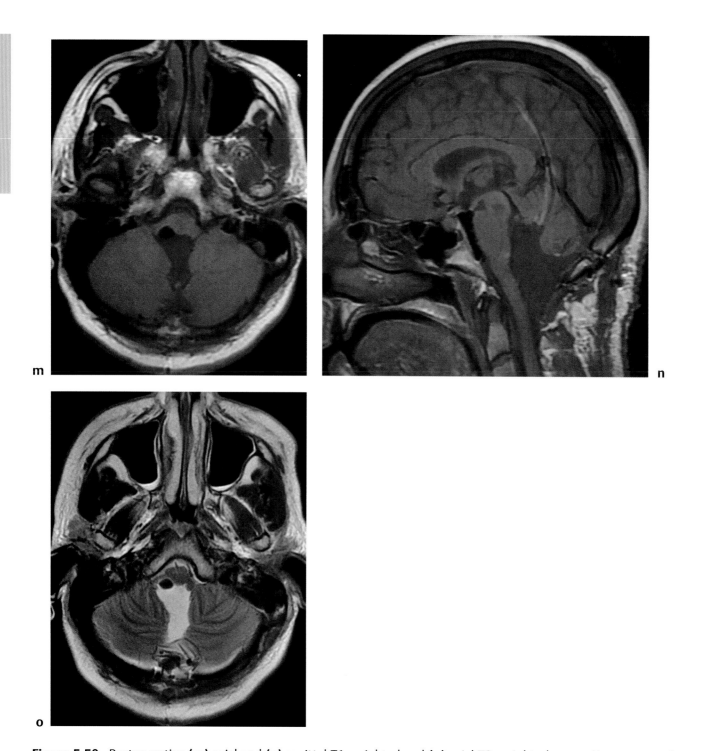

Figure 5.50. Postoperative **(m)** axial and **(n)** sagittal T1-weighted and **(o)** axial T2-weighted magnetic resonance images confirm expected near-complete resection of the tumor. A small remnant is preferable to causing any neurological deficit.

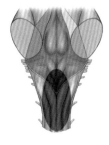

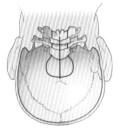

Case 5.51

- Diagnosis: Cervicomedullary juvenile pilocytic astrocytoma (related anatomy: pp. **32, 71, 73**)

- Preoperative examination: Neurologically intact

- Approach: Midline suboccipital and multilevel cervical laminectomies (related approach: p. **248**)

- Positioning: Prone

- Monitoring: Somatosensory evoked potentials and motor evoked potentials

- Outcome: Complete removal of lesion; mild postoperative hemiparesis; patient improved to baseline neurologic status by postoperative day 3.

See Video 5.51

Figure 5.51. A 4-year-old girl presented with neck pain.

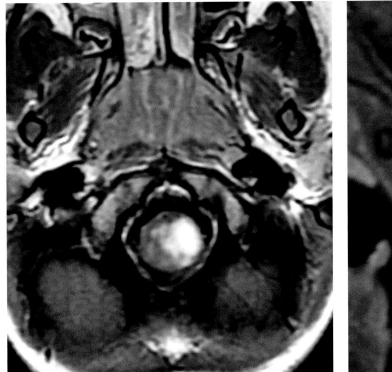

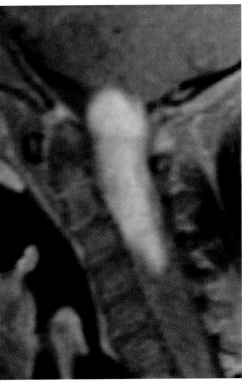

a

b

Figure 5.51. (a) Axial and **(b)** sagittal T1-weighted magnetic resonance images demonstrate a large expansile lesion in the cervicomedullary junction.

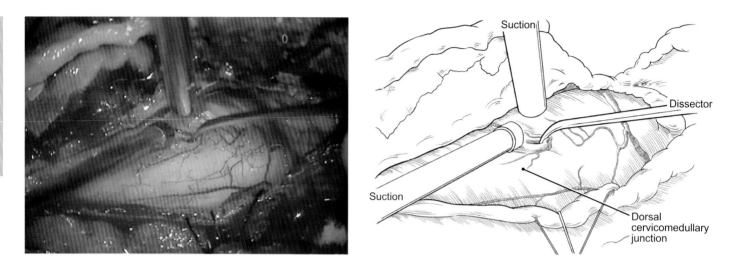

Figure 5.51. (c) The lesion is accessed dorsally using a midline approach. After the dura is opened, the tumor is visualized and a biopsy specimen is obtained. Pathologic analysis of the biopsy specimen identified the lesion as a juvenile pilocytic astrocytoma.

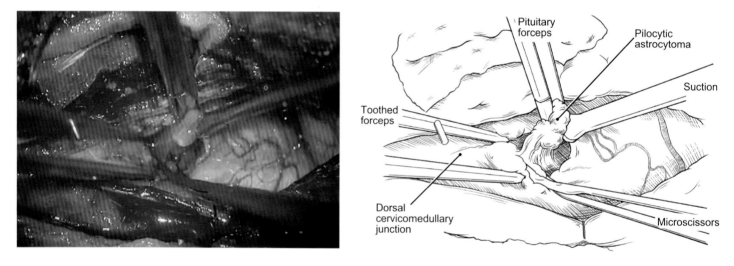

Figure 5.51. (d) The lesion is removed piecemeal using toothed forceps.

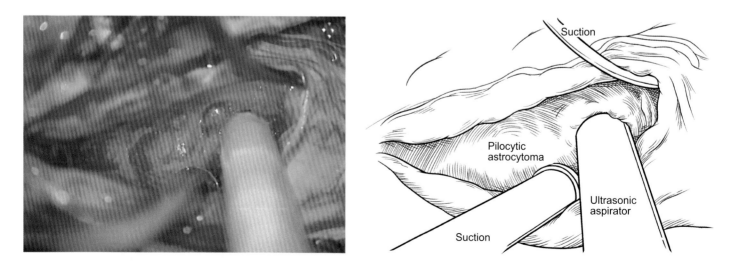

Figure 5.51. (e) An ultrasonic aspirator is used to continue the internal debulking of the lesion.

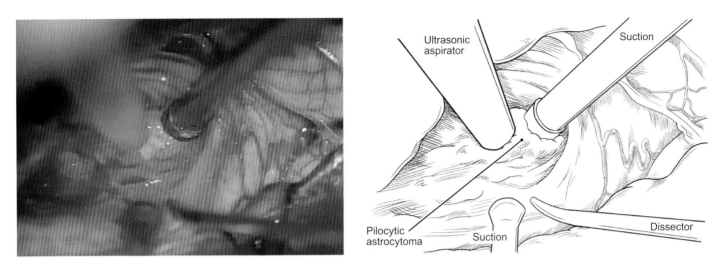

Figure 5.51. (f) In this case, the tumor was distinct from the spinal cord. Thus, it was possible to debulk the tumor to its margins with the normal spinal cord. However, doing so is not possible in every case, especially for high-grade gliomas of the spinal cord, which are infiltrative.

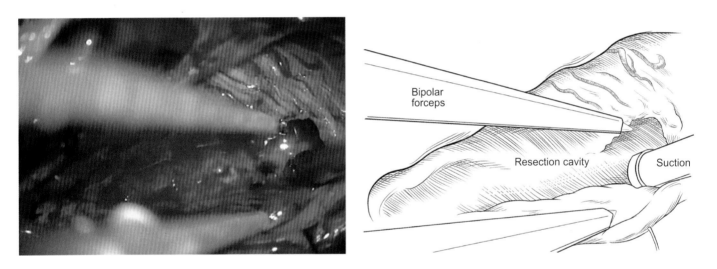

Figure 5.51. (g) After completion of the resection, the cavity is inspected and hemostasis is obtained.

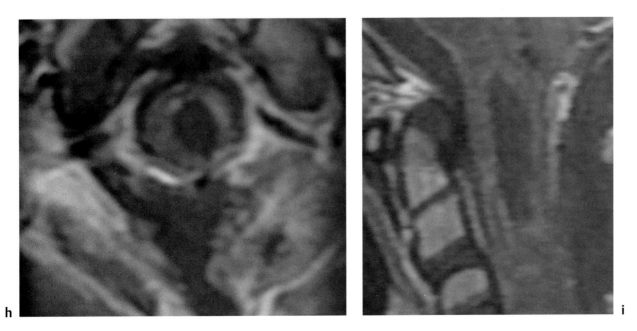

Figure 5.51. Postoperative **(h)** axial and **(i)** sagittal T1-weighted magnetic resonance images demonstrate complete removal of the tumor.

Index